End-Stage Renal Disease

An Integrated Approach

Contributors

Lowanna S. Binkley, R.N.

Richard L. Gibson, M.D.

Patrick E. Hopkins, B.S.

H. Keith Johnson, M.D.

Victoria R. Liddle, R.D.

T. Dwight McKinney, M.D.

George W. McLean, M.D.

Elinor Moores, MSW

Gary D. Niblack, Ph.D.

David Rabin, M.D.

Pauline L. Rabin, M.D.

Robert E. Richie, M.D.

William J. Stone, M.D.

Paul E. Teschan, M.D.

End-Stage Renal Disease

An Integrated Approach

EDITED BY

William J. Stone, M.D.
Pauline L. Rabin, M.D.

School of Medicine
Vanderbilt University
and Veterans Administration
Medical Center
Nashville, Tennessee

1983

ACADEMIC PRESS

A Subsidiary of Harcourt Brace Jovanovich, Publishers

New York   London
Paris   San Diego   San Francisco   São Paulo   Sydney   Tokyo   Toronto

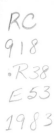
ACADEMIC PRESS, INC.
111 Fifth Avenue, New York, New York 10003

United Kingdom Edition published by
ACADEMIC PRESS, INC. (LONDON) LTD.
24/28 Oval Road, London NW1 7DX

Library of Congress Cataloging in Publication Data
Main entry under title:

End-stage renal disease.

    Includes index.
    1. Renal insufficiency. 2. Renal insufficiency--
Treatment. I. Stone, William J. II. Rabin, Pauline L.
[DNLM: 1. Kidney--Transplantation. 2. Kidney failure,
Chronic--Therapy. 3. Hemodialysis. WJ 342 E55]
RC918.R38E53 1983   616.6'14   82-16399
ISBN 0-12-672280-3

PRINTED IN THE UNITED STATES OF AMERICA

83 84 85 86   9 8 7 6 5 4 3 2 1

Contents

1

Renal Physiology and Pathophysiology of Renal Failure

T. DWIGHT McKINNEY, M.D.

2

The Presentation of the Patient with Chronic Renal Failure

PAUL E. TESCHAN, M.D.

3

Medical Complications of End-Stage Renal Disease

WILLIAM J. STONE, M.D.

4

Endocrine and Metabolic Changes Accompanying End-Stage Renal Disease

G. W. McLEAN, M.D., D. RABIN, M.D., AND W. J. STONE, M.D.

5

Psychiatric Aspects of End-Stage Renal Disease: Diagnosis and Management

PAULINE L. RABIN, M.D.

6

Social Work with Renal Failure Patients:
Roles of the Social Worker

ELINOR MOORES, MSW

7

The Problem of Vascular Access
in the Management of End-Stage Renal Disease:
The Various Possibilities of Producing a Shunt

ROBERT E. RICHIE, M.D.

8

Dialysis

RICHARD L. GIBSON, M.D.

9

Technical Aspects of Dialysis

PATRICK E. HOPKINS, B.S.

10
The Case for Renal Transplantation

*H. KEITH JOHNSON, M.D., ROBERT E. RICHIE, M.D.,
AND GARY D. NIBLACK, Ph.D.*

11
Nursing Care of the Patient with End-Stage Renal Disease

LOWANNA S. BINKLEY, RN

12

The Role of Nutrition in End-Stage Renal Disease

VICTORIA R. LIDDLE, RD

13

End-Stage Renal Disease: An Integrated Approach

WILLIAM J. STONE, M.D. AND PAULINE L. RABIN, M.D.

Contributors

Lowanna S. Binkley, RN, Nephrology Nurse Specialist, Division of Nephrology, Veterans Administration Hospital, Nashville, Tennessee 37203.

Richard L. Gibson, M.D., Assistant Professor of Medicine, Department of Medicine, Division of Nephrology, School of Medicine, Vanderbilt University Hospital, Nashville, Tennessee 37232.

Patrick E. Hopkins, BS, MTASCP, Veterans Administration Hospital, Nashville, Tennessee 37203.

H. Keith Johnson, M.D., Assistant Professor of Medicine, Department of Medicine, Division of Nephrology, Co-director of the Renal Transplant Program, Vanderbilt University Hospital, and Veterans Administration Hospital, Nashville, Tennessee 37232.

Victoria R. Liddle, RD, Dietitian, The Dialysis Clinics, Inc., Nashville, Tennessee 37203.

T. Dwight McKinney, M.D., Assistant Professor of Medicine, School of Medicine, Vanderbilt University Hospital, and Assistant Chief of Nephrology, Veterans Administration Hospital, Nashville, Tennessee 37203.

George W. McLean, M.D., Associate Professor of Medicine, Department of Medicine, University of Tennessee College of Medicine, Chattanooga, Tennessee 37403.

Elinor Moores, MSW, ACSW, Nephrology Social Worker, Social Work Service, Veterans Administration Hospital, Nashville, Tennessee 37203.

Gary D. Niblack, Ph.D., Transplant Immunologist, Department of Surgery, Veterans Administration Hospital, Department of Pathology, Vanderbilt University Hospital, and Director of Histocompatibility, Dia-Clin Laboratories, Nashville, Tennessee 37203.

David Rabin, M.D., Professor of Medicine and Obstetrics and Gynecology, Division of Endocrinology, School of Medicine, Vanderbilt University Hospital, Nashville, Tennessee 37232.

Pauline L. Rabin, M.D., Associate Professor of Psychiatry, School of Medicine, Vanderbilt University Hospital, and Consultant Psychiatrist, Veterans Administration Hospital, Nashville, Tennessee 37232.

Robert E. Richie, M.D., Chief of Renal Transplant Section, Veterans Administration Hospital, Associate Professor of Surgery, Department of Surgery, and Chief of Renal Transplantation Division, Department of

Surgery, Section of Surgical Sciences, School of Medicine, Vanderbilt University Hospital, Nashville, Tennessee 37203.

William J. Stone, M.D., Chief of Nephrology, Veterans Administration Hospital, Professor of Medicine, Department of Medicine, Associate Professor of Medicine, Division of Urology, School of Medicine, Vanderbilt University Hospital, Nashville, Tennessee 37203.

Paul E. Teschan, M.D., Associate Professor of Medicine and Biomedical Engineering, Department of Medicine, Division of Nephrology, School of Medicine, Vanderbilt University Hospital, Nashville, Tennessee 37232

Foreword

The medical specialty of nephrology has enjoyed striking growth during the last two decades. Its practitioners are now concerned with an array of clinical responsibilities that includes, in its most restricted form, the evaluation and care of patients with primary and secondary diseases of the kidneys, hypertension, and disorders of water and electrolyte metabolism. The science of their clinical practice is multifaceted in its origin, deriving from an exciting blend of physiology, morphology and pathology, immunology, biochemistry, microbiology, and pharmacology. But within the broader scope of their clinical purview, it is the care of patients with end-stage renal disease that most often provides the central core of clinical responsibility for the practicing nephrologist. In fact, it was the very advent of kidney transplantation and the various modalities of dialysis in the treatment of such patients that gave rise to the emergence of nephrology as an established medical specialty.

It is therefore appropriate that a book should appear which focuses solely on the care of patients with end-stage renal disease. But why this particular book, and how does it differ from others of a seemingly similar nature that may have appeared recently as part of an ever-growing parade of publications on subjects relevant to nephrology? First, as the population of patients receiving treatment for end-stage renal disease has grown, an ever-increasing number of nonnephrologists have been required to play a role in some facet of such patients, either as a referring physician who first detected the need for nephrological evaluation and treatment or as a later participant in their general supervision once begun on a form of treatment. It is the unusual family practitioner or general internist who has not yet encountered one or more such patients in the course of practice. It has therefore become increasingly important that many physicians should gain a general understanding of the principles and approaches that underlie the care of patients with end-stage renal disease. This book will serve that purpose well for the nonnephrologist, whether he or she should be a medical student, house officer, family practitioner, general internist, or urologist. Second, and even more importantly, it describes an integrated approach to the care of patients with end-stage kidney failure that recognizes the important contribution of nephrologists, dietitians, social workers, psychiatrists, dialysis technicians, surgeons, and other health-care professionals. The care of these patients is best carried out as a coordinated and team effort, and this particular book is among the first to emphasize that point so comprehensively and well.

Lastly, this volume possesses one singular characteristic that is somewhat unique in this era of edited and multiauthored medical books. It has been assembled by a single team of highly experienced professionals who have worked together in the same institution for an extended period as a widely recognized clinical group. Their approach, fully developed through years of close association, can perhaps be labeled appropriately as the "Vanderbilt approach." It reflects the benefit and attraction of effective partnership among differing types of professionals and the smooth continuum of clinical responsibility that can result therein from a single institution. The description of their approach thus avoids a common pitfall of many multiauthored books in which various aspects of a single topic may have been discussed capably by prominent authorities from different institutions, yet the whole of the effort fails to emerge as a cohesive expression of an integrated approach to the topic under consideration.

The volume reads easily. It reflects a timely, highly useful, and comprehensive view of an integrated and practical clinical approach to the management of patients with end-stage renal disease. It will serve as a convenient and valuable reference for the nonnephrologist. The strong clinical and research reputations of most of the authors were known to me before my own arrival at Vanderbilt in 1981. My acquaintance with one dates back to 1958 when we shared a patient with heat-stroke-associated acute renal failure, and I first learned from him of the favorable impact on morbidity of earlier and more frequent hemodialysis without rigid and severe dietary protein restriction. It has taken but a short time to affirm the high standards and clinical excellence of all members of this fine group. They have delivered a useful and timely book.

Roscoe R. Robinson, M. D.
Nashville, Tennessee

Preface

During the past two decades considerable advances have been made in the therapy of chronic renal disease. These advances have resulted in patients being referred to specialized medical centers that have expertise in dialysis and renal transplantation. In consequence, the resident in training, the family practitioner, the internist, and the general psychiatrist often lose touch with this group of patients and feel at a disadvantage when called to treat them on an intermittent basis.

With advances in the treatment of renal disease, a new subset of medical illnesses has become manifest. We are witnessing the medical sequelae of prolonging life by extraordinary means. One striking example is the complex alteration in endocrine function associated with chronic end-stage renal disease (ESRD). Profound changes are observed in the gonads, the thyroid gland, and in the control of calcium and phosphorus metabolism. The patient may develop myriad signs and symptoms, many of which represent a tremendous therapeutic challenge: impotence and sterility in young patients resistant to hormonal replacement therapy; bone disease, a complex amalgam of osteopenia and osteitis fibrosa requiring a delicate regimen that will ameliorate demineralization while not causing hypercalcemia; and a bewildering array of neurologic complications.

Prolonging life artificially has psychological sequelae. Many restrictions accompany the treatment of pre-end-stage, and even more so, end-stage renal disease. The patient and the family must adjust to the ravages of chronic illness. In addition, organic neuropsychiatric complications need to be recognized and not attributed to failure of compliance. The differential diagnosis among organic neuropsychiatric disease, drug-induced psychiatric problems, and depression are often challenging in patients who are struggling with chronic illness, numerous medications, and progressive multisystem disease.

The optimal management of chronic end-stage renal disease requires the skills of many disciplines. Rigorous control of the diet is extremely crucial. The knowledgeable dietitian can present a palatable menu which will assist the patient in adhering to the rigid restrictions of protein and electrolyte intake. Not all patients can work; income is limited; and the prescribed diet may be beyond the means of the family. A new life-style is demanded, and the efforts of an astute social worker can be of inestimable help. For patients on dialysis, nurses are pivotal people in their lives. Nurses dialyze patients in the center, train them in home dialysis, and constantly reinforce adherence to the treatment regimen by supportive care and instruction. The roles of the dietitian, social worker, and nephrology nurse are described in the text.

There is no cure for ESRD, but there is a wide choice of treatment for most patients. Which therapy should be recommended? Dialysis is indispensable, but which form would best fit the needs of the individual patients? How do patients eventually reach a decision to have a kidney transplant? What are realistic expectations for patients choosing this bold new treatment? The authors address these questions and describe the management of rejection phenomena and the long-term effects of the use of immunosuppressants and steroids.

This text has evolved from the extensive experience we have accumulated in the management of chronic end-stage renal disease at the Vanderbilt University Medical Center and Veterans Administration Hospital in Nashville, Tennessee. We have developed an integrated team approach to the diagnosis and day-to-day management of the patient with chronic renal disease. While the book will be valuable to the practicing nephrologist, it is particularly aimed toward helping the medical student, house officer, family practitioner, general internist, surgeon, and psychiatrist who may otherwise feel intimidated when called on to treat this group of patients. The text provides a working knowledge of renal physiology and sets out the pathophysiological changes accompanying the loss of renal function. We attempt to describe clearly the medical complications of ESRD and provide guidelines for differential diagnosis and treatment.

Pauline L. Rabin, M.D.
William J. Stone, M.D.

Renal Physiology
and Pathophysiology
of Renal Failure

T. DWIGHT McKINNEY

1

END-STAGE RENAL DISEASE

I. ANATOMY

A. Gross Anatomy

The kidneys of a normal adult weigh about 150 g each and are approximately 11–14 cm in length. The various anatomical regions of the kidney are shown in Fig. 1. The area nearest the surface is the renal cortex, where the glomeruli are located. However, the bulk of the cortex consists of proximal convoluted tubules. The next region is the renal medulla, which can be divided into an inner and outer zone and the innermost area, the renal papillae. Urine flows from ducts in the papillary tips into a minor calix.

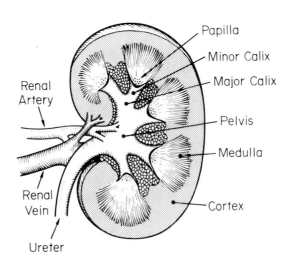

Fig. 1. Gross anatomy of the kidney.

Minor calices unite to form a superior and inferior major calix which join to form the renal pelvis. The pelvis is continuous with the ureter. The renal artery and renal nerves enter and the renal vein, ureter, and lymphatics leave the kidney on its medial aspect in an area known as the renal hilus (*1*).

B. Microscopic Anatomy

The functional unit of the kidney is the nephron (Fig. 2). There are approximately 1,000,000 of these in each adult kidney. A nephron is composed of a glomerulus and in succession a number of tubular segments: proximal convoluted tubule, proximal straight tubule, thin descending limb of Henle's loop, thin ascending limb of Henle's loop, thick ascending limb of Henle, distal convoluted tubule, and the initial portion of a collecting tubule. Collecting tubules from several nephrons progressively unite to form collecting ducts, which join other collecting ducts and ultimately empty their tubular fluid into a minor calix through a duct of Bellini in the papillae.

The glomerulus is composed of a group of capillaries and a covering of epithelial cells. Glomerular capillaries arise from the afferent arteriole and reunite to form the efferent arteriole. The capillaries are covered on their

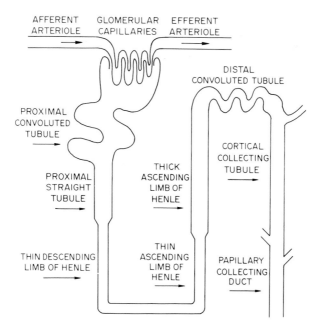

Fig. 2.   Diagramatic representation of a nephron.

external surface by a thin layer of epithelial cells, the visceral layer of Bowman's capsule. This layer of cells is continuous with the epithelium of the proximal convoluted tubule via the parietal layer of Bowman's capsule. The small space between the two layers of Bowman's capsule, Bowman's space, is continuous with the lumen of the proximal convoluted tubule. The process of urine formation begins with filtration of plasma across the glomerular capillaries into Bowman's space.

II. RENAL BLOOD FLOW

The main renal artery undergoes a series of branchings within the kidney until the afferent arterioles are formed. These give rise to the glomerular capillaries, which in turn unite to form the efferent arteriole. The efferent arterioles then break up to form a peritubular capillary network. These join to form small veins, which progressively unite to form the renal vein. Although the kidneys comprise less than 0.5% of body weight, they receive about 20% of the resting cardiac output (2). Blood flow per gram of tissue weight in the kidneys is among the highest of any organ. Renal blood flow has the unique feature of autoregulation. The term autoregulation refers to the ability of renal blood flow to remain relatively constant over a range of mean arterial pressures of about 60–180 mm Hg (2). The mechanisms whereby renal blood flow is kept stable over these wide pressure ranges are not completely understood. However, this feature of the renal circulation is a key factor in maintaining renal excretory function during wide fluctuations in systemic blood pressure.

III. GLOMERULAR FILTRATION

Urine formation begins with passive filtration of plasma across the glomerulus into Bowman's space and, hence, into the proximal convoluted tubule. Glomerular filtration is a selection process that allows water and small non-protein-bound solutes to move from glomerular capillary blood into the urinary space. Larger species, e.g., proteins and blood cells, are restricted in their passage across the glomerular filter.

The factors governing glomerular filtration are the same as those responsible for passive movement of fluid across any capillary: net hydrostatic and osmotic pressure differences across the capillary wall along with the intrinsic permeability properties of the capillary. The principal driving force for glomerular filtration is the hydrostatic (blood) pressure in the glomerular capillaries (P_{gc}). This is opposed by the hydrostatic pressure in the proximal tubule (P_t). The colloid osmotic pressure of blood (π), due to serum proteins, mostly albumin, opposes filtration of fluid across the glomerulus. Since there is a negligible amount of protein in the glomerular filtrate under normal conditions, the colloid osmotic pressure of blood is not opposed by a similar osmotic pressure in the proximal tubule. The rate of filtration in a single glomerulus is equal to

$$kA[(P_{gc} - P_t) - \pi]$$

where k represents the hydraulic permeability of the glomerular capillary. The hydraulic permeability determines how much fluid can be filtered across a specified area of glomerular surface for a given net pressure difference across the capillary and is much larger for glomerular capillaries than for other capillary beds. A is the glomerular capillary surface area (3). The glomerular filtration rate (GFR) for both kidneys is the sum of the individual filtration rates of all the nephrons. The precise values for these determinants of GFR in man are not known. In experimental animals P_{gc} is about 45 mm Hg, P_t is about 10 mm Hg, and the colloid osmotic pressure of blood at the beginning of the glomerular capillary is about 20 mm Hg (3). Thus, at the beginning of the glomerular capillaries there is a net force of approximately 15 mm Hg, which favors glomerular filtration. The high hydrostatic pressure in the glomerular capillaries combined with their high hydraulic permeability and large surface area allows much more fluid to be filtered across them than would be possible in other capillary beds. The other determinant of GFR is renal plasma flow. As mentioned earlier renal blood flow tends to remain relatively constant despite wide variations in systemic blood pressure. As renal plasma (blood) flow increases GFR increases and vice versa.

The GFR of a healthy young man is approximately 125 ml/min and is slightly less in women (4). Clinical measurement of GFR involves the concept of clearance. The term clearance relates the quantity of a substance, x, excreted in the urine per unit time to the volume of plasma which if completely "cleared" of x would yield a quantity of x equal to that excreted in the urine. In order for a substance to be useful as a marker of GFR it should be freely filtered at the glomerulus (small molecular weight and non-protein-bound) and be neither secreted nor reabsorbed by the renal tubules. If a substance has these characteristics its renal clearance will equal GFR. The renal clearance of a substance, C_x, is calculated as follows:

$$C_x = \frac{U_x V}{P_x}$$

In this formula U_x = urinary concentration of x, V = urine flow rate, and P_x = serum concentration of x. Although the clearance of inulin and a number of other substances may be used experimentally to calculate GFR, their use in routine evaluation of patients is limited. Creatinine clearance is the test most frequently used clinically to assess GFR. Creatinine is a small molecule (113 daltons) that is produced at a constant rate from muscles, released into the blood, and excreted in the urine at a constant rate each day (approximately 20 mg/kg body weight each day). It has the aforementioned characteristics necessary for use as a marker of GFR and, for clinical purposes, creatinine clearance, C_{cr}, is equal to GFR. Conventional measurement of C_{cr} usually involves collecting all urine produced in a 24 hr period, measurement of the volume and creatinine concentration of urine, and measurement of the serum creatinine concentration once during the 24 hr period. With these values one may calculate the C_{cr}. For example, if the 24 hr urine volume is 1440 ml, the urine creatinine concentration is 120 mg/dl, and the serum creatinine concentration is 1.0 mg/dl, then

$$C_{cr} = \frac{(120 \text{ mg/dl})(1440 \text{ ml}/1440 \text{ min})}{1.0 \text{ mg/dl}}$$

$$C_{cr} = 120 \text{ ml/min}$$

Since creatinine production and urinary excretion remain constant with constant muscle mass, it is evident from the above formula that if C_{cr} is known for a given serum creatinine concentration future calculations of C_{cr} can be based on serum creatinine concentration measurements alone, provided body weight remains the same. Thus, any doubling of the serum creatinine concentration will reflect a 50% reduction in GFR, etc.

Although measurement of C_{cr} in the above manner should, in theory, be a simple matter, often this is not the case. This is most frequently due to inadequate urine collections, which result in a lower number for the numerator of the above equation and, hence, in a spuriously low C_{cr}. One must, therefore, determine that the urine collection is adequate by measuring the total amount of creatinine excreted during the 24 hr period before concluding that a calculated C_{cr} is valid.

Because of problems associated with improper urine collections it is frequently useful to determine C_{cr} by a method that is independent of urine collections. This may be done by the following formula (5):

$$C_{cr} = \frac{(140\text{-age in years})(\text{edema-free body weight in kg})}{72 \times \text{ serum creatinine in mg/dl}}$$

The correlation between accurate C_{cr} measured in the conventional manner and that estimated by this formula is very good.

With increasing age there is a progressive loss of nephrons and, as a consequence, a decrease in GFR. GFR eventually falls with most types of renal diseases and serial determinations of C_{cr} is the best method of following the course of most patients with progressive renal insufficiency. Many patients will be asymptomatic with C_{cr} in the range of 20–30 ml/min. However, many laboratory abnormalities will be present. Most patients will have some symptoms with C_{cr} of 10–20 ml/min and only the rare patient will not have significant symptoms once C_{cr} is less than 10 ml/min. Once C_{cr} falls to 5–10 ml/min patients are in need of renal replacement therapy in the form of dialysis or renal transplantation.

IV. RENAL HANDLING OF MACROMOLECULES

The glomeruli offer little resistance to filtration of molecules with weights 10,000 daltons or less. However, as molecular weight increases from 10,000 to about 50,000, passage of molecules across the glomerulus becomes more restricted and essentially ceases at the higher molecular weights (4). Molecular weight (and size) is, therefore, a major factor that prevents loss of macromolecules in the urine. Another important factor is the electrical charge on the macromolecule. The glomerulus can be thought of conceptually as consisting of small "pores" lined by negative charges. The negative charges are due to the presence of a sialoprotein coat (6). Thus, for macromolecules of the same molecular weight negatively charged species will encounter more resistance to filtration than neutral species and neutral species will be more restricted than positive species because of electrostatic interactions with the glomerulus (3, 7). The most important macromolecules in blood are the proteins. At normal blood pH most of the serum proteins are negatively charged. This, in addition to their molecular weight, prevents much protein loss in the urine under normal conditions. In certain disease states associated with proteinuria there is loss of this sialoprotein coat, and, thus, of the electronegative charge on the glomerulus. This results in less electrostatic repulsion of negatively charged macromolecules and may account, in part, for the proteinuria seen in these diseases (6).

V. RENAL TUBULAR FUNCTION

Substances whose clearances differ from creatinine are either secreted (clearance greater than creatinine) or reabsorbed (clearance less than creatinine) by the renal tubules. The final urine composition is determined by glomerular filtration, tubular reabsorption of the bulk of glomerular filtrate, and tubular secretion of certain substances.

Quantitatively, the most important tubular functions are those involved in reabsorptive processes. As examples of the magnitude of tubular reabsorption consider the following. With a GFR of 125 ml/min about 180 liters of plasma water are filtered across the glomeruli each day. In that water are about 26,000 mEq of sodium, 4500 mEq of bicarbonate, and 1000 mmol of glucose. Yet, each day only 1–2 liters of urine is excreted, which contains 100–200 mEq of sodium and no bicarbonate or glucose under normal conditions. Most of the metabolic energy expended by the kidneys is attributable to tubular reabsorptive processes.

Substances that are largely reabsorbed by the renal tubules and returned to the blood include sodium, chloride, bicarbonate, calcium, magnesium, inorganic phosphate, glucose, amino acids, water, and other substances in lesser amounts. Substances that are both secreted and reabsorbed by the renal tubules include potassium and uric acid. Substances that are eliminated in the urine primarily because of tubular secretion include drugs such as some of the penicillins and procainamide.

A great deal is now known about the reabsorptive and secretory functions of the various renal tubular segments. These will be discussed briefly in general terms.

A. Proximal Convoluted Tubule

This is the tubular segment where the bulk of glomerular filtrate is reabsorbed. The majority of sodium, chloride, bicarbonate, potassium, calcium, phosphate, amino acids, glucose, and water filtered at the glomerulus is reabsorbed in this location (8). Fluid remains isotonic with blood in the proximal convoluted tubule, i.e., it is neither concentrated or diluted. Most of these reabsorptive processes are ultimately linked to active (energy-requiring) sodium reabsorption. Many of these solutes also have a component of passive (non-energy-requiring) reabsorption by the process of simple diffusion or solvent drag. Active or passive reabsorption of solutes results in diffusion of water out of the tubules into the interstitial space and into the peritubular capillaries. The proximal convoluted tubule is a major site of action of parathyroid hormone. In this location its principal action is to inhibit phosphate reabsorption (9). Organic bases and acids are secreted by proximal convoluted tubules (10, 11).

B. Proximal Straight Tubule

Reabsorption of sodium, chloride, bicarbonate, and phosphate occur in this location (8, 9, 12). The proximal straight tubule is a major site in the nephron where organic acids such as uric acid and penicillins, and organic bases such as procainamide and cimetidine, are secreted into the urine (*8, 10, 13, 14*). A small amount of potassium is secreted into tubular fluid in this location. As in the proximal convoluted tubule parathyroid hormone inhibits phosphate reabsorption in the proximal straight tubule (*9*).

C. Thin Descending and Thin Ascending Limbs of Henle

The thin descending and thin ascending limbs of Henle have not been as thoroughly studied as the other tubule segments. Their main function is in the urinary concentrating and dilution processes.

D. Thick Ascending Limb of Henle

The thick ascending limb of Henle is responsible for reabsorption of most of the sodium chloride remaining in tubular fluid up to this location. The quantity of sodium chloride reabsorbed by the thick ascending limbs is second only to that reabsorbed by the proximal convoluted tubules. The thick ascending limb is an important site of parathyroid hormone-stimulated calcium reabsorption (*15*) and is the major segment where magnesium is reabsorbed (*16*). There is some potassium reabsorbed in this location.

E. Distal Convoluted Tubule

Most of the sodium, chloride, and bicarbonate remaining in tubular fluid as it emerges from the loop of Henle is reabsorbed by the distal convoluted tubule. There is a small amount of calcium reabsorbed in this location. The distal convoluted tubule is a major site where potassium is added to the urine. It is also an important site where hydrogen ions are secreted to form ammonium and titratable acid (see below).

F. Collecting Tubules and Ducts

These segments are responsible for the final regulation of urine volume and composition. A small amount of sodium, chloride, and bicarbonate is reabsorbed by these tubules. These segments are major sites of potassium and hydrogen ion secretion. Sodium reabsorption and potassium and hydrogen ion secretion in this location are increased by aldosterone. Antidiuretic hormone increases water reabsorption in these tubules.

VI. SODIUM

Sodium is the major extracellular cation and total body sodium content is the primary factor that determines extracellular fluid (and blood) volume (*17*). Regulation of sodium balance is, therefore, vital to preservation of normal health. Sodium balance is determined primarily by renal excretion or conservation of sodium salts. The renal handling of sodium is in turn proportional to dietary intake, total body sodium content, and a number of other factors, many of which are mentioned below. The serum sodium concentration, normally maintained in the range of 135–145 mEq/liter, reflects only the balance between relative amounts of sodium and water in the body and is determined principally by the intake and excretion of water. The concentration of sodium in the blood is, therefore, not a reliable indicator of total body sodium content or extracellular fluid volume (*17*). Hypo- or hypernatremia may exist with a normal, low, or expanded extracellular fluid volume. Under normal conditions urinary sodium excretion varies directly with dietary intake and is approximately 200 mEq/day when an average North American diet is ingested.

Sodium handling by the kidneys has been studied extensively in man and experimental animals. Depending on the state of hydration, the amount of sodium reabsorbed from the glomerular filtrate by the various renal tubular segments is as follows: proximal tubules (especially convoluted tubules) 45–65%; ascending limbs of Henle (especially thick ascending limbs) 24–40%; distal convoluted tubules, collecting tubules, and ducts 10% (*18*). The amount of filtered sodium excreted in the urine varies from less than 1% under conditions of sodium depletion to several percent with volume expansion or administration of potent diuretics such as furosemide (*18*).

The mechanisms of reabsorption of sodium salts vary in the different tubular segments. In the initial portion of the proximal convoluted tubule there is preferential (active) reabsorption of sodium bicarbonate and co-transport of sodium salts with other solutes, especially glucose and amino acids. In the latter portions of the convoluted tubule and in the proximal straight tubule the sodium chloride concentration in tubular fluid is greater than and the sodium bicarbonate concentration less than that of blood owing to the preferential reabsorption of sodium bicarbonate in the early proximal convoluted tubule. These anion gradients from tubule fluid to blood are responsible for a large component of passive sodium chloride reabsorption in the latter portions of the proximal tubule (*8*). Also, there is probably a small component of active sodium chloride reabsorption in the proximal tubule. By the time fluid leaves the proximal tubules most of the bicarbonate, phosphate, and organic solutes e.g., amino acids and glucose, have been reabsorbed and returned to the blood and the principal solute remaining in tubular fluid is sodium chloride. A small amount of sodium chloride is reabsorbed in the thin ascending limbs of Henle, by passive processes. The thick ascending limb of Henle is responsible for most of the sodium chloride reabsorbed beyond the proximal tubule. In contrast to other tubule segments where active salt reabsorption occurs because of active sodium reabsorption with chloride being reabsorbed passively, sodium chloride reabsorption in the thick ascending limb of Henle is due to active chloride reabsorption with sodium following passively (19). Finally, sodium reabsorption occurs to a variable extent in the distal convoluted tubules, collecting tubules, and collecting ducts.

A number of factors, many of which are interrelated, affect renal sodium handling. Some of the major ones will be discussed briefly. Tubular reabsorption of sodium increases as the amount of sodium salts delivered to the renal tubules is increased as a consequence of increases in glomerular filtration rate, a process termed glomerulotubular balance (17). The mechanisms responsible for the proportional increase or decrease in the percent of sodium reabsorbed with parallel changes in GFR are not completely understood. The absolute or "effective" blood volume is a major determinant of renal tubular sodium handling. The term low effective blood volume is an operational one that refers to certain states in which total blood volume may be normal, low, or high, but in which the kidneys perceive blood volume to be low, e.g., edematous disorders such as congestive heart failure. A low absolute or effective blood volume increases sodium reabsorption by the renal tubules (17). The amount of sodium reabsorbed by the ascending limb of Henle is proportional to the amount of sodium chloride that escapes reabsorption in the proximal tubule and is delivered to this location. This "load dependency" of sodium reabsorption also occurs, to a lesser extent, in the distal convoluted tubules. Mineralocorticoids stimulate sodium reabsorption by the collecting tubules and ducts and possibly in the distal convoluted tubules (8, 18, 20). Finally, a number of other factors may influence renal sodium handling including renal sympathetic nerves, prostaglandins, vasoactive substances, and ill-defined natriuretic hormones (17).

A.   Renal Sodium Handling in Renal Insufficiency

External sodium balance is usually maintained in chronic progressive renal insufficiency until GFR is severely reduced (21). At a given level of sodium intake if sodium balance is to be preserved, it is necessary for the amount of sodium excreted in the urine, expressed as a fraction of that filtered at the glomerulus, to double when the GFR is reduced by one-half, etc. With average sodium intake normal individuals will excrete less than 1% of sodium filtered at the glomeruli, whereas a person with advanced renal failure may excrete 20% or more (22, 23). This high fractional excretion of sodium appears to result primarily from decreased reabsorption in the distal nephron (24). However, the mechanisms involved have not been fully characterized. Osmotic diuresis in the remaining nephrons and natriuretic hormones, which to date have not been well characterized, are probably important. For example, one group of investigators has identified a substance in the urine of uremic patients which inhibits sodium reabsorption by collecting tubules (25). Although sodium balance may be maintained in advanced renal failure by adjustments in renal sodium excretion, patients cannot adapt rapidly to abrupt changes in sodium intake (22, 23, 26). Therefore, acute increases in sodium intake will not lead to rapid excretion and the consequences of sodium excess, e.g., hypertension and edema, may become evident. Conversely, abrupt decreases in sodium intake may result in varying degrees of sodium depletion with subsequent hypotension and further reduction in GFR (26, 27), whereas a more gradual reduction in sodium intake, even to very low levels, may be tolerated without any evidence of sodium depletion because of decreased renal sodium excretion (28).

Although most patients with chronic renal insufficiency maintain reasonably normal sodium balance by adjustments in renal sodium excretion, patients with diseases affecting primarily the renal tubules tend to be "salt wasters" and patients with chronic glomerulonephritis tend to be "salt retainers."

Finally, even though external sodium balance may appear normal, a subtle (and clinically undetectable) increase in total body sodium content may be an important factor in the pathogenesis of hypertension, which is so frequent in patients with chronic renal insufficiency. In patients with renal failure severe enough to warrent chronic dialysis treatments, the ability to excrete normal amounts of sodium is usually reduced and restriction of dietary sodium intake is usually necessary to avoid the consequences of sodium excess.

VII. POTASSIUM

The serum potassium concentration is normally maintained at approximately 3.5–5.5 mEq/liter, primarily by renal excretion of ingested potassium. The bulk of potassium filtered at the glomerulus is reabsorbed by the proximal convoluted tubules. However, under conditions of excessive intake, potassium clearance may exceed that of creatinine. This occurs primarily because of potassium secretion into tubular fluid of the distal nephron (distal convoluted tubule, collecting tubules, and collecting ducts). The amount of potassium appearing in the urine is largely dependent on this secretion. A number of factors may influence the magnitude of renal tubular potassium secretion. The most important ones are (1) mineralocorticoids; aldosterone increases potassium secretion in the collecting tubules and ducts; (2) tubule fluid flow rate; increased flow rate decreases the concentration gradient against which potassium is secreted and enhances secretion; (3) tubule fluid and cell pH; alkaline pH increases and acid pH decreases secretion; and (4) rate of sodium absorption; in collecting tubules the rate of potassium secretion is proportional to the rate of sodium absorption (29, 30).

Normally, about 100 mEq of potassium are ingested and excreted in the urine each day. However, if renal function is normal much larger quantities may be excreted if intake is increased. In contrast to sodium excretion, which can be reduced to virtually zero under conditions of sodium deprivation, there is an obligatory urinary loss of 10–15 mEq of potassium each day even with severe restriction of intake.

A number of drugs affect renal potassium excretion. The most common of these are the diuretics. The most frequently prescribed diuretics are the thiazide group (including chlorthalidone and metolozone), furosemide, ethacrynic acid, triamterene, and spironolactone. The first three of these increase and the latter two decrease renal potassium excretion. The thiazides, furosemide, and ethacrynic acid may be associated with hypokalemia and triamterene and spironolactone may lead to hyperkalemia, especially in patients with renal insufficiency (31).

Hyperkalemia may be a life-threatening consequence of renal failure (see Chapter 3). However, in most patients the serum potassium concentration does not rise until severe degrees of renal insufficiency are present (32). The mechanisms that account for the higher fractional excretion of potassium in the urine and other factors that maintain normokalemia in the face of declining renal function are incompletely understood. A major factor is increased secretion of potassium by the distal nephron. This may be due, at least in some instances, to increased activity of Na^+, K^+-dependent ATPase, the enzyme necessary for uptake by the cells of the distal nephron (33). Other studies, however, show an adaptive increase in potassium secretion by collecting tubules from uremic animals which is independent of changes in the activity of this enzyme (34). Another important factor is increased fecal loss of potassium. In normal individuals less than 20% of ingested potassium is lost in the stool. However, in severe renal insufficiency fecal potassium excretion may increase markedly (35).

In some patients hyperkalemia may be present, often in association with metabolic acidosis, when the GFR is only modestly reduced. This occurs most often with diabetic, obstructive, or interstitial nephropathies and is frequently due to renin and aldosterone deficiency (36, 37). Although most patients do not become hyperkalemic until severe renal failure is present, patients with lesser degrees of renal insufficiency are more susceptible to the hyperkalemic effects of potassium-sparing diuretics, potassium supplements, trauma, metabolic acidosis, or other factors that increase endogenous or exogenous potassium loads (32).

VIII. CALCIUM AND INORGANIC PHOSPHORUS (PHOSPHATE)

Approximately 500–1000 mg of calcium is ingested each day. About 25% of this is absorbed by the intestine. Gastrointestinal absorption of calcium is increased by vitamin D (38). Renal excretion of calcium is proportional to intake and is normally less than 300 mg/day in men and 250 mg/day in women. The processes of intestinal absorption and renal excretion normally maintain the serum concentration of calcium in the range of 9–11 mg/dl (4.5–5.5 mEq/liter). Of the total amount of calcium in the blood, about 50% is ionized and the remainder is bound to serum proteins (mostly albumin) or complexed with various anions (39). For each 1 g/dl decrease in the serum albumin concentration below normal, the total serum calcium concentration will decrease by approximately 0.8 mg/dl. However, the level of ionized calcium, which is the physiologically important moiety, is not affected by hypoalbuminemia.

Approximately 95% of calcium filtered at the glomerulus is reabsorbed by the renal tubules under normal conditions: 60% by the proximal tubule, 20% by the loop of Henle (especially the thick ascending limb of Henle), 10% by the distal convoluted tubule, and 5% by the collecting tubules and ducts (40). The mechanisms involved in calcium reabsorption have not been totally elucidated. However, in the proximal tubules reabsorption appears to be primarily a passive process occurring as a consequence of active sodium reabsorption. In the distal nephron there is evidence for both active and passive reabsorption (40). Parathyroid hormone enhances calcium reabsorption in the distal nephron (especially thick ascending limb of Henle) (15, 40). Other factors that increase tubular reabsorption of calcium and, hence, reduce urinary excretion include hypocalcemia, hypomagnesemia, blood volume depletion, decreased sodium intake and excretion, and thiazide diuretics. Factors that inhibit tubular reabsorption and increase urinary excretion include hypercalcemia, hypermagnesemia, hypophosphatemia, acidosis, immobilization, high sodium intake and excretion, blood volume expansion, corticosteroids, furosemide, ethacrynic acid, and carbonic anhydrase inhibitor diuretics (40, 41).

The serum phosphate concentration is normally maintained in the range of 2.5–4.5 mg/dl (0.8–1.4 mmol/liter) in adults and slightly higher in children by a combination of intestinal absorption and urinary excretion. About 1000 mg of elemental phosphorus is ingested each day. The majority of this is absorbed, primarily in the small intestines. Absorption is increased by vitamin D. Renal excretion is proportional to intestinal absorption and is usually about 300–700 mg/day (42, 43).

Under normal conditions more than 80% of phosphate filtered at the glomerulus is reabsorbed by the renal tubules. Reabsorption occurs primarily in the proximal convoluted and proximal straight tubule and, to a lesser extent, in the distal convoluted tubules (9). Renal phosphate handling is largely regulated by parathyroid hormone. Phosphate reabsorption is inhibited (and urinary excretion increased) by the hormone (9). Other factors, under certain conditions, may also increase urinary phosphate excretion. These include blood volume expansion, diuretics such as furosemide and thiazides, and osmotic diuresis, e.g., associated with hyperglycemia, hypomagnesemia, and thyrocalcitonin. Factors that increase phosphate reabsorption and, hence, decrease urinary phosphate excretion include phosphate depletion, growth hormone, and vitamin D (9, 41, 42, 44).

A. Effects of Renal Failure on Calcium and Phosphate Metabolism

Alterations in calcium and phosphate metabolism are universal in severe renal insufficiency. There are several consequences of these changes, the major one being metabolic bone disease(see Chapter 3).

The serum phosphate concentration usually remains normal in mild to moderate renal insufficiency. However, once the glomerular filtration rate falls to less than about 25 ml/min, most patients will have some degree of hyperphosphatemia (45). In chronic dialysis patients some degree of hyperphosphatemia is often present. The maintenance of a relatively normal serum phosphate concentration in the presence of declining renal function is due to an increase in the fractional urinary excretion of phosphate primarily as a consequence of increased levels of parathyroid hormone and possibly other factors (44, 46–48). Parathyroid hormone levels are elevated in patients with moderate renal insufficiency (GFR less than 50 ml/min) and are uniformly (and usually markedly) elevated in patients with renal failure severe enough to warrant chronic dialysis treatments (44, 49, 50).

Multiple abnormalities may occur in calcium metabolism in renal insufficiency. In the absence of calcium and vitamin D therapy, most patients with end-stage renal disease are hypocalcemic prior to the institution of chronic dialysis treatments. Many, but not all patients, will have low normal calcium concentrations after the institution of chronic dialysis treatments. Successful renal transplantation usually results in normal values of serum phosphate and calcium after renal function has been restored for several months. (*50*). There are several potential causes for the hypocalcemia of renal failure. First, if the serum phosphate concentration is extremely elevated the solubility of calcium and phosphate in blood will be exceeded. This results in precipitation of calcium phosphate salts and lowering of the serum calcium concentration (*44*). Second, the abnormally low level of 1,25-dihydroxy-vitamin D_3 in renal failure is associated with decreased intestinal absorption of calcium (*38, 44, 51, 52*). Therapy with this vitamin leads to elevation of the serum calcium in these patients (*53*). Finally, there is a resistance to the calcemic action of parathyroid hormone in renal failure, possibly due to low levels of 1,25-dihydroxy-vitamin D_3 and/or uremia per se (*44, 54, 55*).

Hypercalcemia is distinctly unusual in uremic patients prior to the institution of chronic dialysis treatments or therapy with vitamin D or calcium supplements and its presence should suggest a primary hypercalcemic disorder such as multiple myeloma. In chronic dialysis patients hypercalcemia is unusual, but may occur as a consequence of severe secondary hyperparathyroidism, high dialysate calcium concentration, or overtreatment with calcium and vitamin D supplements (*56*). Hypercalcemia may occur in the posttransplant period. Often this is transient, but may persist for several months and is usually due to severe secondary hyperparathyroidism (*50, 56*).

IX. RENAL REGULATION OF ACID–BASE BALANCE

One of the more important functions of the kidneys is regulation of acid–base balance. Arterial blood pH is normally maintained in a very narrow range (7.35–7.45). Blood pH is dependent on the concentration of bicarbonate and partial pressure of CO_2 in blood as described by the Henderson–Hasselbalch equation

$$\text{arterial blood pH} = 6.1 + \frac{\log HCO_3^-}{0.03 \times pCO_2}$$

The kidneys are responsible for maintaining a normal blood HCO_3^- concentration and the lungs for maintaining a normal pCO_2. The kidneys regulate the blood HCO_3^- concentration by (1) reclaiming bicarbonate filtered at the glomerulus and returning this to the blood and (2) excretion of net acid in the form of titratable acid and ammonium (*57*). The processes of HCO_3^- reabsorption and titratable acid and ammonium excretion depend on active secretion of hydrogen ions (protons) by the renal tubules into tubular fluid. The vast majority of HCO_3^- ions filtered at the glomerulus are reabsorbed in the proximal tubules through a sodium–hydrogen ion exchange process as depicted in the following scheme (modified from *57*):

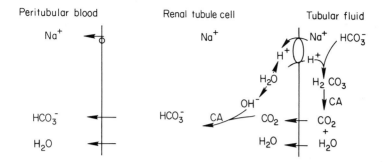

The enzyme carbonic anhydrase (CA in the scheme) is important in catalyzing the reactions involved in hydrogen ion secretion and HCO_3^- reabsorption. Under normal conditions HCO_3^- reabsorption from the glomerular filtrate is complete, i.e., no HCO_3^- appears in the urine. This prevents loss of HCO_3^- from the body which would result in a lower number for the numerator of the above equation and, hence, in a low pH.

When a typical American acid–ash diet is metabolized a number of strong acids are liberated, e.g., phosphoric, sulfuric, organic acids, and others. Since these are strong acids they are virtually completely dissociated at normal blood pH values. The protons released from these acids are buffered in large part by HCO_3^- in blood and extracellular fluid by the following reactions

$$H^+ + HCO_3^- \rightarrow H_2CO_3 \rightarrow H_2O + CO_2 \text{ (expired)}$$

If these reactions continued unabated HCO_3^- stores would be rapidly exhausted since there is normally about 1 mEq per kg body weight of strong acid generated from metabolism of foodstuffs each day that must be buffered (57). HCO_3^- depletion is prevented by the net renal excretion of hydrogen ions and regeneration of HCO_3^- in amounts needed to replenish that decomposed by the above reactions. This occurs by excretion of titratable acid and ammonium by the following scheme:

Ammonium and titratable acid formation occur primarily in the distal convoluted tubules, collecting tubules, and collecting ducts because this is where the tubule fluid pH reaches its lowest values; a low pH is necessary for formation of ammonium and titratable acid in maximal amounts (57). The major form of titratable acid (HA in the above scheme) is monobasic phosphate ($H_2PO_4^-$) which results from addition of a proton to dibasic phosphate (HPO_4^-) (58). For each 1 mEq of ammonium and titratable acid excreted, 1 mEq of "new" HCO_3^- is generated and returned to blood to replenish that decomposed by the buffering processes described earlier. Net urinary acid excretion (the sum of titratable acid and ammonium excretion minus any HCO_3^- lost in the urine) is about 1 mEq per kg body weight per day. Approximately 60% of net acid excretion is in the form of ammonium and 40% in the form of titratable acid. The amount of titratable acid that can be excreted is limited by the amount of buffer anion (A^-) present in tubular fluid. Therefore, if it is necessary to excrete more net acid, e.g., in states of increased acid production such as diabetic ketoacidosis, titratable acid excretion can increase only slightly. Ammonium excretion, however, can increase severalfold by the synthesis of additional ammonia by the renal tubules. Therefore, increased ammonium excretion is the principal way additional acid loads are excreted in the urine (59).

A. Metabolic Acidosis and Renal Insufficiency

Like hyperkalemia, metabolic acidosis does not usually occur until GFR is markedly reduced. However, most patients with GFR less than 25 ml/min will have some degree of metabolic acidosis (60). There are two primary reasons for the metabolic acidosis of renal failure (61, 62). In some patients there is incomplete tubular reabsorption of HCO_3^- by the remaining nephrons. This results in bicarbonaturia. This may be due, at least in some instances, to excessively high levels of parathyroid hormone (63). Second, renal failure results in decreased urinary ammonium excretion (60, 62, 64).

Metabolic acidosis, like hyperkalemia, may develop in some patients whose GFR is only modestly depressed. This occurs primarily in patients with diabetic, obstructive, or interstitial nephropathy (36, 37, 64).

X. URINARY DILUTION AND CONCENTRATION

Normal man can excrete a urine with an osmolality ranging from approximately 50–1000 mOsm/kg H_2O under conditions of water loading and water deprivation, respectively (65). This enables man to vary his urine volume from a few hundred milliliters to several liters each day. In turn, this allows for maintenance of serum osmolality between 280 and 290. The ability to vary urine concentration (and volume) depends on the so-called renal countercurrent system and antidiuretic hormone. A brief description of the processes of urinary concentration and dilution follows. Comprehensive reviews may be found elsewhere (65–67).

The renal cortex is isosmotic to blood. However, there is a progressive increase in the osmolality going from the outer medulla to the papillary tip. The highest osmolality is reached in the latter location (up to about 1000–1200 mOsm/kg H_2O). As will become evident, this progressive increase in tissue osmolality is crucial to the process of urinary concentration. Sodium chloride and urea contribute in about equal amounts to the interstitial osmolality of the medulla. Tubular fluid remains isosmotic to blood as it emerges from the proximal tubules in the renal cortex. As fluid courses through the thin descending limbs of Henle it becomes progressively more concentrated, owing largely to diffusion of water out of the tubule lumen into the interstitium. By the time tubular fluid reaches the bend of the loop of Henle, the osmolality (especially in those nephrons whose loops penetrate into the medulla) is quite high and equal to that of the surrounding interstitium. The composition of tubular fluid and interstitial fluid is different, however. The major solute in tubular fluid at this location is sodium chloride, whereas the interstitial osmolality is due to sodium chloride and urea as noted above. Therefore, as fluid reaches the ascending limb of Henle a concentration gradient exists from tubule lumen to interstitium for sodium chloride and from interstitium to lumen for urea. The thin ascending limb of Henle is poorly permeable to water, moderately permeable to urea, and most permeable to sodium chloride. As a consequence of these permeabilities and concentration gradients sodium chloride diffuses out of tubule fluid and urea diffuses into tubule fluid in lesser amounts. There is little water movement in either direction. The net result of these processes is that fluid in the thin ascending limb becomes hypotonic relative to the surrounding interstitium. As fluid reaches the thick ascending limb of Henle more sodium chloride is reabsorbed and, since this tubule segment is poorly permeable to water, tubular fluid becomes more dilute. Fluid entering the distal convoluted tubule is hypotonic relative to blood regardless of whether the final urine is concentrated or dilute. In the distal convoluted tubule fluid remains dilute or approaches the osmolality of blood. In the absence of antidiuretic hormone the collecting tubules and ducts are impermeable to water. In this situation fluid entering the collecting tubules from the distal convoluted tubules remains dilute (and becomes even more dilute because of continued sodium chloride reabsorption) and a hypotonic urine is excreted.

The process for urinary concentration is the same as that for urinary dilution up to the collecting tubules. In the presence of antidiuretic hormone the collecting tubules and ducts are permeable to water. As fluid courses through these tubules in the presence of the hormone water diffuses out of the tubule lumen and tubular fluid equilibrates with the osmolality of the surrounding hypertonic interstitium. By the time fluid reaches the papillary tip it is maximally concentrated (up to $1000-1200$ mOsm/kg H_2O) and is thus excreted.

The ability to excrete a dilute urine, therefore, depends primarily on sodium chloride absorption in the ascending limb of Henle in the absence of water absorption and on impermeability of the collecting tubules and ducts to water. The ability to excrete a concentrated urine depends principally on the presence of a hypertonic medullary interstitium, the presence of antidiuretic hormone, and collecting tubules and ducts that are capable of increasing their permeability to water in response to the hormone. The maintenance of a hypertonic medullary interstitium ultimately depends on active sodium chloride reabsorption by the thick ascending limb of Henle and on urea recycling from the collecting ducts into the medullary interstitium and from here into the ascending limb of Henle. The details of the urinary concentrating mechanism are beyond the scope of this discussion. However, these are reviewed elsewhere as are the details of medullary blood flow which is very important to this aspect of renal function (2, 66–69).

A. Influence of Chronic Renal Failure on Urinary Concentration and Dilution

Progressive renal insufficiency results in an inability to maximally concentrate the urine. The maximal urinary osmolality of patients with severe renal insufficiency is approximately the same or frequently less than that of serum (isosthenuria and hyposthenuria, respectively) (21, 22, 70, 71). Furthermore, there is little or no increase in urine osmolality when exogenous antidiuretic hormone is administered (22, 70, 71). Decreased concentrating ability may be present with only modestly impaired renal function in diseases involving primarily the renal medulla or associated with hypercalcemia or hypokalemia (65, 71, 72). However, concentrating defects are present regardless of the type of renal disease when severe renal failure is present. The mechanisms responsible for the decreased concentrating ability observed in renal failure are not totally understood and are probably multifactorial. They possibly include (1) decreased production of cyclic AMP by uremic collecting tubules in response to antidiuretic hormone and decreased responsiveness of tubules to the hormone beyond the step of cyclic AMP generation (73), (2) osmotic diuresis in the remaining functioning nephrons, (3) anatomical derangements in the renal countercurrent system (21), and (4) other factors, possibly including inhibitors of antidiuretic hormone (72). Inability to concentrate the urine and decrease urine volume to a minimum results in nocturia. This is often one of the first signs of chronic renal insufficiency.

In contrast to the impairment of urinary concentration, the ability to dilute the urine is reasonably well preserved even in severe renal failure (74).

XI. RENAL ENDOCRINE FUNCTION

The kidneys are both a producer of numerous hormones and a site of action of various hormones which are produced in the kidneys or elsewhere. Many aspects of renal endocrinology are discussed in subsequent sections. However, the present comments are intended to provide a tabulation and brief discussion of the major hormones produced in the kidneys or which have the kidneys as their major site of action. These are shown in Table I.

A. Erythropoietin

Erythropoietin is a polypeptide hormone produced in response to tissue hypoxia which stimulates the bone marrow to produce red blood cells. The kidneys are necessary for normal erythropoietin production. Although there is some controversy, it appears that the kidneys are the major site where the hormone is produced (75, 76). Serum erythropoietin levels are not appropriately elevated in anemic patients with renal failure and are much lower in anephric patients than in those whose kidneys have not been surgically removed (77). The anemia of chronic renal failure is clearly multifactorial.

TABLE I

Renal Endocrine System

Hormones produced by the kidneys
  Erythropoietin
  "Renin"
  1,25-Dihydroxy-vitamin D_3
  Prostaglandins
  Others
Hormones having the kidneys as a major site of action
  Parathyroid hormone
  Antidiuretic hormone
  Aldosterone
  Prostaglandins
  1,25-Dihydroxy-vitamin D_3
  Others

However, a major cause is certainly inappropriate production of erythropoietin.

B. Renin

Renin is an enzyme produced in specialized myoepithelial cells of the afferent arteriole near the glomerulus, the juxtaglomerular cells. Renin is released into the circulation in response to numerous stimuli including decrease in blood pressure in the afferent arteriole, stimulation of the renal sympathetic nerves, epinephrine, norepinephrine, hypokalemia, hyponatremia, and increased delivery of solutes to a specialized part of the distal convoluted tubule, the macula densa, which is located adjacent to the juxtaglomerular cells (78). Renin release in response to many of these stimuli is evidently mediated by prostaglandins (see below). Renin converts a circulating plasma globulin to angiotensin I. This small peptide is cleaved further to a smaller peptide, angiotensin II, primarily in the lungs. Angiotensin II has two principal actions. It is the most potent vasoconstrictor known and is the primary stimulus to the adrenal glands to secrete aldosterone. Activation of the renin–angiotensin–aldosterone system is a major consequence of blood volume depletion or hypotension. If these are the stimuli for renin release, they are restored toward normal by angiotensin II-induced vasoconstriction and aldosterone-induced renal sodium conservation which subsequently expands the blood volume (79). Also, changes in the composition of fluid reaching the macula densa may be important in controlling the glomerular filtration rates of individual nephrons via local activation of the renin–angiotensin system, so-called tubuloglomerular feedback (80). Even though renin is an enzyme and not a hormone per se, it assumes a major role in the regulation of an important hormone, aldosterone, and in the control of blood pressure and possibly glomerular filtration rate.

C. Prostaglandins

Several prostaglandins are synthesized by the kidneys by conversion of the fatty acid arachidonic acid to numerous metabolites. The major ones are prostaglandin E_2 (PGE_2), $PGF_{2\alpha}$, PGD_2, PGI_2, and thromboxane A_2. Although the functions of these various compounds have not been totally elucidated, arachidonic acid derivatives seem to have several important physiological functions including regulation of renal blood flow, sodium and water excretion, and erythropoietin release (81).

D. Vitamin D

The first step in the synthesis of vitamin D is conversion in the skin of 7-dehydrocholesterol to vitamin D_3 under the influence of ultraviolet light. Vitamin D_3 is converted in the liver to 25-OH-vitamin D_3 and is further metabolized to 1,25-dihydroxy-vitamin D_3 in the kidneys. This latter compound is the most active form of vitamin D and the kidneys seem to be the only site of its synthesis. 1-Hydroxylation of vitamin D_3 by the kidneys is stimulated by parathyroid hormone (parathyroid hormone secretion is stimulated by a low concentration of ionized calcium in the blood) and hypophosphatemia. 1,25-Dihydroxy-vitamin D_3 has several important functions. The major ones are to increase intestinal absorption of calcium and, in combination with parathyroid hormone, to mobilize calcium from the bones. Because of these functions normal vitamin D metabolism and production are necessary for the maintenance of normal calcium levels in the blood and for proper bone mineralization (*82*).

E. Parathyroid Hormone

Parathyroid hormone (PTH) has several effects on the kidneys. Renal phosphate excretion is largely regulated by PTH (*9*). The hormone inhibits reabsorption of phosphate in all tubular segments in which phosphate is reabsorbed, especially the proximal tubule and, hence, increases phosphate excretion. Renal calcium handling is also influenced by PTH. In the distal nephron, especially the thick ascending limb of Henle, calcium absorption is increased by PTH (*15*). Bicarbonate reabsorption in proximal tubules may also be inhibited by PTH (*83*, *84*). While this latter effect probably is of little importance in normal individuals, very high levels of PTH may result in bicarbonaturia in certain pathological conditions, including renal failure (*63*). Finally, as noted earlier, PTH is a major factor regulating the renal synthesis of the most active form of vitamin D.

The renal actions of PTH result from activation of adenyl cyclase and subsequent production of 3′,5′-cyclic adenosine monophosphate (cyclic AMP) in the renal tubule cells (*85*). The renal actions of PTH can be mimicked by cyclic AMP analogues.

F. Aldosterone

Aldosterone is the major mineralocorticoid of mammalian species. The hormone is synthesized by the adrenal cortex and secreted into the blood in response to a number of stimuli. The major ones are angiotensin II (or a metabolite of angiotensin II), hyperkalemia and/or total body potassium excess, and, to a lesser extent, adrenocorticotropic hormone, and hyponatremia (86).

Aldosterone increases sodium reabsorption and potassium and hydrogen ion secretion by the renal tubules (85). This results in decreased excretion of sodium and increased excretion of potassium and hydrogen ions in the urine. The major, if not sole, locus of action in the kidney is in part of the distal nephron (collecting tubules and possibly distal convoluted tubules) (20, 87, 88). There is little evidence to suggest that aldosterone has any direct effect on the proximal tubules. Similarly, the molecular mechanism whereby aldosterone alters ion transport by renal tubules is uncertain. The effect on sodium handling seems to require protein synthesis, whereas the effects on hydrogen and potassium ions do not (87, 89).

G. Antidiuretic Hormone

In order to reduce urine volume to a minimum under conditions of water deprivation, a concentrated urine must be excreted. As noted earlier, a concentrated urine depends on the presence of antidiuretic hormone (ADH) and its effect on the collecting tubules and collecting ducts. ADH is synthesized in the hypothalamus and transported down specialized neurons to the neurohypophysis where it is stored (90). When ADH is released from its storage site into the blood it travels to the kidneys where it is bound to the surface of the collecting tubules and ducts and activates adenyl cyclase. The subsequent increase in intracellular cyclic AMP levels ultimately leads to increased water permeability of the tubules, an effect that can be mimicked by exogenous cyclic AMP (91). The normal stimulus for ADH release from the neurohypophysis is an increase in the osmolality of the blood. Blood osmolality is normally maintained in the range of 280–290 mOsm/kg H_2O by a balance of water intake and urinary water excretion, the former regulated by the thirst mechanism and the latter by ADH. The threshold for ADH release is a blood osmolality of about 280 mOsm/kg H_2O and the maximal osmotic stimulus for release is attained at an osmolality of about 295 (92). Although the blood osmolality is normally the stimulus for ADH release, a number of nonosmolar factors such as blood volume depletion, hypotension, pain, various drugs, and lung diseases may also cause ADH release. These may, under certain conditions, be very potent stimuli and may result in ADH release despite a low blood osmolality which would normally prevent ADH release. When this occurs there is failure to excrete adequate amounts of water in the urine and, hence, a total body excess of water develops with attendant hyponatremia and hypoosmolality. This is the so-called syndrome of inappropriate secretion of antidiuretic hormone (*93, 94*).

H. Other Hormones

In addition of the aforementioned hormones other hormones may have effects on the kidneys. For some of these their precise physiological role has not been totally defined, e.g., thyrocalcitonin. For others, e.g., "natriuretic hormones," little is known about their physical properties, sites of production, and site or mechanism of action in the kidney.

GENERAL REFERENCES

Brenner, B. M., and Rector, F. C., Jr., eds., "The Kidney," 2nd ed. Saunders, Philadelphia, Pennsylvania, 1981.

Earley, L. E., and Gottschalk, C. W., eds., "Strauss and Welt's Diseases of the Kidney." Little, Brown, Boston, Massachusetts, 1979.

Pitts, R. F., ed., "Physiology of the Kidneys and Body Fluids," 3rd ed. Year Book Med. Publ., Chicago, Illinois, 1974.

Schrier, R. W., ed., "Renal and Electrolyte Disorders, "2nd ed. Little, Brown, Boston, Massachusetts, 1980.

REFERENCES

1. Pitts, R. F. "Physiology of the Kidneys and Body Fluids," 3rd ed., pp. 1–10. Year Book Med. Publ., Chicago, Illinois, 1974.
2. Stein, J. H. The renal circulation. *In* "The Kidney" (B. M. Brenner and F. C. Rector, Jr., eds.), pp. 215–250. Saunders, Philadelphia, Pennsylvania, 1976.
3. Maddox, D. A., and Brenner, B. M. Glomerular filtration of fluid and macromolecules: The renal response to injury. *Annu. Rev. Med.* **28**, 91–102 (1977).
4. Renkin, E. M., and Robinson, R. R. Glomerular filtration. *N. Engl. J. Med.* **290**, 785–792 (1974).
5. Cockcroft, D. W., and Gault, M. H. Prediction of creatinine clearance from serum creatinine. *Nephron* **16**, 31–41 (1976).
6. Venkatachalam, M. A., and Rennke, H. G. The structural and molecular basis of glomerular filtration. *Circ. Res.* **43**, 337–347 (1978).
7. Brenner, B. M., Bayliss, C., and Deen, W. M. Transport of molecules across renal glomerular capillaries. *Physiol. Rev.* **56**, 502–534 (1976).
8. Burg, M. B. The renal handling of sodium, chloride, water, amino acids, and glucose. *In* "The Kidney" (B. M. Brenner and F. C. Rector, Jr., eds.), 2nd ed. pp. 328–370. Saunders, Philadelphia, Pennsylvania,
9. Dennis, V. W., Stead, W. W., and Myers, J. L. Renal handling of phosphate and calcium. *Annu. Rev. Physiol.* **41**, 257–271 (1979).

10. Woodhall, P. B., Tisher, C. C., Simonton, C. A., and Robinson, R. R. Relationship between para-aminohippurate secretion and cellular morphology in rabbit proximal tubules. *J. Clin. Invest.* **61**, 1320–1329 (1978).

11. McKinney, T. D., and Speeg, K. V. Heterogeneity for organic base transport in rabbit proximal tubules. *Clin. Res.* **29**, 850 (abstr.) (1981).

12. McKinney, T. D., and Burg, M. B. Bicarbonate and fluid absorption by renal proximal straight tubules. *Kidney Int.* **12**, 1–8 (1977).

13. McKinney, T. D., Myers, P., and Speeg, K. V., Jr. Cimetidine secretion by rabbit renal tubules in vitro. *Am. J. Physiol.* **241**, F69–F76 (1981).

14. McKinney, T. D., and Speeg, K. V., Jr. Cimetidine and procainamide secretion by proximal tubules in vitro. *Am. J. Physiol.* **242**, F672–F680 (1982).

15. Bourdeau, J. E., and Burg, M. B. Effect of PTH on calcium transport across the cortical thick ascending limb of Henle's loop. *Am. J. Physiol.* **239**, F121–F126 (1980).

16. Quamme, G. A., and Dirks, J. H. Magnesium transport in the nephron. *Am. J. Physiol.* **239**, F393–F401 (1980).

17. Schrier, R. W. Renal sodium excretion, edematous disorders, and diuretic use. *In* "Renal and Electrolyte Disorders" (R. W. Schrier, ed.), pp. 65–114. Little, Brown, Boston, Massachusetts, 1980.

18. Lassiter, W. E. Disorders of sodium metabolism. *In* "Strauss and Welt's Diseases of the Kidney" (L. E. Earley and C. W. Gottschalk, eds.), pp. 1507–1541. Little, Brown, Boston, Massachusetts, 1979.

19. Burg, M. B., and Green, N. Function of the thick ascending limb of Henle's loop. *Am. J. Physiol.* **224**, 659–668 (1973).

20. Schwartz, G. J., and Burg, M. B. Mineralocorticoid effects on cation transport by cortical collecting tubules in vitro. *Am. J. Physiol.* **235**, F576–F585 (1978).

21. Depner, T. A., and Gulyassy, PF. Chronic renal failure. *In* "Strauss and Welt's Diseases of the Kidney" (L. E. Earley and C. W. Gottschalk, eds.), pp. 211–262. Little, Brown, Boston, Massachusetts, 1979.

22. Kleeman, C. R., Okun, R., and Heller, R. J. The renal regulation of sodium and potassium in patients with chronic renal failure and the effect of diuretics on the excretion of these ions. *Ann. N.Y. Acad. Sci.* **139**, 520–539 (1966).

23. Slatopolsky, E., Elkan, I. O., Werts, C., and Bricker, N.S. Studies on the characteristics of the control system governing sodium excretion in uremic man. *J. Clin. Invest.* **47**, 521–530 (1968).

24. Hayslett, J. P. Functional adaptation to reduction in renal mass. *Physiol. Rev.* **59**, 137–164 (1979).

25. Fine, L. G., Bourgoignie, J. J., Hwang, K. H., and Bricker, N. S. On the influence of the natriuretic factor from patients with chronic uremia on the bioelectric properties and sodium transport of the isolated mammalian collecting tubule. *J. Clin. Invest.* **58**, 590–597 (1976).

26. Schrier, R. W., and Regal, E. M. Influence of aldosterone on sodium, water, and potassium metabolism in chronic renal disease. *Kidney Int.* **1**, 156–168 (1972).

27. Levin, D. M., and Cade, R. Influence of dietary sodium on renal function in patients with chronic renal disease. *Ann. Intern. Med.* **42**, 231–245 (1965).

28. Danovitch, G. M., Bourgoignie, J., and Bricker, N. S. Reversibility of the "salt losing" tendency of chronic renal failure, *N. Engl. J. Med.* **294**, 14–19 (1977).

29. Wright, F. S., and Giebisch, G. Renal potassium transport: Contributions of individual nephron segments and populations. *Am. J. Physiol.* **235**, F515–F527 (1978).

30. Stokes, J. B. Potassium secretion by cortical collecting tubule: Relation to sodium absorption, luminal sodium concentration, and transepithelial voltage. *Am. J. Physiol.* **241**, F395–F402 (1981).

31. Kunau, R. T., and Stein, J. H. Disorders of hypo and hyperkalemia. *Clin. Nephrol.* **7**, 173–190 (1977).

32. van Ypersele de Strihou, C. Potassium homeostasis in renal failure. *Kidney Int.* **11**, 491–504 (1977).

33. Schon, D. A., Silva, P., and Hayslett, J. P. Mechanism of potassium excretion in renal insufficiency. *Am. J. Physiol.* **227**, 1323–1330 (1974).

34. Fine, L.G., Yanagawa, N., Schultze, R. G., Tuck, M., and Trizna, W. Functional profile of the isolated uremic nephron. Potassium adaptation in the rabbit cortical collecting tubule. *J. Clin. Invest.* **64**, 1033–1043 (1979).

35. Hays, C. P., McLeod, M. E., Robinson, R. R., and Stead, E. A. An extrarenal mechanism for the maintenance of potassium balance in severe chronic renal failure. *Trans. Assoc. Am. Physicians* **80**, 207–216 (1967).

36. Batlle, D. C., Arruda, J. A. L., and Kurtzman, N. A. Hyperkalemic distal renal tubular acidosis associated with obstructive uropathy. *N. Engl. J. Med.* **304**, 373–380 (1981).

37. Schambelan, M., Stockigt, J. R., and Bigleri, E. G. Isolated hypoaldosteronism in adults: A renin deficiency syndrome. *N. Engl. J. Med.* **287**, 573–578 (1972).

38. Lemann, J., Adams, N. D., and Gray, R. W. Urinary calcium excretion in human beings. *N. Engl. J. Med.* **301**, 535–541 (1979).

39. Ladenson, J. H., Lewis, J. W., McDonald, J. M., Slatopolsky, E., and Boyd, J. C. Relationship of free and total calcium in hypercalcemic conditions. *J. Clin. Endocrinol. Metab.* **48**, 393–397 (1978).

40. Suki, W. N. Calcium transport in the nephron. *Am. J. Physiol.* **237**, F1–F6 (1979).

41. Massry, S. G., Friedler, R. M., and Coburn, J. W. Excretion of phosphate and calcium: Physiology of their renal handling and relation to clinical medicine. *Arch. Intern. Med.* **131**, 828–859 (1973).

42. Knochel, J. P. The pathophysiology and clinical characteristics of severe hypophosphatemia. *Arch. Intern. Med.* **137**, 203–220 (1977).

43. Fitzgerald, F. Hypophosphatemia. *Annu. Rev. Med.* **29**, 177–189 (1978).

44. Slatopolsky, E., Rutherford, W. E., Rosenbaum, R., Martin, K., and Hruska, K. Hyperphosphatemia. *Clin. Nephrol.* **7**, 138–146 (1977).

45. Slatopolsky, E., Rutherford, W. E., Hruska, K., Martin, K., and Klahr, S. How important is phosphate in the pathogenesis of renal osteodystrophy? *Arch. Intern. Med.* **138**, 848–852 (1978).

46. Bank, N., Su, W. S., and Aynedjian, H. S. A micropuncture study of renal phosphate transport in rats with chronic renal failure and secondary hyperparathyroidism. *J. Clin. Invest.* **61**, 884–894 (1978).

47. Slatopolsky, E., Caglar, S., Gradowska, L., Canterbury, J., Reiss, E., and Bricker, N. S. On the prevention of secondary hyperparathyroidism in experimental chronic renal disease using "proportional reduction" of dietary phosphorus intake. *Kidney Int.* **2**, 147–151 (1972).

48. Swenson, R. S., Weisinger, J. R., Ruggeri, J. L., and Reaven, G. M. Evidence that parathyroid hormone is not required for phosphate homeostasis in renal failure. *Metab., Clin. Exp.* **24**, 199–204 (1975).

49. Reiss, E., Canterbury, J., and Kanter, A. Circulating parathyroid hormone concentration in chronic renal insufficiency. *Arch. Intern. Med.* **124**, 417–422 (1969).

50. Katz, A. I., Hampers, C. L., and Merrill, J. P. Secondary hyperparathyroidism and renal osteodystrophy in chronic renal failure. *Medicine (Baltimore)* **48,** 333–374 (1969).

51. Stanbury, S. W. Bone disease in uremia. *Am. J. Med.* **44,** 714–724 (1968).

52. Coburn, J. W., Koppel, M. J., Brickman, A. S., and Massry, S. G. Study of intestinal calcium absorption in patients with renal failure. *Kidney Int.* **3,** 264–272 (1973).

53. Berl, T., Berns, A. S., Huffer, W. E., Hammill, K., Alfrey, A. C., Arnaud, C. D., and Schrier, R. W., 1,25-dihydroxycholecalciferol effects in chronic dialysis: A double-blind controlled study. *Ann. Intern. Med.* **88,** 774–780 (1978).

54. Massry, S. G., Stein, R., Garty, J., Arieff, A. I., Coburn, J. W., Norman, A. W., and Friedler, R. M. Skeletal resistance to the calcemic action of parathyroid hormone in uremia: Role of 1,25 (OH)$_2$ D$_3$. *Kidney Int.* and **9,** 467–474 (1976).

55. Massry, S. G., Coburn, J. W., Lee, D. N. B., Jowsey, J., and Kleeman, C. R. Skeletal resistance to parathyroid hormone in renal failure. Studies in 105 human subjects. *Ann. Intern. Med.* **78,** 357–364 (1973).

56. David, D. S. Calcium metabolism in renal failure. *Am. J. Med.* **58,** 48–56 (1975).

57. Rector, F. C., Jr. Renal acidification and ammonium production; chemistry of weak acids and bases; buffer mechanisms. *In* "The Kidney" (B. M. Brenner and F. C. Rector, Jr., eds.), pp. 318–343. Saunders, Philadelphia, Pennsylvania, 1976.

58. Simpson, D. P. Control of hydrogen ion homeostasis and renal acidosis. *Medicine (Baltimore)* **50,** 503–541 (1971).

59. Pitts, R. F. The role of ammonia production and excretion in regulation of acid-base balance. *N. Engl. J. Med.* **284,** 32–38 (1971).

60. Sebastian, A., McSherry, E., and Morris, R. C., Jr. Metabolic acidosis with special reference to the renal acidoses. *In* "The Kidney" (B. M. Brenner and F. C. Rector, Jr., eds.), pp. 615–660. Saunders, Philadelphia, Pennsylvania, 1976.

61. Schwartz, W. B. Hall, P. W., Hays, R. M., and Relman, A. S. On the mechanism of acidosis in chronic renal disease. *J. Clin. Invest.* **38,** 39–52 (1959).

62. Relman, A. S. The acidosis of renal disease. *Am. J. Med.* **44,** 706–713 (1968).

63. Muldowney, F. P., Donohoe, J. F., Carroll, D. V., Powell, D., and Freany, R. Parathyroid acidosis in uremia. *Q. J. Med.* **41,** 321–342 (1972).

64. Wrong, O., and Davies, H. E. F. The excretion of acid in renal disease. *Q. J. Med.* **28,** 259–313 (1959).

65. Harrington, J. T., and Cohen, J. J. Clinical disorders of urine concentration and dilution. *Arch. Intern. Med.* **131,** 810–825 (1973).

66. Wirz, H., and Diriz, R. Urinary concentration and dilution. *In* "Handbook of Physiology" (J. Orloff and R. W. Berliner, eds.), Sect. 8, pp. 415–430. Physiol. Soc., Washington, D.C., 1973.

67. Jamison, R. L. Urine concentration and dilution. *In* "The Kidney" (B. M. Brenner and F. C. Rector, Jr., eds.), pp. 495–550. Saunders, Philadelphia, Pennsylvania, 1981.

68. Kokko, J. P., and Rector, F. C., Jr. Countercurrent multiplication system without active transport in inner medulla. *Kidney Int.* **2,** 214–223 (1972).

69. Stephenson, J. L. Concentration of urine in a central core model of the renal counterflow system. *Kidney Int.* **2,** 85–94 (1972).

70. Tannen, R. L., Regal, E. M., Dunn, M. J., and Schrier, R. W. Vasopressin-resistant hyposthenuria in advanced renal disease. *N. Engl. J. Med.* **280,** 1135–1141 (1969).

71. Holliday, M. A., Egan, T. J., Morris, C. R., Jarrah, A. S., and Harrah, J. L. Pitressin-resistant hyposthenuria in chronic renal disease. *Am. J. Med.* **42,** 378–387 (1967).

72. Berl, T., Anderson, R. J., McDonald, K. M., and Schrier, R. W. Clinical disorders of water metabolism. *Kidney Int.* **10,** 117–132 (1976).

73. Fine, L. G., Schlondorff, D., Trizna, W., Gilbert, R. M., and Bricker, N. S. Functional profile of the uremic nephron. Impaired water permeability and adenylate cyclase responsiveness of the cortical collecting tubule to vasopressin. *J. Clin. Invest.* **61,** 1519–1527 (1978).

74. Kleeman, C. R., Adams, D. A., and Maxwell, M. H. An evaluation of maximal water diuresis in chronic renal disease. I. Normal solute intake. *J. Lab. Clin. Med.* **58,** 169–184 (1961).

75. Fried, W. Erythropoietin and the kidney. *Nephron* **15,** 327–349 (1975).

76. Erslev, A. J., and Shapiro, S. S. Hematologic aspects of renal failure. *In* "Strauss and Welt's Diseases of the Kidney" (L. E. Earley and C. W. Gottschalk, eds.), pp. 277–306. Little, Brown, Boston, Massachusetts, 1979.

77. Radtke, H. W., Erbes, P. M., Schippers, E., and Koch, K. M. Serum erythropoietin concentrations in anephric patients. *Nephron* **22,** 361–365 (1978).

78. Davis, J. O., and Freeman, R. H. Mechanisms regulating renin release. *Physiol. Rev.* **56,** 1–56 (1976).

79. Laragh, J. H., Baer, L., Brunner, H. R., Buhler, F. R., Sealey, J. E., and Vaughn, E. D. Renin, angiotensin, and aldosterone system in pathogenesis and management of hypertensive vascular disease. *Am. J. Med.* **52,** 633–652 (1972).

80. Stowe, N., Schnermann, J., and Hermle, M. Feedback regulation of nephron filtration rate during pharmacologic interference with the renin-angiotensin and adrenergic system in rats. *Kidney Int.* **15,** 473–486 (1979).

81. Dunn, M. J., and Hood, V. L. Prostaglandins and the kidney. *Am. J. Physiol.* **233,** F169–F184 (1977).

82. De Luca, H. F. Vitamin D endocrinology. *Ann. Intern. Med.* **85,** 367–377 (1976).

83. McKinney, T. D., and Myers, P. Bicarbonate transport by proximal tubules: Effect of parathyroid hormone and dibutyryl cyclic AMP. *Am. J. Physiol.* **238,** F166–F174 (1980).

84. McKinney, T. D., and Myers, P. PTH inhibition of bicarbonate transport by proximal convoluted tubules. *Am. J. Physiol.* **239,** F127–F134 (1980).

85. Chase, L. R., and Aurbach, G. D. Parathyroid function and the renal excretion of 3′,5′-adenylic acid. *Proc. Natl. Acad. Sci. U.S.A.* **58,** 518–525 (1967).

86. Bravo, E. L. Regulation of aldosterone secretion: Current concepts and newer aspects. *Adv. Nephrol.* **7,** 105–120 (1978).

87. Paillard, M. Effects of aldosterone on renal handling of sodium, potassium, and hydrogen ions. *Adv. Nephrol.* **7,** 83–104 (1978).

88. Gross, J. B., and Kokko, J. P. Effects of aldosterone and potassium-sparing diuretics on electric potential differences across the distal nephron. *J. Clin. Invest.* **59,** 82–89 (1977).

89. Fimognari, G. M., Fanestil, D. D., and Edelman, I. S. Induction of RNA and protein synthesis in the action of aldosterone in the rat. *Am. J. Physiol.* **213,** 954–962 (1967).

90. Zimmerman, E. A., and Robinson, A. G. Hypothalamic neurons secreting vasopressin and neurophysin. *Kidney Int.* **10,** 12–24 (1976).

91. Grantham, J. J., and Burg, M. B. Effect of vasopressin and cyclic AMP on permeability of isolated collecting tubules. *Am. J. Physiol.* **211,** 255–259 (1966).

92. Robertson, G. L., Shelton, R. L., and Athar, S. The osmoregulation of vasopressin. *Kidney Int.* **10,** 25–37 (1976).

93. Zerbe, R., Stropes, L., and Robertson, G. Vasopressin function in the syndrome of inappropriate antidiuresis. *Annu. Rev. Med.* **31,** 315–327 (1980).

94. Schrier, R. W., and Berl, T. Nonosmolar factors affecting renal water excretion. *N. Engl. J. Med.* **292,** 81–88, 141–145 (1975).

The Presentation of the Patient
with Chronic Renal Failure

PAUL E. TESCHAN

I. A SUMMARY OF PATIENTS' INITIAL MODES
OF PRESENTATION

The patients' initial modes of presentation are summarized in Table I. A
fuller discussion now follows:

Copyright © 1983 by Academic Press, Inc.
ISBN 0-12-672280-3

END-STAGE RENAL DISEASE

TABLE I

Patients' Initial Modes of Presentation

A. *The patient is sick*, with clinical disability due to:
  1. Certain rather nonspecific clinical symptoms
  2. Fluid volume overload
  3. Other symptoms or illness
  4. Illness or injury with apparent acute renal failure
B. *The patient is not sick*, but seeks medical advice because of:
  1. Family history
  2. An observed abnormality
  3. An accidentally discovered abnormality

A. The Patient Is Sick

1. Due to Certain Rather Nonspecific Clinical Symptoms

These symptoms are listed in the order of decreasing renal function, or increasing severity.

Mild exertion fatigue
Sense of malaise, sluggishness, weakness
Shortened attention span
Diminished ability to pursue a cognitive mental task
Insomnia and daytime drowsiness
Anorexia, weight loss
Erratic memory
Vague headaches, slurred speech
Emotional irritability, reduced sociability
Diminished libido and sexual performance
Episodic nausea, vomiting
Itching, dry skin
Hypothermia, sensations of coldness
Subtle myoclonus, restlessness including "restless legs"
Hiccoughs, flapping tremor
Muscle jerks and cramps, tics
Paranoid and compulsive personality changes, anxiety,
Bizarre behavior
Disorientation, confusion, hallucinations
Mumbling speech, unsteady gait, variable paresis
Meningismus, transiently impaired vision or hearing
Torpor, coma, convulsions, death

Certain characteristics of these symptoms in a patient with chronic renal failure deserve special emphasis (*1–7*):

a. As chronic, progressive renal disease reduces the number of functioning nephrons and so produces progressive renal failure, the symptoms are at first subtle, often progress insidiously but ultimately produce overt disability.

b. The patient's degree of disability, the number and severity of his symptoms, tends to be greater (i) at lower levels of glomerular filtration; (ii) when renal function declines rapidly; or (iii) when dietary excesses, illness, or injury induce increased catabolism of body tissues with accelerated accumulation of metabolites in the body water.

c. As these symptoms progress from subtle, virtually "subclinical" levels to cause overt disability they also typically wax and wane in number and severity to produce an undulating clinical course.

d. By inspection these symptoms appear *primarily* to reflect abnormal function of the *central nervous system*.

c. These disabling symptoms are promptly reversed and suppressed by means of carefully initiated dialysis treatment. For this reason they are often attributed to renal excretory failure, i.e., the failure of the kidney to excrete one or more dialyzable, toxic solutes.

2. Due to Fluid Volume Overload

The patient may seek medical attention because of ankle edema, ascites, exertional dyspnea, dyspnea at rest, and orthopnea. In these cases the intrinsic renal disease is severe enough to cause progressive renal excretory failure, this time of *volume*. Both salt and water gradually accumulate in excess of concurrent intake. When the cumulative, positive salt and water balance is sufficiently great, alveolar edema, peripheral edema, pleural or pericardial effusions, and ascites will occur.

These symptoms and physical findings of fluid volume overload may be reversed by bulk removal of extracellular fluid. This may be accomplished gradually by restricting salt and water intake while administering the more potent diuretics to produce a negative salt and water balance. Bulk removal of extracellular fluid may be achieved very rapidly by means of controlled ultrafiltration (*convective* transport) across a dialyzer membrane in the direction of a transmembrane pressure gradient. The latter is typically achieved by applying a negative pressure (vacuum) to the dialysate chamber of the dialyzer, and the volume of the collected extracellular fluid (ultrafiltrate) may be measured directly. Since dialysate is not flowing, the reversal of the patient's symptoms is not attributable to dialysis (*diffusive* transport) across the dialyzer membrane. Noncolloidal solute concentrations in the body water change very little during the ultrafiltration process.

Differential diagnostic considerations necessarily include heart disease with congestive heart failure; hepatic cirrhosis with anasarca and "hepatorenal syndrome"; and the nephrotic syndrome with anasarca. However, the higher levels of azotemia associated with fluid retention due to chronic renal failure, among other features, will aid in the differentiation.

3. Due to Other Symptoms or Illnesses

Several examples will illustrate this type of presentation:

a. A patient seeks relief from increasingly severe, recurrent headaches. The workup reveals severe, accelerated, or malignant hypertension with the azotemia of chronic renal failure due to nephrosclerosis or other chronic renal or renovascular lesion.

b. A patient with known or unrecognized diabetes mellitus notes gradual visual impairment. In addition to diabetic retinopathy further investigations provide evidence of diabetic nephropathy and chronic renal failure.

c. Following an accidental or elective surgical injury the catabolic stress produces disproportionately abnormal levels of azotemia or acidemia, revealing the underlying reduced ability of chronically diseased kidneys to maintain the chemical composition of the plasma and the extracellular fluid within normal limits.

d. Similarly, in patients with chronic renal failure, the reduced renal excretion of many drugs, if given in "usual doses," may reproduce many of the symptoms listed in Section I,A,1 (see also Chapter 4).

4. Due to Illness or Injury and Appears
to Develop Acute Renal Failure

The "acute" renal failure in these instances may initially be considered as a "complication" of the injury or intercurrent illness, but may in fact represent exacerbation or "clinical decompensation" of preexisting chronic renal failure. In other examples of acute renal failure, renal function occasionally does not recover sufficiently to normalize the measured chemical composition of the extracellular fluid. Such chronic renal failure may persist.

B. The Patient Is Not Sick

Although the patient is not sick, he may seek medical advice because of the following reasons:

1. Family History

A person seeks a "medical checkup" because renal disease, diabetes mellitus, or other chronic illness has been discovered in other members of his family. Subsequent examination may reveal evidence of renal disease and a degree of chronic renal failure.

2. An Observed Abnormality

An otherwise asymptomatic person, his family, or his physician may note and seek the cause of his pallor, easy bruising, or tawny discoloration of the skin. Chronic renal failure may be discovered in the subsequent workup.

3. Accidentally Discovered Abnormality

Abnormal urinary findings or serum chemical determinations may be discovered accidentally in the course of routine examinations for school, employment, insurance, or military service. Further investigations may document chronic renal disease and the renal functional impairment.

C. Modifiers of Clinical Disability That Influence the Assessment of Patients and the Choice and Intensity of Treatment

Particularly with respect to the disabling symptoms cited in Section I,A,1, certain other characteristics of chronic renal disease and failure influence patients' clinical behavior and practical requirements for treatment as follows:

1. Isosthenuric Polyuria

At comparable low rates of glomerular filtration, patients with interstitial nephritis who maintain a higher urinary flow and fixed specific gravity (isosthenuric polyuria) tend to have fewer and milder symptoms (Section I,A,1) than those with glomerulonephritis or nephrosclerosis who may excrete a smaller proportion of glomerular filtrate. "Symptomatic decompensation" occurs if rates of water and salt intake fall behind concurrent obligatory rates of excretion, or if blood pressure and therefore renal perfusion are significantly reduced (see Section I,B,2).

2. Reversibility

Patients with chronic renal disease and failure sometimes present with symptoms that develop more rapidly than one would expect from the known average progression of the patient's renal disease itself. Their previously asymptomatic state "decompensates," becoming symptomatic and often disabling. This frequent experience reveals that the degree of renal failure in many patients has at least three components: (a) rapidly reversible, (b) slowly reversible, and (c) fixed or gradually progressive. It is critically important and often very helpful to approach treatment of all chronic renal failure patients with these three components clearly in mind.

a. THE RAPIDLY REVERSIBLE COMPONENT. See Chapter 1. Whatever the basic renal disease, the level of residual renal function still depends on (a) the renal blood flow and glomerular filtration rate, which in turn depend on the effective circulating blood volume, the extracellular fluid volume, cardiac pump function, arterial blood pressure, and the vasomotor (constrictor) tone of the renal vasculature; and (b) an unobstructed postrenal urinary tract. The degree of renal failure in any patient with chronic renal disease may well include a circulatory (functional) and/or an obstructive component. These in turn will serve to exacerbate some of the symptoms listed in Section I,A,1. When treatment succeeds in expanding the reduced plasma or extracellular fluid volumes, improving cardiac output, normalizing blood pressure, and blocking renal vasoconstrictor responses or removing obstructions to urinary flow, renal function may again recover and the symptoms may rapidly improve or disappear.

b. THE SLOWLY REVERSIBLE COMPONENT (8). Again, regardless of the chronic parenchymal renal lesion, both renal function and symptoms may be improved by alleviating such concurrent contributors of functional damage as urinary tract obstruction (calculi; sloughed renal papillae; retroperitoneal mass or fibrosis; prostatic or other bladder neck obstruction); active pyelonephritis due to infection; analgesic abuse; or poisoning with such heavy metals as lead or cadmium; renal artery stenosis; accelerated or malignant hypertension; lesions of lupus erythematosus or of Wegener's granulomatosis; or the nephropathy of hypercalcemia, hyperuricemia, hypokalemia (potassium depletion), or of nephrotoxic drugs. Recovery is usually more gradual as these intercurrent dysfunctional conditions are relieved by appropriate treatment.

c. THE FIXED OR SLOWLY PROGRESSIVE COMPONENT. This component is typically determined by the basic lesion in the kidney itself, the number of residual functioning nephrons, amount and location of scar tissue, and involvement of blood vessels or various nephron (tubule) segments. Renal excretory capacity will progressively decrease as the renal disease itself progresses, but at varying, usually slow rates in different patients.

Note: As previously stated, the foregoing discussion is cast in terms of renal *excretory* function and failure. The other functions of the kidney, including the endocrine and metabolic functions, do not always decline in parallel with excretory function. For example, as renal failure progresses, renin secretion may increase in some patients, producing more severe hypertension; or in the case of polycystic renal disease, the relatively high levels of hemoglobin and hematocrit suggest that renal erythropoietin secretion is preserved while excretory function declines. Peptide hormone degradation, a normal function of the kidney, may be affected as well; and each of these phenomena may indirectly modify the patient's symptom profile and the design of his treatment program.

D.   The Problem of Mistaken Identity

*1.   Syndromes That Mimic the Illness of Chronic Renal Failure:
The "False Positive" Case (9)*

The clinical symptoms cited in Section I,A,1 are nonspecific in that one or more of them also occurs in other disease states in which renal failure is absent or too minimal to contribute to significant symptoms. However, when they do occur they notably cause one or a few, but not usually the entire spectrum of the disabling symptoms listed in Section I,A,1. Moreover they may be further differentiated from symptoms attributable to renal failure per se by (a) specific historical features, collateral laboratory tests, or physical findings, (b) their usual response to appropriate, specific therapy, and (c) their usual failure to respond to dialysis treatment.

Among the conditions that may mimic to some extent the illness of renal failure, and that must be identified and differentiated from it, are

1.   Hypertensive encephalopathy, usually associated with accelerated or malignant hypertension

2.   "Toxemia" of sepsis

3.   Water intoxication, e.g., serum sodium concentrations usually less than 115 mEq/liter with evidence of recent, rapid water load and expansion of the total body water

4.   Severe hypernatremia, e.g., serum sodium concentrations greater than 155 mEq/liter

5.   Drug effects: primary effects of sedatives, narcotics, and tranquilizers, and secondary effects of antihypertensives and other drugs (see Chapter 3)

6.   Reactive depression, acute anxiety reactions and certain psychotic states (see Chapter 5)

7.   Severe anemia

8.   Hypocalcemia tetany

9.   Hypercalcemia

10.   Certain nutritional and vitamin deficiencies

11.   Liver disease with failure, hepatic encephalopathy, and "hepato-renal syndrome"

12.   Other medical conditions such as diabetic ketoacidosis, hypoxemia, respiratory acidosis or alkalosis, hyperosmolar coma

TABLE II

Examples of Complaints and Incomplete Diagnosis and Treatment

Locus or organ system	Complaint or finding	"Operational diagnoses"	Possible treatment erroneously limited by incomplete or incorrect diagnoses
Head, oral	Loose teeth, halitosis	Same	Dental extractions, mouth washes
CNS	"Cannot concentrate," nervousness, insomnia	Anxiety	Tranquilizers, sedatives
	Myoclonic jerks, convulsions	Epilepsy	Anticonvulsants
	Blurred, reduced vision	Refractive error, cataracts	New spectacles Cataract surgery
Lungs	Cough with pulmonary infiltrates by X-ray	Tuberculosis, mycosis, cancer	Antimicrobials, supportive care
Cardiovascular	Hypertension	Essential hypertension	Diuretics, antihypertensives
	Breathlessness	Congestive heart failure	Digitalis, diuretics
Gastrointestinal	Nausea, vomiting, weight loss	Dyspepsia, peptic ulcer disease	Antacids, etc.
Genitourinary	Increased urinary frequency	Prostatism	Antibiotics, reduced fluid intake
	Impotence	Anxiety, situational dysfunction	Reassurance, psychotherapy
Skin	Itching	Dry skin	Lotions
Bones	"Osteoporosis" (demineralization) by X-ray	Osteoporosis	Diet, minerals, vitamins, exercise, hormones
Joints	Pain; swelling	Gout, rheumatoid arthritis, collagen disease	Colchicine, uricosurics, steroids
Blood	Anemia	Iron deficiency, refractory anemia	Iron, vitamins, transfusions
Systemic	Fatigue, weight loss, muscle wasting	Anxiety state, undernutrition,	Reassurance, diet, vitamins, minerals, supportive care, antimicrobials, steroids

13. Specific neurological or neurovascular lesions: cerebral atrophy, angiitis, epilepsy, brain tumors, encephalitis or meningitis, etc.

It should be noted that all these conditions may also occur in patients with chronic renal failure, some perhaps more readily than in persons with more normal renal function; and some of these conditions may themselves acutely exacerbate the degree of renal failure and so indirectly induce the entire spectrum of symptoms in Section I,A,1. This latter circumstance represents a reversible component with clinical decompensation (Section C,2) and may be impossible to differentiate clearly from the foregoing inter-current conditions.

2. *Manifestations of Chronic Renal Failure That May Mimic*
   Other Diseases and Lead to Misdirected Treatment:
   The "False Negative" Case

When patients seek specialized health care according to self-perceived complaints rather than through a general medical workup, both they and the health professionals they consult are at some risk of misdiagnosis. If one reviews the symptoms in Section I,A,1, and recognizes that all organ systems sustain functional and/or structural injury in most patients at some time during the course of chronic renal failure, one can readily imagine the examples of diagnostic and treatment errors listed in Table II. Most of these have occurred, by anecdote at least and some have occurred more often than others.

E. The Organ Systems Involved in Chronic Renal Failure,
Their Contribution to Presenting Symptoms,
and Their Response to Dialysis Treatment

The principal presenting symptoms in patients with chronic renal failure are usually identifiable as signals generated or mediated by the central nervous system (CNS; see Section I-A) in the absence of such intercurrent symptomatic states as fluid volume overload and the conditions listed in Section I,D (*1–3, 7*). In time, as chronic renal failure persists or progresses, encephalopathic symptoms may be joined by various clinical "signals" of damage from most of the other organ systems of the body together with generalized wasting and evidence of undernutrition. These latter "signals" from cutaneous, cardiovascular, pulmonary, erthropoietic, musculoskeletal, endocrine, gastrointestinal, or peripheral nervous systems contrast with the

CNS-generated encephalic or neurobehavioral symptoms in the following ways:

1. They are usually detected in the course of medical workup as physical findings, laboratory determinations or X-ray changes rather than as presenting symptoms

2. While they are frequently (and some of them uniformly) detectable in most patients at some time in the clinical course, they infrequently result in significant clinical disability

3. They tend to appear "late" in the progressive clinical course associated with longer systemic exposure to more severe grades of renal failure, i.e., usually after many of the presenting neurobehavioral symptoms have already appeared

4. Dialysis influences these non-CNS abnormalities (and the symptoms they produce) sluggishly or not at all

In many discussions, including this text, these several systemic findings in patients with end-stage renal disease are considered as "medical complications" of chronic renal failure. Accordingly the reader should consult Chapter 3 for an extended discussion of these manifestations.

II. THE UREMIC ILLNESS

A. The Definition of "Uremic Illness"

If the words *uremia* or *uremic* were used carefully and consistently by most authors according to precise definitions, they might be useful terms. Such is not the case. Some common usages of *uremia* which too often appear interchangeably in individual discussions are as follows:

1. Usage according to the root meaning, "urine in the blood," usually relates to increased concentrations in the blood of mainly nitrogenous and acidic solutes which normal kidneys excrete, i.e., the common kinds of blood chemical abnormalities in patients with renal failure, regardless of how large or small their deviations from normal may be. Example: "uremic serum," in which urea and creatinine concentrations are increased to any level above the range of concentrations in populations of normal individuals, and without regard to whether there is clinical illness in the patient (7, 10).

2. "Uremia" is used to refer to a patient's disabling symptoms (e.g., as listed in Section I,A,1), which comprise the "bedside" clinical illness of renal failure, especially when the other conditions given in Section I,D do not exist in the patient. Example: "He looks uremic" (1–3, 7).

3. Most frequently, "uremia" is used apparently to include all of the bodily abnormalities which can occur at any time in patients with renal failure of any severity (*11*). Examples: "uremic bone disease"; "uremic odor to the breath"; "uremic lung." "Uremic serum" (*1*, above) and "uremic symptoms" or "uremic patients" (*2*, above) are likely to be included here as well. This usage is further illustrated in the text of Chapter 3.

Since the disordered composition of the patient's body fluids, the disabling neurobehavioral symptoms and the abnormalities in the other organ systems (Section I,E) are not pathogenetically related in any known, defined way (*12, 13*), and since contemporary usages of the word are various, and hence untrustworthy and likely to be misleading, the term "uremia" was deliberately avoided in the foregoing Section I. This treatment allowed us to introduce Section I,D (mimicking syndromes) and Section I,E (other systemic involvement) as differentiable for the patient's practical benefit even in the presence of renal failure, rather than permitting the tempting but ambiguous label "uremia" to obscure further options for both diagnosis and treatment. Among the benefits of such precise definitions to clinicians' thinking and patients' health is the separation of dialysis-responsive from dialysis-unresponsive symptoms and findings. Thus, dialysis treatment in reference to the listed usages of "uremia" is fairly successful if it refers to blood chemical abnormalities (Section II,A, paragraph 1), is very successful if it refers to disabling symptoms (Section II,A, paragraph 2), or is a mixture of some successes and many failures if used in terms of all bodily abnormalities in renal failure Section II,A, paragraph 3). Hence in the *following* discussion our use of the term "uremia" will be restricted to the clinical "uremic illness" consisting of the symptoms in Section I,A,1, manifested in a patient with chronic (or acute) renal failure when the mimicking syndromes of Section I,D are absent.

B. Symptoms, Solutes, and Neurobehavioral Measurements

A review of the symptoms comprising the uremic illness as listed in Section I,A,1 and their known response to treatment reveals that they share the following general characteristics (*1, 2, 7*):

1. They are generated by (or mediated via) the nervous system, and are recognizable as cognitive, neuromuscular, sensory or autonomic impairments

2. They represent integrated illness behaviors in whole organisms

3. They define and characterize the uremic illness (or syndrome) clinically; i.e., they are the manifestations by which clinicians identify the clinical uremic illness

4. They disable patients

5. Especially the encephalopathic symptoms are readily ameliorated and controlled by means of dialysis treatment, and are therefore among the principal indications for dialysis

6. They are further improved or eliminated by successful and uncomplicated renal transplantation

7. They are descriptive words written by clinicians in medical records to record their subjective impressions of the patient's clinical state

The foregoing facts are expressed more dynamically in the diagram shown in Fig. 1. Several considerations serve to explicate the diagrammed relationships in Fig. 1.

1. The arrows at locus 2 denote *abnormal deviations* in solute concentration, either up (e.g., azotemia) or down (e.g., pH or bicarbonate ion concentration). Deviations are produced by increased metabolic production (locus 1) or reduced renal excretion (locus 3), and are reduced by inverse changes in locus 1 and locus 3 or by the interventions 4 or 5.

2. The solutes are not specified beyond the implicit assumption that they are likely to be dialyzable, water-soluble crystalloids rather than colloids (*14*).

3. The solutes are also not specified because evidence is still insufficient to implicate any measured or detectable chemical moiety (singly or in combination) in the pathogenesis of the symptomatic uremic illness (*12, 13, 15*).

4. The solute mass–balance relationships 1–5 have been quantified and have been made accessible to simple mathematical analysis for urea, creati-

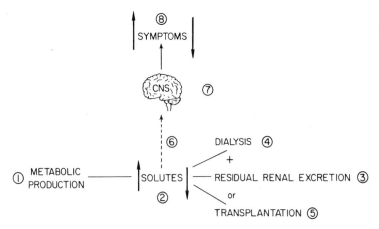

Fig. 1. Outline of relationships between solute flux and clinical illness with renal failure. See text. (Modified from Fig. 12, ref. 7, *Kidney International*, **15**, 1979, p. 690, with permission.)

nine, and acid–base equilibria (*16, 17*). Calculations employing the easily measured urea marker are most widely used on the assumptions that (a) some small molecule(s) (not necessarily urea) may participate in producing the uremic illness; and (b) all small molecules are likely to exhibit similar kinetic behavior (*15*).

5. The steps (locus 6) are unknown by which abnormal solute composition of the body fluids influences the CNS function (locus 7) to produce the symptoms of the uremic illness (locus 8). However, the severity of symptoms *tends* to vary directly with the abnormalities in the solute concentrations.

6. Certain CNS functions may be objectively quantified. Measurable CNS dysfunction was found to vary directly with the degree of chronic renal failure and, in parallel with the symptoms of the uremic illness, to respond to treatment by means of dialysis or renal transplantation.

7. Thus, the numerical neurobehavioral indices provide quantitative outcome measures by which the "chemical axis" (loci 1–5) may be related specifically to the "clinical axis" (loci 2–6–7–8), i.e., by which solute composition may be quantitatively related to the more critical, clinically significant issue: the control of patients' symptomatic and disabling clinical uremic illness.

As a concluding note to this section, the foregoing statements (2 and 3) require further elaboration because they may imply to the reader a topic which is even more problematical and semantically treacherous, if possible, than the term "*uremia*": namely, "uremic toxins," or "uremic toxicity," or "toxemia." To illustrate, Table III presents an incomplete list of putative uremic toxins, substances that have been discovered in "uremic serum" and/or dialysates from "uremic subjects" in abnormal concentrations. It is therefore sometimes implied that these compounds are "toxic" in the sense that they "cause" any one or more of the systemic abnormalities in patients with renal failure. *However, no experimental system has existed heretofore* (and hence no convincing evidence has appeared) by which a damaging "neurotoxicity" has been established for any of these substances *in the concentrations* in which they are found in patients who manifest the presenting, mainly neurobehavioral symptoms of the clinical uremic illness. The further formulations in this chapter appear to suggest possibilities for such an experimental system (*3*).

Meanwhile, the numbing size and diversity of the list of proposed, potential substances itself subverts further progress in this area. The task to establish a believable chemical basis for any of the clinical abnormalities is therefore commonly perceived to be "multifactorial" (*43*). By this it is usually and probably wrongly implied that the task is beyond productive investigation.

TABLE III

A Partial List of Proposed "Uremic Toxins"

1.	Urea (*18, 19*)
2.	Cyanate (*20*)
3.	Guanidines; guanidinosuccinic acid (*21–23*)
4.	Indoles (*24, 25*)
5.	"Middle molecules" (*26–28*)
6.	Myoinositol (*29*)
7.	Ions: H^+; K^+ (*10*)
8.	Parathyroid hormone (*30*)
9.	Aliphatic amines (*31*)
10.	ATP deficiency (*32, 33*)
11.	Tryptophan (*34*)
12.	Urinod (*35*)
13.	Acetoin; 2,3-butylene glycol (*32*)
14.	Carbonyl chloride (*36*)
15.	Peptides; conjugated amino acids (*37*)
16.	Free amino acids (*24, 38*)
17.	Phenols (*24, 39*)
18.	Aromatic amines (*40*)
19.	Aromatic acids (*41*)
20.	See references *24, 37*, and *42* for many more candidates and detailed discussion

C. Quantitative Studies of the Uremic Illness

1. Methods

On the premise that measurements of CNS function might yield quantitative estimates of clinically relevant (symptomatic) impairments in patients with renal failure, as well as their responses to treatment, both electrophysiological and psychometric measures were employed. Electrophysiological indices included (a) the quantified power spectrum of the spontaneous EEG; (b) the visually evoked response latency; and (c) the power distribution of the response to photic driving (see Fig. 1, locus 7).

Psychometric measures of certain cognitive functions (reaction time, short-term memory, and sustained vigilance) were employed as probes of the integrated illness behaviors that are represented in such early symptoms (Section I,A,1) as "malaise," "sluggishness," "shortened attention span," "inability to pursue a cognitive mental task" (such as subtracting serial 7's from 100), "insomnia" and "daytime drowsiness," and "erratic memory" (see Fig. 1, locus 8). The reader is invited to consult references for details of methods and the results of both clinical studies and the prior investigations in laboratory animals (*3, 7*).

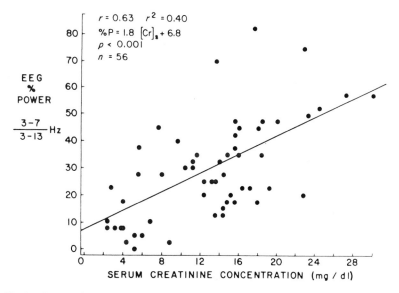

Fig. 2. Percent slow-wave-associated $(3-7)/(3-13)$ Hz EEG power versus concurrent serum creatinine concentrations in 56 azotemic patients with chronic renal failure prior to onset of maintenance hemodialysis. (Reprinted from ref. 7, *Kidney International*, **15**, 1979, p. 681, with permission.)

2. Effects of Renal Failure, Dialysis, and Transplantation

Slowing of EEG wave frequencies is an early finding in renal failure. Figure 2 reveals that more (occipital) EEG power tends to appear in the slower wave frequencies between 3 and 7 Hz in patients with more severe renal failure. This effect is again seen in Fig. 3 in comparisons of average 3–7 Hz power levels among normals, "low-azotemics" (serum creatinine concentrations, Cr_s, less than 10 mg/dl) and "high-azotemics" (Cr_s greater than 10 mg/dl). The EEG slowing induced by renal failure (A) is ameliorated by dialysis (D) treatment and transplantation (T). This effect is seen both in the group means and in the individual data $A \rightarrow D$ and $D \rightarrow T$.

Figure 4 presents data from a test of cognitive function, a reaction time test requiring rapid choice of response according to the color of a stimulus light. The results are similar to those elicited by the EEG probe.

This similarity was noted in four additional measures in the same groups of patients, as summarized in Fig. 5. The average value among normal subjects for each measure was set at 0 and the difference between the means of each successive pair of patient groups (e.g., Normal–High Azotemic–Dialyzed–Transplanted) were factored by the averaged standard errors (SEM) of each pair. Thus, the differences between average test results for each clinical group and each measure are plotted as multiples of the averaged

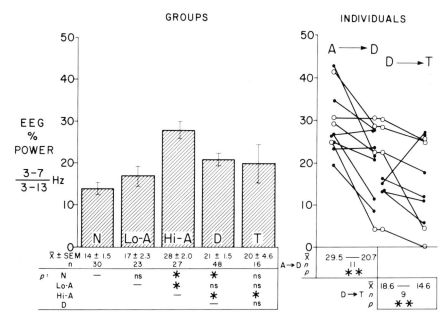

Fig. 3. Slow-wave-associated EEG power in five clinical *groups* and in *individuals* contributing data to more than one treatment group. In the *group* data, bars represent means (X) and brackets ± standard error of the mean for the number (*n*) of individuals in the group. N = normals; Lo-A = azotemia, serum creatinine less than 10 mg/dl; Hi-A = serum creatinine greater than 10 mg/dl; D = during stable maintenance hemodialysis; T = following successful renal transplantation. For *individuals* contributing data to more than one treatment situation (A, D, or T), each data point represents the single value or the mean of 2–25 separate values from each patient in each treatment situation. Open circles identify four patients who traversed and were studied in all three clinical situations: A (Hi-A), D, and T. Levels of statistical significance (*p*) are shown for the indicated comparisons: NS = not significant; * = *p* < 0.05; ** = *p* < 0.01. (Reprinted from ref. 7, *Kidney International*, **15**, 1979, p. 684, with permission.)

standard errors of the adjacent group means. Figure 5 reveals that the three EEG-related electrophysiological measures and the three cognitive function tests (a) varied congruently in response to dialysis treatment, and further improvement following successful renal transplantation; (b) varied in parallel with the symptomatic clinical uremic illness in these patients; and (c) provided objective, quantitative outcome data instead of subjective, imprecise, verbal guesswork for the medical record.

3.   Assessing the "Adequacy of Dialysis"

First, the meaning of "adequacy of dialysis" needs clarification. We shall take it to mean that dialysis is adequate when it suppresses the disabling

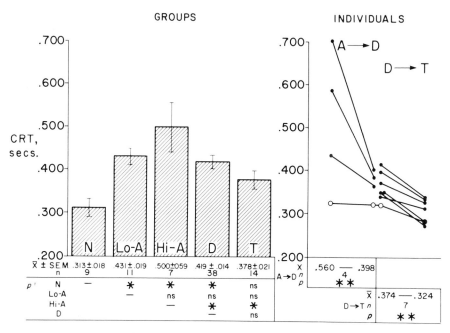

Fig. 4. Choice reaction time (sec) in five clinical *groups* and in *individuals* contributing data to more than one treatment group. See Fig. 3 for designations. (Reprinted from ref. 7, *Kidney International*, **15**, 1979, p. 688, with permission.)

clinical uremic illness, i.e., when it optimizes the function of the CNS generator of the illness behaviors (symptoms) by reversing the impairments induced by renal failure. By way of contrast, from Sections I,E and II,A, the reader correctly infers that dialysis treatment is inevitably inadequate *if* it is *expected* to correct *all* of the abnormalities associated with renal failure. Failure to draw these distinctions has resulted in encumbering several studies of the "effects of dialysis" with measurements that dialysis affects very little, while ignoring measurements of the CNS functions that dialysis affects very much.

In view of the experimental data summarized in Section II,C,2, a reexamination of Fig. 1 (and paragraph 7 following it) reveals an opportunity for the design of prospective experiments to assess the adequacy of dialysis. Thus, the "chemical axis" (loci 1–5) may be viewed as a set of measurable and/or controllable *independent* variables with solute concentrations 2 as *intermediate* rather than as dependent variables. The true, clinically relevant and now quantifiable *dependent* variables are seen in the "clinical axis" (loci 2–6–7–8).

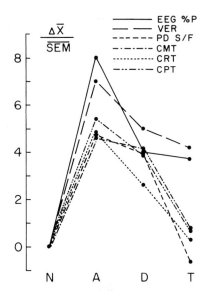

Fig. 5. Congruence of neurobehavioral responses in normal subjects (N) matched in age to azotemic patients (A, serum creatinine concentrations greater than 10 mg/dl before onset of chronic maintenance hemodialysis treatment), dialyzed patients (D) after stabilization on chronic maintenance hemodialysis, and patients following successful renal transplantation (T). The three EEG-related measures are "EEG % Power" as in Fig. 3; "VER," latency (sec) of the major negative deflection of the visual evoked response; and "PD S/F," the ratio of EEG spectral power in the subharmonic (S) to that in the fundamental (F) frequency bands. The three psychometric measures are "CMT," continuous memory test; "CRT," choice reaction time, as in Fig. 4; and "CPT," continuous performance test (see ref. 7). The difference between each adjacent pair of means is factored by their averaged standard errors. [Reprinted from Teschan (2), with permission.]

Figure 6 summarizes the results in nine patients of one such experiment (44). During the initial control period of the study, a standard amount of *combined* (dialyzer plus residual renal) *urea clearance* was prescribed in each patient to be *numerically* equal to 10% of normal glomerular filtration rate per week per liter of body water.* This formulation recognized that patients with chronic renal failure are generally asymptomatic until GFR falls below the 10% level, and that the dialysis prescription should take into account the size of the pool from which urea was being cleared.

---

* 3000 ml/week/liter. This estimate of "dialysis dose" was based on urea kinetics. Hence, residual *urea* clearance was used rather than the average of simultaneous urea and creatinine clearances which more closely approximates other estimates of GFR at low rates of glomerular filtration. The amount of dialysis thus varied inversely with the average level of residual renal urea clearance during each experimental period.

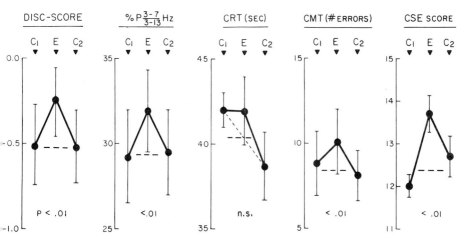

Fig. 6. Neurobehavioral responses to reduced dialysis. "Disc-score" = discriminant function score (see ref. *44*); % power (3–7)/(3–13)Hz = slow-wave associated power in occipital EEG leads, as in Figs. 2 and 3; "CRT" = choice reaction time (latency) in seconds as in Fig. 4; "CMT" = continuous memory test, number of errors; and "CSE Score" = clinical self-evaluation score on a questionnaire concerning patients' own symptoms. C_1 = first control period, average combined urea clearance, 3000 ml/week/liter, 3 months; E = experimental period, average combined urea clearance, 2000 ml/week/liter, 6 months; C_2 = final control period, average combined urea clearance, 3000 ml/week/liter, 3–6 months. P = significance level by paired *t* test of the difference between the average of values in $C_1 + C_2$ and the most abnormal 3-month average of values in E. See text. [Reprinted from ref. *44*, with permission from *Artificial Organs: Proceedings of the Third Meeting of the International Society for Artificial Organs*, Volume 5 (Supplement), 1981.]

Urea generation was treated as an intermediate variable to detect its response to changes in dialysis prescription.

After 3 months, this control level was followed by an experimental period of 6 months during which the combined urea clearance was reduced to two-thirds of the control level. During a final 3–6 month control period, the combined urea clearance was reestablished at the initial level. Figure 6 reveals that the experimental reduction of dialysis treatment produced measurable systematic slowing in the EEG power spectrum, whether measured as percentage power in the slow, 3–7 Hz range, or by the discriminant function. Right and left frontal and occipital 3–7 Hz power and the frequencies at which the maximal spectral power occurred were measured (*45*). Similar, statistically significant deterioration occurred in the continuous memory test and the average scoring of questions assessing the subjective severity of the patients' symptoms (Clinical Self-Evaluation). Average results of the Choice Reaction Time test were different between the control periods, so that the small deviation during the experimental period did not reach statistical significance.

To conclude this section, certain experimental data have been presented to establish and illustrate that when the uremic illness is recognized *as* a neurobehavioral syndrome, then both the illness and its response to treatment can be studied objectively by means of quantitative neurobehavioral probes. A dialysis prescription to achieve a combined urea clearance of 3000 ml/week/liter appeared to assure symptom-related, neurobehavioral stability. Reductions below this level produced measurable neurobehavioral abnormalities. It remains to be shown experimentally whether further neurobehavioral improvement can be evoked by *increasing* the prescription above the 3000 ml/week/liter level or whether optimized neurobehavioral function depends not only on dialysis prescription but interactively on the concurrent metabolic rates as may be indexed by urea generation.

Finally, quantitative measurement of the independent, intermediate, and dependent variables and the control of the independent set the stage for dialysis research with meaningful clinical value: assessing the adequacy of dialysis is just one arena for future studies.

D.   Brain–Mind–Behavior: Implications of
the Presenting Symptoms and Their Response to Treatment
for Rehabilitation and the Quality of Life

The foregoing sections have (a) outlined the major ways by which patients with chronic renal failure reach medical attention, (b) identified the aggregated sequence of common, nonspecific presenting ("uremic") symptoms *as* a syndrome expressing neurobehavioral (mainly encephalic) impairments, and (c) examined the results of certain quantitative measurements of such functional impairments of the brain, at the electrophysiological level and at the level of patients' cognitive performance, including their responses both to differing amounts of dialysis and to successful renal transplantation.

However, the significance of all of this for the patient is in terms of (a) the practical disabilities imposed by the symptomatic uremic illness as renal function deteriorates, and (b) the disabilities inherent in the interactions between the patient and his treatment program even as the treatment relieves his disabling uremic illness. The latter dimension extends beyond the hospital and clinic into the patient's own arena of daily living, and may be introduced by the following statement: We need to understand what renal failure and maintenance dialysis do to the patient's brain in the comprehensive terms of what the brain does for the patient.

Figure 7 outlines this larger concept of *brain* functions as a servant–executor of the processes of the *mind* and as the orchestrator and executor of

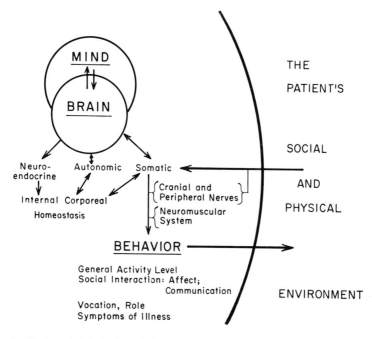

Fig. 7. Brain–mind–behavior relationships that participate in the illness of renal failure and its response to treatment. (Reprinted from ref. *1*, with permission.)

behavior, including those abnormal illness behaviors or clinical signals by which we perceive that the patient is sick (*1, 2*). In this concept, the *mind* or *mental function* refers (a) to a patient's conscious, subjective perceptions of his environment, body, environment–self interactions (including the adequacy and appropriateness of those interactions), memory, thinking, expectations, feelings, and emotions; and (b) to the processes by which he organizes these ingredients in terms of their significance for him and translates them into overt behavior. Of course, the existence and efficiency of these processes are not directly accessible to us, but may be inferred by observing (or measuring) a patient's overt behavior.

These functions of *mind* are characterized in the work of Chapman and Wolfe as "the highest integrative functions of man" and are related by the authors both to the mass of functioning brain tissue on one hand and to the observed behavioral impairments of these patients on the other (*46*). Thus, Table IV uses the Chapman–Wolfe formulation to illustrate vividly the manner and extent to which the illness behaviors of symptomatic uremia impair patients' functioning at the highest integrative level. Conversely,

TABLE IV

Highest Integrative Functions of Man and Illness Behaviors of the Uremic State[a]

A. Highest integrative functions of man

1. To express needs, purposes, and to engage in goal-directed activity; to express affect; interact with environment, pursue values, maintain purposive activity, and to satisfy simple biological needs.

2. To maintain mental and physical mechanisms for goal achievement, including associative capacity; alertness or vigilance; appropriate inhibition of unsuitable behavior; appropriate initiative of activity; capacity for abstraction; orientation to time, place, person and situation; memory; learning ability; ability to extinguish previously appropriate responses; sensory-motor efficiency and skilled actions; ability to fulfill social, vocational, and community responsibilities; ability to perceive self and self-environment relationships; and ability to perceive environmental stimuli.

3. To initiate, organize, and maintain appropriate and effective adaptive reactions, including adequate defenses with acceptable levels of anxiety, depression, and compensatory behavior.

4. To maintain adaptive organization during stress and to recover promptly from the effects of stress (physical, situational) including appropriate displays of defenses and rates of recovery.

B. Illness behaviors of the uremic state

1. Lassitude, lethargy, sluggishness; emotional irritability and withdrawal; euphoria and depression; paranoid and compulsive personality changes; exertional fatigue; insomnia and daytime drowsiness; restlessness; decreased appetite; waning sexual interest and potentia.

2. Impaired ability to focus or sustain attention, to perform mental arithmetic, or to express ideas in more than simple language; sluggishness; drowsiness; muttering and mumbling; disorientation; confusion; erratic memory; delusions; hallucinations; torpor; coma.

3. Anxiety; paranoid and compulsive personality trends, bizarre behavior; catatonia.

4. Chronic, variable, and worsening disorder when untreated; exacerbations sometimes induced by complications in the course of single or multiple dialyses.

[a] Summary of outline according to Chapman and Wolfe (46). (Reprinted from Ref. 1, with permission).

this construct also reveals the significance for normal living which is inherent in an effective regimen of dialysis, diet, and medication, or of uncomplicated renal transplantation. If the patient without other cerebral disease can be freed from dialysis-responsive impairments, integrative capacities of the brain and possibilities for useful behavioral outcomes are largely restored.

The attractive inference to be drawn from this discussion so far is that good dialysis restores patients to normal living; but more than 20 years accumulated experience worldwide suggests instead that relief of symptoms and chemical restoration by dialysis are *necessary* but sometimes *insufficient* for satisfactory living. Instead, several further influences too often appear to prevent patients' "second life" from being an altogether good life *(47)*:

1. The stresses of self-discipline required to "comply" with a relatively complex regimen of medications-diet-dialysis
2. The lurking threat of "living on borrowed time"
3. The limitations on time, travel and choice of job, recreational, and community activities
4. Conflicts between self-images: (a) a *sick* person continuously reminded by frequent contacts with health professionals of his dependence on them and on complex technology for life; and (b) a *well* person, who ought to work and be active along with all other well persons, according to encouragements by the same health professionals
5. Diminished self-image and perceptions in terms of a sense of fitness, physical appearance, exercise tolerance and endurance, sexual performance and enjoyment, employability, earning power, and standard of living
6. Conflicts with spouse and other family members deriving consciously or subconsciously from any of the above
7. Financial burdens of care, and the governmentally imposed loss of financial support (Medicare and Medicaid eligibility) if one continues to work and "earn too much"
8. Others

Despite these personal and environmental stresses, most patients appear to cope exceedingly well, and provide inspiring examples of human adaptability.

Yet, actual behavioral outcomes among patients in the open systems of daily living are rarely quantified, as for example in scores reflecting achieved rehabilitation. Table 5 presents an attempt at such quantitation in terms of the criteria and scoring system adopted in 1979 by the European Dialysis and Transplant Association. Such criteria and scoring could be more widely used, especially to compare outcomes of different modalities of treatment.

The reader is referred to more complete discussions in Chapter 5 in which we are invited to consider in more detail the psychiatric and psychosocial

TABLE V

Rehabilitation to Potential Occupation of Full-Time Work
or Full-Time Housework

			Class number
Able to work	Working	Full-time	1
		Part-time	2
	Not yet working	No work available	3
		Earning capacity less than pension/benefits	4
Unable to work		Living at home	5
		Requires equivalent to hospital care	6

dimensions of patients' adaptational stresses. Indeed these stresses may seriously compromise the potential benefits of any sound medical regimen. Nevertheless, a sound medical regimen including an effective dialysis prescription when indicated, remains the fundamental, essential basis for all other options for quality of life which patients may wish to exercise.

ACKNOWLEDGMENTS

The author wishes to acknowledge the support of commanders and colleagues in the Research and Development Command, United States Army Medical Corps, the Vanderbilt University School of Medicine, the Artificial Kidney-Chronic Uremia Program of the NIADD-KD, and the Dialysis Clinics, Inc., who over the years have made this present contribution possible.

GENERAL REFERENCES

Drukker, W., Parsons, F. M., and Maher, J. F., eds. "Replacement of Renal Function by Dialysis." Martinus Nijhoff, The Hague, 1978.
Levy, N. B., ed. "Psychonephrology I. Psychological Factors in Hemodialysis and Transplantation." Plenum, New York, 1981.
Massry, S. G., and Sellers, A. L., eds. "Clinical Aspects of Uremia and Dialysis." Thomas, Springfield, Illinois, 1976.
Schreiner, G. E., and Maher, J. F. "Uremia, Biochemistry, Pathogenesis and Treatment." Thomas, Springfield, Illinois, 1961.

REFERENCES

1. Teschan, P. E., and Ginn, H. E. The nervous system. In "Clinical Aspects of Uremia and Dialysis" (S. G. Massry and A. L. Sellers, eds.), pp. 3–33. Thomas, Springfield, Illinois, 1976.

2. Teschan, P. E. Measurement of neurobehavioral responses to renal failure, dialysis and transplantation. *In* "Psychonephrology I. Physiological Factors in Hemodialysis and Transplantation" (N. B. Levy, ed.), pp. 13–18. Plenum, New York, 1981.

3. Teschan, P. E. Pathogenesis of uremia. *Am. J. Med.* **48,** 671–677 (1970).

4. Bright, R. Cases and observations illustrative of renal disease accompanied by the secretion of albuminous urine. *Guy's Hosp. Rep.* **1,** 338–379 (1836).

5. Addison, T., On the disorders of the brain connected with diseased kidneys. *Guy's Hosp. Rep.* **4,** 1–7 (1839).

6. Schreiner, G. E. Mental and personality changes in the uremic syndrome. *Med. Ann. D. C.* **28,** 316–323 (1959).

7. Teschan, P. E., Ginn, H. E., Bourne, J. R., Ward, J. W., Hamel, B., Nunnally, J. C., Musso, M., and Vaughn, W. K. Quantitative indices of clinical uremia. *Kidney Int.* **15,** 676–697 (1979).

8. Schreiner, G. E., and Maher, J. F. "Uremia, Biochemistry, Pathogenesis, and Treatment," pp. 24–28. Thomas, Springfield, Illinois, 1961.

9. Schreiner, G. E., and Maher, J. F. "Uremia, Biochemistry, Pathogenesis, and Treatment," pp. 29–35. Thomas, Springfield, Illinois, 1961.

10. Gotch, F. A. A quantitative evaluation of small and middle molecule toxicity in therapy of uremia. *Dial. Transplant.* **9,** 183–194 (1980).

11. Schreiner, G. E., and Maher, J. F. "Uremia, Biochemistry, Pathogenesis, and Treatment," pp. 55–380. Thomas, Springfield, Illinois, 1961.

12. Gordon, A., Bergström, J., Fürst, P., and Zimmerman, L. Separation and characterization of uremic metabolites and biologic fluids: A screening approach to the definition of uremic toxins. *Kidney Int.* **7,** Suppl. 2, S45–S51 (1975).

13. Schreiner, G. E. The search for the uremic toxins. *Kidney Int.* **7,** Suppl. 3, S270–S271 (1975).

14. Schreiner, G. E., and Maher, J. F. "Uremia, Biochemistry, Pathogenesis, and Treatment," pp. 50–51. Thomas, Springfield, Illinois, 1961.

15. Sargent, J. A. Which mathematical model to guide clinical dialysis? *In* "Replacement of Renal Function by Dialysis" (W. Drukker, F. M. Parsons, and J. F. Maher, eds.), pp. 208–213. Martinus Nijhoff, The Hague, 1978.

16. Gotch, F. A. Solute transport and ultrafiltration and hemodialysis. *In* "Clinical Aspects of Uremia and Dialysis" (S. G. Massry and A. L. Sellers, eds.), pp. 639–658. Thomas, Springfield, Illinois, 1976.

17. Gotch, F. A., and Sargent, J. A. Principles and biophysics of dialysis. *In* "Replacement of Renal Function by Dialysis" (W. Drukker, F. M. Parsons, and J. F. Maher, eds.), pp. 38–68. Martinus Nijhoff, The Hague, 1978.

18. Schreiner, G. E., and Maher, J. F. "Uremia, Biochemistry, Pathogenesis, and Treatment," pp. 52–213. Thomas, Springfield, Illinois, 1961.

19. Johnson, W. J., Hagge, W. W., Wagoner, R. D., Dinapoli, R. P., and Rosevear, J. W. Toxicity arising from urea. *Kidney Int.* **7,** Suppl. 3, S288–S293 (1975).

20. Gilboe, D. D., and Javid, M. J. Breakdown products of urea and uremic syndrome. *Proc. Soc. Exp. Biol. Med.* **115,** 633–637 (1964).

21. Cohen, B. D., Handelsman, D. G., and Pai, B. N. Toxicity arising from the urea cycle. *Kidney Int.* **7,** Suppl. 3, S285–S287 (1975).

22. Barsotti, G., Bevilacqua, G., Morelli, E., Cappelli, P., Balestri, P. L., and Giovannetti, S. Toxicity arising from guanidine compounds: Role of methylguanidine as a uremic toxin. *Kidney Int.* **7,** Suppl. 3, S299–S301 (1975).

23. Shainkin, R., Giatt, Y., and Berlyne, G. M. The presence and toxicity of guanidinopropionic acid in uremia. *Kidney Int.* **7,** Suppl. 3, S302–S305 (1975).

24. Hicks, J. M., Young, D. S., and Wooton, I.D.P. Abnormal blood constituents in acute renal failure. *Clin. Chim. Acta* **7,** 623–633 (1962).
25. Ludwig, G. D., Senesky, D., Bluemle, L. W., Jr., and Elkinton, J. R. Indoles in uremia: Identification by countercurrent distribution and paper chromatography. *Am. J. Clin. Nutr.* **21,** 436–450 (1968).
26. Scribner, B. H., and Babb, A. L. Evidence for toxins of "middle" molecular weight. *Kidney Int.* **7,** Suppl. 3, S349–S351 (1975).
27. Funck-Brentano, J. L., Man, N. K., Sausse, A., Cueille, G., Zinfraff, J., Drueke, T., Jungers, P., and Billion, J. P. Neuropathy and "middle" molecule toxins. *Kidney Int.* **7,** Suppl. 3, S352–S356 (1975).
28. Babb, A. L., Ahmad, S., Bergström, J., and Scribner, B. H. The middle molecule hypothesis in perspective. *Am. J. Kidney Dis.* **1,** 46–50 (1981).
29. Liveson, J. A., Gardner, J., and Bornstein, N. B. Tissue culture studies of possible uremic neurotoxins: Myoinositol. *Kidney Int.* **12,** 131–136 (1977).
30. Massry, S. G. Is parathyroid hormone a uremic toxin? *Nephron* **19,** 125–130 (1977).
31. Simenhoff, M. L. Metabolism and toxicity of aliphatic amines. *Kidney Int.* **7,** Suppl. 3, S314–S317 (1975).
32. Thölen, V. H., and Bigler, F. Die pathogenese des urämie syndroms. *Schweiz. Med. Wochenschr.* **94,** 65–69 (1964).
33. Hutchings, R. H., Hughstrom, R. W., and Scribner, B. H. Glucose intolerance in patients on long-term intermittent dialysis. *Ann. Intern. Med.* **65,** 275–285 (1966).
34. Gulyassy, P. F., and de Torrente, A. Tryptophan metabolism in uremia. *Kidney Int.* **7,** Suppl. 3, S311–S313 (1975).
35. Hartman, F. A. The symptoms of urinod poisoning. *Arch. Intern. Med.* **16,** 98–108 (1915).
36. Sen, D. K. Carbonyl chloride cycle in uraemia. *Nature* (*London*) **205,** 908–909 (1965).
37. Lubash, G. D., Stenzel, K. H., and Rubin, A. L. Nitrogenous compounds in hemo-dialysate. *Circulation* **30,** 848–852 (1964).
38. Muting, D., and Dishuk, B. D. Free amino acids in serum, csf and urine in renal disease with and without uremia. *Proc. Soc. Exp. Biol. Med.* **126,** 754–758 (1967).
39. Muting, D. Studies on the pathogenesis of uremia. Comparative determinations of glucuronic acid indican, free and bound phenols in the serum, csf and urine of renal diseases with and without uremia. *Clin. Chim. Acta* **12,** 551–554 (1965).
40. Morgan, R. E., and Morgan, J. M. Plasma levels of aromatic amines in renal failure. *Metab., Clin. Esp.* **15,** 479–481 (1966).
41. Kramer, B., Seligson, H., Baltrush, H., and Seligson, D. The isolation of several aromatic acids from the hemodialysis fluids of uremic patients. *Clin. Chim. Acta* **11,** 363–371 (1965).
42. Drukker, W., Parsons, F. M., and Maher, J. F., eds. "Replacement of Renal Function by Dialysis," Chapter 18. Martinus Nijhoff, The Hague, 1978.
43. Luke, R. G. Uremia and the BUN. *N. Engl. J. Med.* **305,** 121–125 (1981).
44. Teschan, P. E. Assessing the adequacy of dialysis. *Artif. Organs* **5,** Suppl., 65–67 (1981).
45. Bourne, J. R., Hamel, B., and Ward, J. W. A discriminant-analysis-based scoring system for the electroencephalogram. *Proc. IEEE, Southeast Conf., 1980* pp. 257–261 (1980).
46. Chapman, L. F., and Wolfe, H. G. The cerebral hemispheres and the highest integrative functions of man. *Arch. Neurol.* (*Chicago*) **1,** 357–424 (1959).
47. Ginn, H. E., and Teschan, P. E. The quality of life of the chronic dialysis patient. *In* "Replacement of Renal Function by Dialysis" (W. Drukker, F. M. Parsons, and J. F. Maher, eds.), pp. 685–694. Martinus Nijhoff, The Hague, 1978.

3

Medical Complications
of End-Stage Renal Disease

WILLIAM J. STONE

I. INTRODUCTION

End-stage renal disease (ESRD) leaves no organ spared. It is a systemic illness that challenges the therapist to the utmost. Each attempt by physicians to intervene creates a new series of problems. Drug toxicity is rampant. While

57

ISBN 0-12-672280-3

methods of dialysis ameliorate certain complications and afford symptomatic relief in some areas, the patient often becomes subjected to progressive
bone disease, access-related infections, and insidious encephalopathies.
Renal transplantation is best tolerated by the young, is accompanied by a
totally different set of complications, and carries with it a high risk of graft
failure.

Yet, there is a great deal positive about this illness. To the knowledgeable
physician most of the complications are able to be diagnosed and successfully
treated. Long survivals of apparently hopelessly ill patients are possible. In
some patients a reversible cause of uremia will be found and much suffering
averted. Renal replacement therapy remains the most favorable example of
our ability to substitute for the function of a vital organ.

In this chapter the major reversible aspects and medical complications of
ESRD will be reviewed. Guidelines for therapy of each are emphasized. The
important role of drug toxicity in this illness and appropriate drug dosing
information are stressed.

II. REVERSIBLE ASPECTS OF RENAL FAILURE

Before considering the pathophysiology of advanced renal failure, it is
important to list factors that may be reversible and return the patient to a
better level of kidney function (Table I). This presupposes that the patient
does not have acute renal failure from a base line of normal renal function.
First, in established renal disease a superimposed obstructive uropathy may
worsen renal function. A residual urine volume will check lower urinary tract
function but requires a cooperative patient who can stand or sit to void. Less
than 50 ml would be a reasonably normal value although there should be
almost none. Obstruction of the ureters or pelves may be evaluated by renal

TABLE I

Reversible Factors that May Worsen
the Degree of Renal Insufficiency

1. Obstruction of the urinary tract
2. Uncontrolled hypertension
3. Depletion of body fluids
4. Drug-induced interstitial nephritis superimposed
   on another renal disease
5. Hypercalcemia
6. Hyperphosphatemia
7. Analgesic overuse
8. Untreated congestive heart failure

ultrasonography. Dilatation of collecting structures indicates obstructive nephropathy. Relief of obstruction is followed by improvement, which may not become maximal for 6 months. Second, severe elevation of blood pressure may lead to malignant nephrosclerosis. Treatment is mandatory with restoration of blood pressure to normal levels as soon as possible. Again, recovery of function is not rapid and may not achieve a maximum for months. Third, depletion of body fluids by vomiting, diarrhea, diuretics, or renal salt wasting may temporarily worsen renal function. Correction of deficits will almost immediately return renal function to a base line level. Other aggravating factors include untreated congestive heart failure, hypercalcemia, hyperphosphatemia, and a superimposed interstitial nephritis due to drugs. Finally, many nephrology patients have headache or other nonspecific complaints, causing them to ingest great quantities of over-the-counter analgesics such as salicylates, acetaminophen, and phenacetin. Dose-related analgesic nephropathy can cause renal insufficiency. Cessation of analgesics, particularly if large doses have been taken for a prolonged period, can lead to striking recovery of renal function (1). Patient education is extremely important in prevention as well, since many patients do not consider over-the-counter products as "medicine" and will not inform physicians of their use of these drugs.

III. ORGAN SYSTEM INVOLVEMENT AND OTHER COMPLICATIONS

A. Anemia

The anemia of chronic renal failure patients has several basic characteristics: (1) it is directly related to level of renal function; (2) it is worse in surgically anephric individuals; and (3) its etiology is multifactorial. Decline in hematocrit (values below 40%) begins when the creatinine clearance (C_{cr}) falls below 30–40 ml/min and progresses linearly to approximately 20% by the time that the C_{cr} is 5–10 ml/min. Institution of chronic dialysis regimens at this point will often improve the hematocrit (2). More severe anemia than indicated above usually represents another process superimposed on the major causes of uremic anemia: failure of erythropoietin production and accumulation of inhibitors of erythropoiesis (3, 4). Many of the other causes are listed in Table II. The bleeding diathesis of uremia due to decreased platelet agregation is rarely of clinical significance in the well-dialyzed patient. The chronic hemodialysis patient is most at risk of anemia because of dialysis-related problems: dialysance of iron and vitamins; introduction of copper, oxidants, or excessive heat into the hemodialysate;

TABLE II

Factors that May Contribute to Uremic Anemia

---

1. Blood loss
   a. Gastrointestinal hemorrhage
   b. Laboratory tests (venipuncture)
   c. Residual erythrocytes in hemodialyzer and lines postdialysis
   d. Other (e.g., retroperitoneal hemorrhage)
2. Deficiencies of vitamins and minerals
   a. Iron
   b. Vitamins B_6 and B_{12}
   c. Folate
3. Hemolysis
   a. Hexose monophosphate shunt deficit causing sensitivity to oxidants
   b. Hypersplenism
   c. Copper intoxication during dialysis
   d. Uremic toxins
   e. Overheated dialysate
   f. Other
4. Secondary hyperparathyroidism
5. Primary failure of erythropoiesis
   a. Erythropoietin deficiency
   b. Inhibitors of erythropoiesis: uremic toxins

---

and blood loss (leaks through rents in the dialyzer membrane, blood remaining in the lines and dialyzer at the termination of dialysis, frequent venipuncture for laboratory tests, and anticoagulant-related hemorrhage). The contribution of the anephric state is illustrated by our hemodialysis patients. Those who are nephric (residual renal tissue) have an average hematocrit of 29% and require 0.1 blood transfusions per month. However, our anephric patients need 2.1 transfusions per month to maintain a hematocrit of 20%. The most valuable diagnostic tests in evaluating the anemia of these patients are the serum ferritin and bone marrow examination (for iron stores, megaloblastic changes).

The following therapeutic approach has evolved at our center:

1. Provide iron and water soluble vitamins as daily oral supplements.

2. Deionize and/or provide reverse osmosis water in preparation of hemodialysate.

3. Rinse dialyzers and lines as completely of blood as possible at the termination of each hemodialysis. As much as 3000 ml per year may be routinely lost in this manner.

4. Minimize laboratory tests requiring blood samples and withdraw only the least volume required. Application of assay methods pioneered by neonatologists using small quantities of blood would further diminish losses.

5. Regularly check the patient's stools for occult blood and monitor serial hematocrits.

6. Androgens will increase erythropoietin production. Nephric patients almost always increase hematocrit values during androgen therapy while anephric subjects are usually refractory. Parenteral testosterone (men) and parenteral nandrolone (women) provide a better response than oral preparations in our experience. Nandrolone is preferred in women because its masculinizing effects are less.

7. Iron deficiency may develop even during oral iron therapy. Primary iron malabsorption or antacid–iron interaction in the gut may be responsible for this phenomenon. This may be successfully treated with parenteral iron dextran during hemodialysis (1000 mg of elemental iron given slowly into the venous line over 2 hr).

B. Immunity: Leukocyte Function

Blood immunoglobulin and leukocyte concentrations are preserved in ESRD patients unless underlying diseases or administered drugs are immunosuppressive. Mild alterations in immune function are observed and relate to defective skin barriers to infection, abnormal granulocyte motility and phagocytosis and depressed cell-mediated immunity (5). However, even serious infections such as vascular access-related bacteremia will usually rapidly respond to antibiotic therapy. Chronic dialysis patients do not become infected with opportunistic pathogens, unlike renal transplant recipients, and will develop normal antibody responses to immunization (6). Blood leukocyte levels do fall in the first few hours of each hemodialysis, but are restored to normal by the end of the treatment. Pulmonary sequestration may play a role in the leukopenia. The clinical significance of either event is unclear (7). Peripheral blood eosinophilia is commonly observed in chronic hemodialysis patients but is unexplained.

C. Common Acid–Base and Electrolyte Abnormalities

1. Metabolic Acidosis

Due to loss of excretory function inorganic and organic anions accumulate in renal failure. A "high anion gap" (serum $Na - Cl - HCO_3$ greater than 16 mEq/liter) metabolic acidosis is commonly observed. With the exception of patients having renal tubular acidosis, lowering of the serum bicarbonate concentration due to dietary acid retention is not seen until the C_{cr} drops below 20 ml/min (8). A typical Western diet contains 1 mEq acid/kg body weight/day. Protein restriction may modify this acid load somewhat in ESRD patients. Dietary supplementation with sodium bicarbonate or sodium citrate in a quantity equal to the acid load will restore the serum bicarbonate to normal levels. Uremic metabolic acidosis is not a cause of severe acidemia (pH < 7.20). If severe acidemia is present in a uremic patient, a mixed acidosis (respiratory + metabolic, two or more kinds of metabolic) will be present. Chronic hemodialysis ameliorates uremic acidosis by providing an acetate, lactate, or bicarbonate load. However, it is often necessary to supplement chronic dialysis patients with sodium bicarbonate or citrate to maintain a normal concentration of serum bicarbonate. A maximum of 1 mEq/kg body weight/day will usually suffice.

TABLE III

Factors Worsening Hyperkalemia

---

1. Intra- to extracellular shifts
   a. Acidemia
   b. β-Adrenergic blockade
   c. Insulin deficiency
   d. Barium poisoning
   e. Digitalis glycosides
   f. Succinyl choline and similar drugs
   g. Arginine HCl
2. Increased load
   a. Devitalized tissue
      (1) Ischemic, traumatized, or necrotic areas
      (2) Hematomas
      (3) Gastrointestinal hemorrhage
      (4) Hemolysis
      (5) Lysis of neoplastic cells
      (6) Rhabdomyolysis
      (7) Burns
   b. Drugs and other products
      (1) Oral and parenteral K-containing agents including penicillin G, potassium iodide (SSKI), Alka-Seltzer, Ringer's lactate, parenteral alimentation fluids
      (2) Blood and blood products
      (3) Potassium-sparing diuretics
      (4) Geophagia
      (5) Salt substitutes
      (6) Drugs causing hypoaldosteronism $\pm$ hyporeninemia (heparin, nonsteroidal anti-inflammatory agents)
   c. Recipients of renal transplants perfused in Collins' solution (141 mEq K/liter)
   d. Foods rich in potassium

---

2. Hyperkalemia

Barring potassium secretory defects such as seen in hypoaldosteronism, elevation of the serum potassium due to retention of dietary potassium is rarely a problem until the C_{cr} approaches 10 ml/min or less. Factors that can augment hyperkalemia at any level of renal function, but especially in renal failure, are listed in Table III (9). Poor dietary compliance is almost always a major contributor to hyperkalemia. Renal diets often must be restricted to 60 mEq of potassium per day. Salt substitutes may contain potassium chloride and must be avoided.

The electrocardiogram and absolute serum concentration are good indicators to use in determining the severity of potassium excess and its treatment. The more rapidly hyperkalemia has developed, the worse the cardiac and neuromuscular effects. Prior chronic mild hyperkalemia has some protective action at any given level of serum potassium elevation. Any degree of hyperkalemia will have more severe neuromuscular effects if the patient is also hyponatremic, hypocalcemic, or hypermagnesemic. Therapy may be classified according to rapidity of onset (Table IV).

If the serum potassium is 7.0 mEq/liter or greater or if there are any severe EKG changes indicative of hyperkalemia (AV block or QRS widening), immediate measures must be initiated (intravenous calcium or sodium bicarbonate) and may be followed by a glucose–insulin infusion. At lesser degrees (5.5–6.9 mEq/liter) of hyperkalemia, exchange resins, dialysis, and repeat dietary instruction will usually correct the problem. Undertreatment is to be avoided at all costs.

TABLE IV

Therapy of Hyperkalemia

1. Immediate (seconds to minutes)
a. Intravenous calcium salts
b. Intravenous sodium bicarbonate
c. Intravenous hypertonic saline (if hyponatremia is present)
2. Slower (30 minutes or more to be instituted or to have an appreciable effect)
a. Intravenous insulin and glucose
b. Hemodialysis versus zero potassium dialysate
3. Slow (several hours or more)
a. Oral and/or rectal sodium polystyrene sulfonate resin
b. Potassium intake restriction
c. Gastric suction
d. Kaliuretic diuretic drugs (requires residual renal function)
e. Peritoneal dialysis

3. Hypocalcemia–Hyperphosphatemia

There are three major factors in the hypocalcemia of renal failure: (1) prescribed protein–phosphate restricted diets are low in calcium; (2) vitamin D deficiency is frequent and progressive; (3) hyperphosphatemia accompanies C_{cr} values below 30 ml/min (10). Demineralization of bone (osteomalacia), secondary hyperparathyroidism (osteitis fibrosa), and muscular weakness intensify as renal dysfunction worsens. Tetany is unusual probably due to the accompanying acidosis. Therapy begins with the normalization of the serum phosphate by oral phosphate-binding agents (aluminum salts). Thereafter, the serum calcium can be increased with dietary calcium supplements and vitamin D analogues. The major benefit is the prevention of renal osteodystrophy (osteomalacia and/or osteitis fibrosa) and extraskeletal calcification. Persistent hyperphosphatemia in the face of a normal serum calcium appears to be a common cause of metastatic calcification (11). Extreme care must be directed toward avoidance of phosphate-containing cathartics and enemas in uremic patients. Adequate doses of oral aluminum hydroxide or carbonate must be given with meals to normalize the serum phosphate. Dialysis alone almost never is sufficient in controlling hyperphosphatemia. Hypercalcemia in a newly diagnosed patient with severe renal insufficiency raises suspicion that a hypercalcemic state (primary hyperparathyroidism, multiple myeloma, occult carcinoma) has produced the renal damage. Hypercalcemia is not unusual in established chronic dialysis patients, either due to overuse of calcium–vitamin D supplements or to secondary hyperparathyroidism.

4. Hypermagnesemia

Hypermagnesemia has many clinical features in common with hyperkalemia. To produce this state both renal insufficiency and the administration of magnesium-containing agents are required unless massive parenteral doses are given (12). Antacids, laxatives, and other agents that contain magnesium are available over-the-counter (OTC) as well as by prescription. Patients regard OTC drugs as benign and may not inform physicians of their use. Patient counseling and physician awareness are mandatory in preventing hypermagnesemia, since either may be ignorant of the potential problem.

5. Hyponatremia

Water retention bedevils most patients with renal failure. A powerful thirst unrelated to hypovolemia is a common finding. Hyperosmolality may be a critical factor in creating thirst. Reduction of fluid intake to match urinary and insensible losses will restore order but is often difficult to achieve. Rarely, hyperlipidemic or paraproteinemic states may produce spurious hyponatremia. Accumulation of glucose, mannitol, or sorbitol in excess in extracellular fluid can produce a true hyponatremia resulting from a shift of water out of cells. Emergency levels of hyponatremia (less than 115 mEq/liter) may be successfully treated with hemodialysis or by "loop diuretics" and replacement of excreted NaCl by hypertonic solutions if there is residual renal function.

D. Abnormal Drug Metabolism

As renal dysfunction worsens, the elimination of many drugs and their metabolites decreases. If usual doses are given, higher blood and tissue concentrations of both drugs and metabolites result and are frequently toxic. Knowledge of the metabolism of drugs by renal failure subjects is often preliminary, nonexistent, or limited to the parent drug. The major causes of drug toxicity in uremic patients are listed in Table V. The first and third have been well emphasized, but metabolite toxicity is a "sleeping dragon." Abnormal drug metabolism has not yet been shown to be clinically significant. If the patient requires some form of dialysis therapy, this new route of elimination of drugs must be considered.

Fortunately, encyclopedic references have become available to help in the dosing of drugs to renally impaired subjects (13, 14). Common drugs to avoid because of heightened toxicity or ineffectiveness are listed in Table VI. Drugs that require particular care are found in Table VII. Many of these can be given safely by taking into account the linearity of the elimination constant (K_{el}) to creatinine clearance (C_{cr}) as illustrated in Fig. 1 (15). K_{el} is proportional to the reciprocal of the half-life $(t_{1/2})$ during the elimination phase of drug disposition. If one knows K_{el} for anephrics and for normals, a simple graph of K_{el} versus C_{cr} will allow determination of K_{el} at any C_{cr} (Fig. 1).

TABLE V

Causes of Drug Toxicity in Renal Failure

1. Retention of parent drug
2. High blood and tissue levels of renally excreted metabolites
3. Metabolic load accompanying the drug
4. Abnormal drug degradation
5. Abnormal drug binding by plasma proteins
6. Alterations in target organs induced by uremia

TABLE VI

Drugs Requiring Major Dosage Revision
in Uremic Patients

Antimicrobials	Cardiac glycosides
Aminoglycosides[a]	Digoxin
Cephalosporins[a]	Digitoxin
Penicillins[a]	Arthritis, gout
Polymyxins	Allopurinol
Vancomycin	Antineoplastics
Flucytosine[a]	Bleomycin
Cotrimoxazole[a]	Cyclophosphamide[a]
Amantadine	Methotrexate
Analgesics, narcotics	Mithramycin
Salicylates[a]	Neuromuscular agents
Meperidine	Neostigmine
Morphine	Miscellaneous
Antiarrhythmics	Insulin
Procainamide[a]	Cimetidine[a]
Quinidine[a]	Clofibrate
N-Acetylprocainamide[a]	Methimazole
Antihypertensives	Nicotinic acid
Clonidine	Propylthiouracil
Diazoxide[a]	
Nitroprusside[a]	

[a] Dialyzed significantly.

This is invaluable because the daily maintenance dose of a drug at any level of abnormal renal function ($D*$) is to the usual dose (D) as are the ratios of the respective K_{el} values

$$\frac{D*}{D} = \frac{K_{el}^*}{K_{el}}$$

or

$$D* = \frac{K_{el}^*}{K_{el}} D$$

or

$$D* = \frac{t_{1/2}}{t_{1/2}^*} D$$

The dose fraction ($D*/D$) can also be graphed against C_{cr} (Fig. 2) and a series of lines drawn from normal ($D*/D = 1.0$ at a $C_{cr} = 100$ ml/min) to

TABLE VII

Drugs to Avoid in Uremic Patients

Antimicrobials	Diuretics
Methenamine mandelate	Acetazolamide
Nalidixic acid	Mercurials
Nitrofurantoin	Triamterene
Tetracyclines (other than	Spironolactone
doxy- or minocycline)	Thiazides (alone)
Neomycin	Amiloride
Analgesics, narcotics	Arthritis, gout
Salicylates	Gold salts
Acetaminophen	Probenecid
Phenacetin	Phenylbutazone
Phenazopyridine	Antineoplastics
Meperidine	Nitrosourea
Morphine	Cisplatin
Sedatives, tranquilizers	Neuromuscular agents
Barbiturates	Gallamine
Glutethimide	Pancuronium
Lithium	Succinylcholine
Ethchlorvynol	Antiarrhythmics
Methaqualone	Bretylium
Phenothiazines	Others
Antacids, laxatives	Terbutaline
Magnesium-containing	Acetohexamide
Phosphate-containing	Chlorpropamide
Mineral oil	
Antihypertensives	
Methyldopa	
Guanethidine	
Reserpine	

selected points of dose fraction values at zero renal function (*16*). These lines are lettered and form convenient "dosing lines" that need never be changed. However, the best available information about the elimination of a particular drug in anephrics and normals is of critical importance in calculating the dose ratio at zero renal function. The correct dosing line may then be selected to determine maintenance dose at any level of renal function. It is usually a good idea to give a loading dose in patients with abnormal renal function. The first dose advised in the package insert for patients with normal renal function may be used as the loading dose. The calculated maintenance dose (from the dose fraction derived from the nomogram) begins one dosage interval later. With experience and particularly in drugs with slow elimination in renal impairment, the dosage interval may be lengthened with

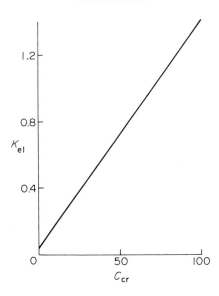

Fig. 1. Elimination rate constant (K_{el}) for a theoretical drug excreted in the urine plotted against creatinine clearance (C_{cr}). There is also a small amount of extrarenal metabolism since K_{el} is not zero at a C_{cr} of zero.

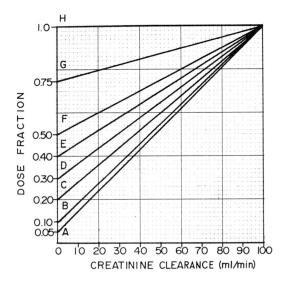

Fig. 2. Dose fraction for all possible drugs is graphed against creatinine clearance. Convenient dosing lines are drawn (see text). (Reproduced from ref. 9, p. 83, with permission.)

TABLE VIII

Dose Fraction Line for Maintenance Dose of Antimicrobials

Amikacin A	Cloxacillin F	Nafcillin E
Amphotericin-B G	Colistimethate B	Nalidixic acid A
Amoxicillin B	Cotrimoxazole E	Nitrofurantoin D
Ampicillin C	Dicloxacillin E	Oxacillin F
Carbenicillin B	Doxycycline G	Oxytetracycline C
Cefaclor D	Erythromycin E	Penicillin-G B
Cefadroxil A	Ethambutol E	Piperacillin D
Cefamandole B	Flucytosine B	Polymixin-B B
Cefazolin A	Gentamicin A	Rifampin H
Ceforanide B	Isoniazid F	Streptomycin A
Cefoxitin A	Kanamycin A	Sulfisoxazole F
Cephalothin A	Lincomycin E	Tetracycline B
Cephalexin A	Methicillin B	Thiabendazole H
Cephapirin C	Metronidazole H	Ticarcillin B
Cephradine B	Mezlocillin D	Tobramycin A
Chloramphenicol G	Miconazole H	Trimethoprim F
Clindamycin G	Minocycline F	Vancomycin A

preservation of the same maintenance dose per unit time, e.g., in enterococcal endocarditis in an ESRD patient instead of giving penicillin G, 250,000 units q 4 hrs, 750,000 q 12 hr may be administered.

A list of antimicrobial agents commonly in use along with the current dosing line employed at this center is appended (Table VIII). It is important to realize the universality of this nomogram, which may be used for any drug once elimination data are known for normal subjects and for anephrics. To reiterate, the nomogram will not have to be changed but the dosing line may need to be altered as new data are accumulated.

E. Special Senses

1. Eyes

Many renal failure patients have normal vision for their age. Hypertensive and diabetic retinopathy are common because of the prevalence of these conditions as causes of renal impairment. If there is poor control of hyperphosphatemia or hypercalcemia, metastatic calcification of the eyes is frequent. This may present as "red eyes" due to conjunctival deposits of calcium phosphate or as band keratopathy (17). Pingueculae, subconjunctival hemorrhages, and cataracts are not uncommon. Less frequent complications include bacterial and candidal endophthalmitis, spontaneous hyphema, dialysis-induced glaucoma, spontaneous retinal detachment, and exophthalmos. Alport's syndrome causes renal failure and is associated with a number of ocular problems.

2. Ears

Hearing loss is frequent in renal failure patients, particularly in the high frequencies. Deafness does not appear to worsen due to chronic dialysis regimens (*18*). Aminoglycoside antibiotics, furosemide, ethacrynic acid, erythromycin, vancomycin, and other drugs may cause deafness or vestibular toxicity. This effect is often heightened in renal failure patients because drug levels tend to be greater due to improper dosing. Administration of more than one ototoxic drug can be a problem. Rare cases of idiopathic uremic deafness have responded to renal transplantation.

Taste–Smell

As renal function declines to C_{cr} values below 10 ml/min, patients often complain that "all food tastes the same" or that "meat tastes terrible" (*19*). Disordered olfaction may also accompany uremia. Smells that once stimulated the appetite now result in nausea and vomiting. Some reports have linked uremic hypogeusia to zinc deficiency, but the relationship is controversial. These defects are usually corrected by adequate dialysis.

F. Gastrointestinal Tract

The most frequent symptom complex leading to initiating dialysis therapy of stable chronic renal failure patients involves some combination of anorexia, nausea, vomiting, and weight loss. Malnutrition is frequently present and must be corrected at all costs. Endoscopic studies have demonstrated up to a 60% incidence of inflammation and hypertrophic folds in the stomach and duodenum of chronic hemodialysis patients. Biopsies have confirmed a 40–50% incidence of gastritis and duodenitis, sometimes in asymptomatic individuals (*20*). Chronic gastrointestinal hemorrhage is also common, but peptic ulceration is not. Acute or chronic pancreatitis is not unusual; however, elevated serum amylase concentrations are even more frequent. In a study of 37 asymptomatic chronic hemodialysis patients at this center, 40% had elevated serum amylase values and the mean concentration for all subjects was twice the upper limit of normal. Presumably this asymptomatic hyperamylasemia is the result of decreased renal excretion of the enzyme. Determination of the percentage of pancreatic isoenzyme may be helpful in the diagnosis of acute pancreatitis in uremia (*21*). Serum gastrin values also rise in proportion to renal insufficiency and may be of significance in the pathogenesis of gastritis and gastrointestinal bleeding. Other gastrointestinal hormones that are frequently elevated in fasting renal failure subjects include cholecystokinin, glucagon, gastric inhibitory peptide, and vasoactive intestinal peptide (22). Small bowel function is usually normal. Chronic hepatitis B afflicts approximately 10% of all chronic hemodialysis patients, mainly due to transmission by blood products. Non-A non-B hepatitis is also seen. Both often cause prolonged carrier states in uremic patients (23). Cholecystitis and cholelithiasis occur at a normal rate. Apparent hyperbilirubinemia without alterations in other liver function tests can result from administration of greater than 200 mg of propranolol daily to an ESRD patient (24). Retention of a propranolol metabolite interferes with the determination of bilirubin by diazotization reactions. "Hyperbilirubinemia" abates when propranolol is withdrawn. Serum transaminase levels in ESRD patients vary in the opposite direction toward subnormal values by the SMA 12/60 method (25). Knowledge of the patient's baseline SGOT is critical in the assessment of myocardial infarction and hepatic injury. Less common complications include subcapsular hepatic and bowel mucosal hematomas, spontaneous retroperitoneal hemorrhage, ileus, diverticular disease, gastroparesis, and spontaneous colonic perforation. Constipation is the most nettling bowel complaint due to its frequency in otherwise well ESRD patients and to its resistance to therapy. Drug bezoars and high fecal impactions have had to be extracted at laparotomy (26). The efficiency of the uremic colon in removing water from its lumen is legendary, possibly related to hypomotility. High fiber renal failure diets are available. If added fiber does not improve the situation, single agents in the category of softeners, fiber, or stimulants may be employed (27). ESRD patients should assiduously avoid all phosphate- and magnesium-containing cathartics or enemas.

G. Hypertension

Hypertension is found in nearly every ESRD patient at one time or another (28). In about 60–70% of affected individuals removal of excess extracellular fluid by diuretics or dialysis will result in a return to normotension. The rest will be extremely sensitive to fluid withdrawal, rapidly changing from hyper- to hypotension. Drug therapy is always necessary in these latter patients for control of elevated blood pressure. Once volume overload has been corrected, the use of β-adrenergic blocking agents (propranolol, nadolol, metoprolol) and vasodilators (hydralazine, minoxidil) has been most suitable in our center. Diuretics are discontinued once chronic dialysis is initiated. A new drug, captopril, that blocks the renin–angiotensin system may prove useful in some patients. Clonidine is another alternative to β blocker, vasodilator therapy; however, lower initial doses and dosage increments than in nonuremic patients are recommended. Impotence may

be worsened on any regimen. Unpredictable hypotension and a high incidence of impotence in male patients have limited the utility of methyldopa
and guanethidine in uremia. The high incidence of depression in uremic
patients has eliminated reserpine as a useful agent.

Accelerated hypertension may be treated by the usual drug regimens.
Nitroprusside therapy must be monitored closely because its metabolite,
thiocyanate, accumulates. Thiocyanate may be removed by dialysis if toxic
concentrations are discovered.

H. Lungs

Most respiratory symptoms in renal failure patients result from pulmonary
edema related to salt and fluid overload or heart failure. Treatment is
straightforward. Ultrafiltration without dialysis is particularly useful. About
1% of all ESRD patients develop a refractory pleuritis that is often hemorrhagic and may lead to entrapment of a lobe and pulmonary restriction (29).
Surgical removal of this fibrous peel is commonly required. Metastatic
pulmonary calcification occurs in patients with chronic hyperphosphatemia.
Its roentgenographic appearance mimics pulmonary edema (30). Abnormalities of diffusion and vital capacities are seen. Radionuclide scans with
technetium pyrophosphate ("bone scan") are diagnostic since normal lungs
do not usually appear on such scintigrams. Prevention and treatment
involve normalization of the serum phosphate level. Pulmonary thrombo-
and air embolism, originating in the dialyzer or vascular access, are not
unusual in hemodialysis patients.

A final unresolved problem concerns hypoxemia seen in the first hour of
virtually all hemodialyses (31). Cardiopulmonary arrests, dyspnea, and
other pulmonary allergic-like events may rarely be observed at this time in
hemodialysis patients. There seems little doubt that any patient may have
acute pulmonary edema when hemodialyzed on a new membrane system.
Cardiopulmonary arrest may follow. Therapy is supportive including
removal of the patient from the system. The common finding of hypoxemia,
neutropenia, and activation of complement in the first hours of hemodialysis
is unexplained and the three major components may not be related to one
another. Alveolar hypoventilation induced by dialysis-related hypocapnia
could be responsible for hypoxemia. In the compliant patient, the lungs seem
to be one of the best preserved organ systems in uremia.

I. Muscle

Muscle weakness is a common accompaniment of incompletely treated
ESRD. Hyperkalemia, hyponatremia, hypocalcemia, and hypermagnesemia

cause acute weakness. Anorexia and vomiting lead to malnutrition and muscle wasting. Long-term dialysis patients may develop a proximal myopathy closely allied to the progression of secondary hyperparathyroidism and osteodystrophy (*32*). Type 2 fiber atrophy is seen. Therapy directed toward restoration of normal serum calcium, phosphate, and parathyroid hormone levels is usually corrective. Renal transplantation may also help, although glucocorticoid therapy necessitated to prevent rejection can worsen the myopathy. Muscle weakness has also been shown to correlate with a low muscle transmembrane potential difference and with adequacy of dialysis (*33*). Initiation of or conversion to adequate dialysis regimens corrects both the abnormal transmembrane potential difference and muscle weakness. A troublesome acute problem occurs in many hemodialysis patients during ultrafiltration to remove excessive fluid accumulation. Sudden, severe cramping of the leg muscles begins toward the end of the procedure and causes severe pain. Intravenous infusion of hyperosmotic solutions of sodium chloride, mannitol, or glucose has been helpful. The etiology remains obscure. Muscles may calcify in patients with ectopic calcification elsewhere. Clofibrate therapy of uremic hyperlipidemia has caused myotoxicity at doses considered safe in patients with normal renal function. Dosage of clofibrate must be reduced. Finally, many (19–42%) chronic dialysis patients will show persistent elevations in serum creatine kinase (CPK) activity that may correlate with myopathy (*34*). The CPK is not useful in diagnosing myocardial infarction unless the uremic patient's baseline values are known. There is no uniform agreement as to which CPK isoenzyme is causing increased activity.

J. Joints

Joint pain related to osteodystrophy is common. Attacks of acute monarticular arthritis may be caused by sodium urate (gout), calcium hydroxyapatite or oxalate (uremic pseudogout), or bacterial contamination of the joint space due to sepsis. Gout and pseudogout are treated the same as in nonuremic subjects. "Dialysis elbow" is another frequent complaint. Olecranon bursitis with effusion develops on the extremity used for vascular access. Simple aspiration is usually adequate. Tumoral calcinosis may also be seen in large joints of poorly compliant patients prone to ectopic calcification. Although aseptic necrosis of the hips, shoulders, and knees is very common in renal transplant patients, these difficult problems are virtually never seen in uremic patients who have not received chronic glucocorticoid therapy. However, renal osteodystrophy may create a more conducive setting for aseptic necrosis.

K. Heart and Circulation

Heart disease is the leading cause of death in ESRD patients (*35*). This has been linked to the relatively uniform finding of hypertriglycridemia, an unusual diet, hypertension, and other factors (see Table IX). Cardiac hypertrophy and increased cardiac indices are caused by anemia, arteriovenous shunts and fistulae employed for hemodialysis, and the tendency toward hypertension. Accelerated atherosclerosis is common and relates most to hypertension. Hyperkalemia, hypocalcemia, myocardial or valvular calcification, dialysate acetate, acidosis, and antihypertensive drugs may worsen already compromised cardiac function. A cardiomyopathy unrelated to atherosclerosis is thought to be generated by uremic toxins. Chronic hypotension is not unusual in dialysis populations. If unexplained by other treatable causes, primary myocardial disease may be the etiology of hypotension. Autonomic insufficiency is not a factor (*36*). Endocarditis following access-related sepsis has been reported (*37*). Diastolic murmurs are common in hemodialysis patients without endocarditis and may be related to severe anemia, uncontrolled hypertension, and a very high cardiac output.

Echocardiography has proved to be a singularly useful tool in the evaluation of cardiac performance in uremia (*38*). Wall thickness and

TABLE IX

Factors Contributing to Uremic Cardiac Disease

    1. Hypertension
    2. Fluid overload
    3. Anemia
    4. Arteriovenous shunts for dialysis
        (may be multiple)
    5. Atherosclerosis
    6. Electrolyte and acid–base disorders
    7. Metastatic calcification (valves, myocardium,
        conducting tissue)
    8. Nutritional deficits
    9. Endocarditis
   10. Uremic cardiomyopathy
   11. Antihypertensive drugs
   12. Pericarditis
   13. Cardiorenal diseases
        a. Vasculitides
        b. Amyloidosis
        c. Diabetes mellitus
        d. Oxalosis
        e. Fabry's disease
        f. Scleroderma

motion, chamber size, valve function, calcification, vegetation, and pericardial effusion can be evaluated by this technique. Pericarditis in uremic patients remains elusive as to etiology but affects about 20% of the population (39). It is diagnosed by the presence of a pericardial friction rub. Fever, chest pain, and a pericardial effusion are usually present as well. Treatment is symptomatic. There is no evidence that the initiation of dialysis or an increased duration of dialysis is therapeutic except in patients who have not previously been dialyzed. Slow resolution or development of tamponade are the two end points. Constrictive pericarditis is extremely rare. All patients should be followed with serial echocardiograms and physical examinations until resolution is assured. If tamponade develops, a subxiphoid pericardial window has been the best approach at our center. There has been little morbidity and no mortality. Other cardiac surgery has been performed in uremic patients with varying results including coronary artery bypass and replacement of defective valves (40). Succinyl choline should not be used as an anesthetic in cardiac surgery because severe hyperkalemia often results in the postoperative period.

L. Skin, Nails, and Mucous Membranes

Pruritus is a major problem. There is no current uniformly successful therapy or a good explanation for generalized itching in uremic patients. Ultraviolet phototherapy, phenothiazines, water-holding creams, subtotal parathyroidectomy, topical steroids, intravenous lidocaine, and oral activated charcoal are among the recommended treatments. None is uniformly successful.

Uremic skin is often deeply pigmented, giving the patient the appearance of a "tan all over." The pigmentation also may have a yellowish cast, somewhat mimicking jaundice. There is no scleral pigmentation, however. Theories revolve around excessive hormonal stimulation of melanocytes (lipotropin levels are elevated) and retention of urinary pigments.

Multiple needle punctures for hemodialysis and the use of prosthetic devices protruding through the skin for both hemodialysis and peritoneal dialysis create a portal of entry for infectious agents. Vascular access infections, bacteremia (41), and peritonitis result. Sweat and sebaceous gland functions are also insufficient.

About 1% of chronic dialysis patients have a syndrome indistinguishable from porphyria cutanea tarda. Most are nonalcoholic and not iron overloaded. Huge blisters develop in light-exposed skin, particularly over the hands. High levels of plasma uroporphyrin III have been implicated due to reduced activity of uroporphyrinogen decarboxylase. Treatment consists of diminishing exposure to light and use of sunscreens.

About 10% of dialysis patients show "half and half" fingernails, where the distal portion is brown and the proximal half appears normal. Onycholysis, transverse lines, splinter hemorrhages, and "spoon" nails may also be seen. Severe secondary hyperparathyroidism is particularly associated with loss of nails.

Foul-smelling breath and stomatitis are also part of the uremic syndrome.

M. Osteodystrophy

Structurally deficient bone is a major cause of symptoms in uremic patients (*42, 43*). Secondary hyperparathyroidism, possibly as a result of persistent hypocalcemia and defective removal of parathyroid hormone, leads to increased bone resorption. Vitamin D deficiency develops following loss of renal production of active metabolites of cholecalciferol and aggravates the calcium deficiency associated with poor dietary intake. Chronic metabolic acidosis leaches bone mineral. Retention of magnesium, fluoride, and aluminum in bone tissue due to inadequate excretion may further weaken its structure (*44*). Bone pain and fractures are the inevitable result. Initial therapy consists of the following:

1. Correct hyperphosphatemia with oral phosphate binders (aluminum hydroxide and aluminum carbonate).
2. Give at least 1 g of elemental calcium as a supplement to the daily diet.
3. Most patients will require some form of vitamin D. The 1,25-dihydroxylated metabolite appears to be the most physiological. The 25-hydroxylated metabolite is also useful. Neither 1-α-hydroxy or 24,25-dihydroxycholecalciferol are marketed at present.
4. Cimetidine may help to control hyperparathyroidism, but subtotal parathyroidectomy is frequently necessary in advanced osteitis fibrosa.
5 A subset of patients, having mainly osteomalacia on bone biopsy and a tendency toward hypercalcemia on small doses of 25-hydroxy- or 1,25-dihydroxycholecalciferol, constitutes a tremendous therapeutic problem (*44*). Their bones seem to dissolve before the eyes of concerned physicians, fracturing in multiple sites. All attempts at treatment have been futile. Some ask to be allowed to die because of chronic pain and immobility. If osteodystrophy is refractory to therapy, novel approaches include withdrawal of aluminum-containing phosphate binders with substitution of magnesium hydroxide, combinations of active metabolites of vitamin D, and rapid renal transplantation.

N. Nervous System

It has been estimated that one-third of all neurological symptoms in a uremic population are caused by drug toxicity (45). A wide range of drug classes are involved (Table X). Penicillin and cephalosporins in excessive dosage can cause myoclonic jerks and grand mal seizures. Excessive sedation and/or psychiatric symptoms are seen with many sedatives, hypnotics, and tranquilizers. Anticoagulants may promote spontaneous subdural hematomas. Meperidine metabolites can accumulate and cause seizures. Overdosage of isoniazid or cimetidine can lead to encephalopathy. Uremic patients are very sensitive to morphine and neuromuscular blocking agents. Neuromuscular symptoms may be aggravated by hyperkalemia, hypocalcemia, hyponatremia, hypermagnesemia, and administration of aminoglycoside antibiotics.

TABLE X

Drugs that Cause Unexpected
Neurological Disorders in Uremia

Penicillins
Cephalosporins
Phenothiazines
Cimetidine
Meperidine
Morphine
Isoniazid
Reserpine
Anticoagulants
Cyproheptadine
Benzodiazepines
Barbiturates
Nitrofurantoin
Glutethimide
Ethchlorvynol
Meprobamate
Methaqualone
Haloperidol
Methyldopa
Antihistamines
Neuromuscular blocking agents
β-Adrenergic antagonists
Amantadine
Hypoglycemic agents

Peripheral neuropathy appears to be a less common presenting complaint of ESRD patients in the last decade. The decreased incidence may be related to improved dietary treatment of severe renal insufficiency and earlier initiation of adequate chronic dialysis regimens. The neuropathy is sensorimotor, mainly seen in the extremities, and far worse in the legs (46). Early symptoms are "restless legs" and burning feet, often exacerbated at night. Standard diets, vitamin supplements (B vitamins including B_6 and B_{12}), and dialysis regimens almost always result in slow restoration of normal function over 6–12 months. Biopsies show primary axonal degeneration with secondary segmental demyelinization. The etiology is unproved but most likely is due to dialyzable uremic toxins. Also, the carpal tunnel syndrome commonly occurs in chronic hemodialysis patients, responding to surgical decompression.

Uremic encephalopathy is similar in etiology and pathogenesis to the neuropathy, mainly being seen in patients who are late in reaching treatment by ESRD centers. Clinical manifestations include virtually every neuropsychiatric sign and symptom, although focal defects are unusual. Disordered mentation, neuroses, psychoses, personality changes, coma, myoclonic jerks, seizures, headache, asterixis, tremors, and motor abnormalities are common in affected patients and bear some relationship to the severity and duration of untreated renal failure (46). The EEG shows a pattern typical of metabolic encephalopathy: slowing of background activity with an excess of theta and delta waves. Lumbar punctures are usually normal although protein content may be elevated. Radionuclide brain scans, CT scans, and ultrasound studies are normal. The treatment is ordered toward normalization of the blood chemistry by standard ESRD diets, medications, and dialysis regimens. Recovery usually occurs over several days to weeks.

There are two other diffuse encephalopathies seen exclusively in chronic hemodialysis patients. The first and less significant has been termed the dialysis disequilibrium syndrome. The pathogenesis is straightforward and preventable (47). Some combination of headache, nausea, vomiting, irritability, and somnolence occurs late in the patient's first dialysis or in the initial use of a very efficient dialyzer. In severe cases delirium, coma, and convulsions may be seen. High blood levels of urea and other solutes retained in renal failure have been rapidly dialyzed out of the extracellular compartment. Water shifts intracellularly and intracerebrally. Therefore, acute cerebral edema explains the symptom complex. Restoration of extracellular osmolality with nontoxic solutes (glucose, mannitol) is helpful both as therapy of established dialysis disequilibrium and in preventing its occurrence in susceptible patients. The best preventive mechanism is to initiate dialysis regimens slowly (lower blood flows, less efficient dialyzers, shorter dialysis times) so that solute is removed in a less rapid manner. This syndrome is almost never seen in peritoneal dialysis because of its lower solute clearances.

The second and often fatal encephalopathy has been called dialysis dementia (DD), progressive dialysis encephalopathy, dialysis encephalopathy, and other terms. Four findings, otherwise unexplained, must be present to confirm the diagnosis of dialysis dementia: motor abnormalities (myoclonic jerks, seizures), dementia, abnormal speech (aphasia, dysnomia, verbal dyspraxia), and a characteristic EEG (48). The last demonstrates very slow, high amplitude activity with biphasic or triphasic spikes. The symptoms most often begin in well-dialyzed patients years after the start of the dialysis regimen, although there is a great variability in this feature of the illness. An insidious dementia may be the initial manifestation. Osteodystrophy, severe anemia, and gastrointestinal symptoms often accompany the eventual overwhelming neurological disorder. Epidemics of DD have occurred around the world when aluminum has contaminated dialysate. The incidence of sporadic cases averages about 1–5% and is less well linked to aluminum intoxication. However, the epidemic and sporadic cases are clinically identical. It is our belief that enhanced absorption or sensitivity to aluminum from oral phosphate binders or other aluminum-containing compounds is

TABLE XI

Over-the-Counter Antacids
Containing Aluminum

Alternagel	(Stuart)
Aludrox	(Wyeth)
Amphojel	(Wyeth)
A-M-T	(Wyeth)
Basaljel	(Wyeth)
Camalox	(Rorer)
Creamalin	(Winthrop)
Delcid	(Merrell-National)
Di-Gel	(Plough)
Gaviscon	(Marion)
Gelusil	(Warner-Chilcott)
Kolantyl	(Merrell-National)
Kudrox	(Kremers-Urban)
Maalox	(Rorer)
Mygel	(Geneva)
Mylanta	(ICI)
Riopan	(Ayerst)
Robalate	(Robins)
Rolaids	(Warner-Lambert)
Simeco	(Wyeth)

responsible in patients without aluminum in their dialysate. However, the lack of suitable nontoxic oral phosphate binders and the low prevalence of sporadic cases has caused no general change in treatment regimens to date. At our center early cases are treated by withdrawal of aluminum antacids (see Table XI), substitution of magnesium hydroxide, close monitoring of serum magnesium levels, and use of dialysate containing no magnesium. Renal transplantation may be curative in about half of afflicted patients.

Cervical bruits can be found in most chronic hemodialysis patients by systematic auscultation. However, the majority are generated by a hyperdynamic circulation associated with anemia and arteriovenous fistulae for hemodialysis (49). Care must be taken to avoid invasive diagnostic testing unless there is further evidence of occlusive disease of the carotid arteries.

Although various thrombotic and hemorrhagic stroke syndromes are more common in dialysis populations, the most distinct of these is spontaneous subdural hematoma (50). The prevalence is about 1% in hemodialysis patients. Unrelenting headache is the most consistent symptom. Focal signs are the rule but there are exceptions. Computed tomography of the cranium usually establishes the diagnosis but is not foolproof. Despite early diagnosis and surgical drainage, mortality is often greater than 50%. Craniotomy with removal of the membranes may be necessary for a better outcome.

O. Malignancy

Organ transplantation has been clearly demonstrated to result in an increased frequency of neoplastic diseases. However, chronic dialysis patients are also susceptible to malignant diseases at a rate 3–7 times that of age and sex-matched controls (51, 52). Smoking and advanced age are risk factors, but time on dialysis is not. Unlike renal transplant recipients, the spectrum of malignancies developed by untransplanted ESRD patients is the same as a control population without renal disease (53).

REFERENCES

1. Murray, T. G., and Goldberg, M. Analgesic-associated nephropathy in the U.S.A.: Epidemiologic, clinical and pathogenetic features. *Kidney Int.* **13,** 64–71 (1978).
2. Radtke, H. W., Frei, U., Erbes, P. M. *et al.* Improving anemia by hemodialysis: Effect on serum erythropoietin. *Kidney Int.* **17,** 382–387 (1980).
3. Linton, A. L., Clark, W. F., Driedger, A. A. *et al.* Correctable factors contributing to the anemia of dialysis patients. *Nephron* **19,** 95–98 (1977).
4. Fisher, J. W. Mechanism of the anemia of chronic renal failure. *Nephron* **25,** 106–111 (1980).

5. Goldblum, S. E., and Reed, W. P. Host defenses and immunologic alterations associated with chronic hemodialysis. *Ann. Intern. Med.* **93**, 597–613 (1980).

6. Osanloo, E. O., Berlin, B. S., Popli, S. *et al.* Antibody responses to influenza vaccination in patients with chronic renal failure. *Kidney Int.* **14**, 614–618 (1978).

7. Dumler, F., and Levin, N. W. Leukopenia and hypoxemia. Unrelated effects of hemodialysis. *Arch. Intern. Med.* **139**, 1103–1106 (1979).

8. Emmett, M., and Narins, R. G. Clinical use of the anion gap. *Medicine (Baltimore)* **56**, 38–54 (1977).

9. Kunau, R. T., and Stein, J. H. Disorders of hypo- and hyperkalemia. *Clin. Nephrol.* **7**, 173–190 (1977).

10. Davis, D. S. Calcium metabolism in renal failure. *Am. J. Med.* **58**, 48–56 (1975).

11. Gipstein, R. M., Coburn, J. W., Adams, D. A. *et al.* Calciphylaxis in man. A syndrome of tissue necrosis and vascular calcification in 11 patients with chronic renal failure. *Arch. Intern. Med.* **136**, 1273–1280 (1976).

12. Randall, R. E., Cohen, M. D., Spray, C. C. *et al.* Hypermagnesemia in renal failure. *Ann. Intern. Med.* **61**, 73–88 (1964).

13. Bennett, W. M., Muther, R. S., Parker, R. A. *et al.* Drug therapy in renal failure: Dosing guidelines for adults. *Ann. Intern. Med.* **93**, 62–89, 286–325 (1980).

14. Anderson, R. J., Gambertoglio, J. G., and Schrier, R. W. "Clinical Use of Drugs in Renal Failure." Thomas, Springfield, Illinois, 1976.

15. Dettli, L., Spring, P., and Habersang, R. Drug dosage in patients with impaired renal function. *Postgrad. Med. J.* **46**, Suppl., 32–35 (1970).

16. Spring, P. Calculation of drug dosage regimens in patients with renal disease: A new nomographic method. *Int. J. Clin. Pharmacol.* **11**, 76–80 (1975).

17. Walsh, F. B., and Howard, J. E. Conjunctival and corneal lesions in hypercalcemia. *J. Clin. Endocrinol.* **7**, 644–652 (1947).

18. Henrich, W. L., Thompson, P., Bergström, L. *et al.* Effect of dialysis on hearing acuity. *Nephron* **18**, 348–351 (1977).

19. Ciechanover, M., Peresecenschi, G., Aviram, A. *et al.* Malrecognition of taste in uremia. *Nephron* **26**, 20–22 (1980).

20. Margolis, D. M., Saylor, J. L., Geisse, G. *et al.* Upper gastrointestinal disease in chronic renal failure. A prospective evaluation. *Arch. Intern. Med.* **138**, 1214–1217 (1978).

21. Levitt, M. D., and Ellis, C. Serum isoamylase measurements in pancreatitis complicating chronic renal failure. *J. Lab. Clin. Med.* **93**, 71–77 (1979).

22. Owyang, C., Miller, L. J., DiMagno, E. P. *et al.* Gastrointestinal hormone profile in renal insufficiency. *Mayo Clin. Proc.* **54**, 769–773 (1979).

23. Gahl, G. M., Hess, G., Arnold, W. *et al.* Hepatitis B virus markers in 97 long-term hemodialysis patients. *Nephron* **24**, 58–63 (1979).

24. Stone, W. J., McKinney, T. D., and Warnock, L. G. Spurious hyperbilirubinemia in uremic patients receiving propranolol. *Clin. Chem. (Winston-Salem, N.C.)* **25**, 1761–1765 (1979).

25. Warnock, L. G., Stone, W. J., and Wagner, C. Decreased aspartate aminotransferase (SGOT) activity in serum of uremic patients. *Clin. Chem. (Winston-Salem, N.C.)* **20**, 1213–1216 (1974).

26. Townsend, C. M., Remmers, A. R., and Sarles, H. E. Intestinal obstruction from medication bezoar in patients with renal failure. *N. Engl. J. Med.* **288**, 1058–1059 (1973).

27. Stone, W. J. Therapy of constipation in patients with chronic renal failure. *Dial. Transplant.* **6** (July), 30–32 (1977).

28. McDonald, W. J. The use of antihypertensive drugs in chronic renal failure. *In* "Drugs and Renal Disease" (W. M. Bennett, G. A. Porter, S. P. Bagby, and W. J. McDonald, eds.), pp. 113–128. Churchill-Livingstone, Edinburgh and London, 1978.

29. Galen, M. A., Steinberg, S. M., Lowrie, E. G. *et al.* Hemorrhagic pleural effusion in patients undergoing chronic hemodialysis. *Ann. Intern. Med.* **82**, 359–361 (1975).

30. Faubert, P. F., Shapiro, W. B., Porush, J. G. *et al.* Pulmonary calcification in hemodialyzed patients detected by technetium-99m diphosphonate scanning. *Kidney Int.* **18**, 95–102 (1980).

31. Craddock, P. R., Fehr, J., Brigham, K. L. *et al.* Complement and leukocyte-mediated pulmonary dysfunction in hemodialysis. *N. Engl. J. Med.* **296**, 769–774 (1977).

32. Lazaro, R. P., and Kirshner, H. S. Proximal muscle weakness in uremia. Case reports and review of the literature. *Arch. Neurol. (Chicago)* **37**, 555–558 (1980).

33. Cotton, J. R., Woodard, T., Carter, N. W. *et al.* Resting skeletal muscle membrane potential as an index of uremic toxicity. *J. Clin. Invest.* **63**, 501–506 (1979).

34. Ma, K. W., Brown, D. C., Steele, B. W. *et al.* Serum creatine kinase MB isoenzyme activity in long-term hemodialysis patients. *Arch. Intern. Med.* **141**, 164–166 (1981).

35. Lazarus, J. M., Lowrie, E. C. *et al.* Cardiovascular disease in uremic patients on hemodialysis. *Kidney Int.* **2**, Suppl., S167–S175 (1975).

36. Nies, A. S., Robertson, D., and Stone, W. J. Hemodialysis hypotension is not the result of uremic peripheral autonomic neuropathy. *J. Lab. Clin. Med.* **94**, 395–402 (1979).

37. Cross, A. S., and Steigbigel, R. T. Infective endocarditis and access site infections in patients on hemodialysis. *Medicine (Baltimore)* **55**, 453–466 (1976).

38. Friedman, H. S., Shah, B. N., Kim, H. G. *et al.* Clinical study of the cardiac findings in patients on chronic maintenance hemodialysis: The relationship to coronary risk factors. *Clin. Nephrol.* **16**, 75–85 (1981).

39. Luft, F. C., Gilman, J. K., and Weyman, A. E. Pericarditis in the patient with uremia: Clinical and echocardiographic evaluation. *Nephron* **25**, 160–166 (1980).

40. Haimov, M., Glabman, S., Schupak, E. *et al.* General surgery in patients on maintenance hemodialysis. *Ann. Surg.* **179**, 863–867 (1974).

41. Dobkin, J. F., Miller, M. H., and Steigbigel, N. H. Septicemia in patients on chronic hemodialysis. *Ann. Intern. Med.* **88**, 28–33 (1978).

42. Coburn, J. W. Renal osteodystrophy. *Kidney Int.* **17**, 677–693 (1980).

43. Katz, A. I., Hampers, C. L., and Merrill, J. P. Secondary hyperparathyroidism and renal osteodystrophy in chronic renal failure. *Medicine (Baltimore)* **48**, 333–374 (1969).

44. Hodsman, A. B., Sherrard, D. J., Wong, E. G. C. *et al.* Vitamin D-resistant osteomalacia in hemodialysis patients lacking secondary hyperparathyroidism. *Ann. Intern. Med.* **94**, 629–637 (1981).

45. Richet, G., Lopez de Novales, E., and Verroust, P. Drug intoxication and neurological episodes in chronic renal failure. *Br. Med. J.* **2**, 394–395 (1970).

46. Raskin, N. H., and Fishman, R. A. Neurologic disorders in renal failure. *N. Engl. J. Med.* **294**, 143–148, 204–210 (1976).

47. Rodrigo, F., Shideman, J., McHugh, R. *et al.* Osmolality changes during hemodialysis. Natural history, clinical correlations, and influence of dialysate glucose and intravenous mannitol. *Ann. Intern. Med.* **86**, 554–561 (1977).

48. Dewberry, F. L., McKinney, T. D., and Stone, W. J. The dialysis dementia syndrome: Report of fourteen cases and review of the literature. *ASAIO J.* **3**, 102–108 (1980).

49. Duncan, G. W., Kirshner, H. S., and Stone, W. J. Cervical bruits in hemodialysis patients. *Stroke* **11**, 672–674 (1980).

50. Leonard, A., and Shapiro, F. L. Subdural hematoma in regularly hemodialyzed patients. *Ann. Intern. Med.* **82**, 650–658 (1975).

51. Lindner, A., Farewell, V. T., and Sherrard, D. J. High incidence of neoplasia in uremic patients receiving long-term hemodialysis. *Nephron* **27,** 292–296 (1981).
52. Matas, A. J., Kjellstrand, C. M., Simmons, R. L. *et al.* Increased incidence of malignancy during chronic renal failure. *Lancet* **1,** 883–886 (1975).
53. Jacobs, C., Reach, I., and Degoulet, P. Cancer in patients on hemodialysis. *N. Engl. J. Med.* **300,** 1279–1280 (letter) (1975).

4

Endocrine and Metabolic Changes Accompanying End-Stage Renal Disease

G. W. McLEAN, D. RABIN, and W. J. STONE

I. INTRODUCTION

The kidney is intimately linked with the endocrine system. This chapter examines the effects of disordered renal function on the thyroid, gonads,

85

END-STATE RENAL DISEASE

pancreas, adrenal, and pituitary glands. Since the kidney generates, activates, and degrades many different hormones, it is not surprising that profound changes in endocrine function accompany end-stage renal disease (ESRD). The kidney itself functions as an endocrine organ; it synthesizes and secretes erythropoietin and renin and activates vitamin D. The kidney also degrades polypeptide hormones. In addition, some polypeptides and products of steroid hormone metabolism which are water soluble are excreted in the urine.

II. ABNORMALITIES OF BASAL METABOLISM AND THYROID HORMONE ECONOMY

Some patients with advanced uremia have symptoms and signs similar to those of hypothyroidism. The skin is usually dry and sallow yellow in color. Reflexes are slowed or absent. Appetite is decreased. Mental function is dulled and patients complain of easy fatigability. Normocytic and normochromic anemia is frequent. The basal metabolic rate and the body temperature may be subnormal, and cold intolerance is common. Hyperlipidemia occurs in both syndromes, although hypercholesterolemia is common in hypothyroidism, and hypertriglyceridemia more likely in uremia. It is often difficult to distinguish whether the patient's clinical picture is due entirely to ESRD, or whether there is associated independent hypothyroidism. This distinction is rendered more difficult because uremia per se leads to metabolic aberrations resembling those seen in hypothyroidism. Urea itself can induce hypothermia in experimental animals (1). Knochel and Seldin (2) showed that heat production and overall energy utilization in uremic subjects increased after dialysis was initiated, indicating an increase in basal metabolic rate. Because most patients are now begun on dialysis when they reach ESRD, they do not experience the profound hypometabolism characteristic of the syndrome in its most severe and chronic form.

The uremic state influences the metabolism of thyroid hormones. Circulating levels of thyroxine and triiodothyronine not infrequently are low in uremia. This further complicates the distinction between the syndrome of uremic hypometabolism and coincidental hypothyroidism. In the situation of health, iodide is trapped by the thyroid gland and organified into mono- and diiodotyrosines which are subsequently coupled to thyroglobulin rich in triiodothyronine (T_3) and tetraiodothyronine (T_4). The synthesis of thyroglobulin and the release of thyroid hormones, chiefly T_4, into the bloodstream is under the control of pituitary thyrotropin (TSH). The latter is subject to direct feedback inhibition from circulating T_3 and T_4. Most of circulating T_3 is derived from T_4 secreted from the thyroid gland. Under normal conditions, T_4 is monodeiodinated by peripheral tissues at the 5′ position to T_3 which is manyfold more potent as a stimulator of metabolism than is its parent hormone. Under conditions of fasting, carbohydrate restriction, fever, chronic illness, and secondary to certain drugs, the deiodination of T_4 occurs preferentially at the 5 position such that reverse T_3 (rT_3), a metabolically inactive metabolite, accumulates (3, 4). In a teleological sense, these rapid adjustments in thyroid hormone metabolism allow the organism to adapt to circumstances of illness or food deprivation with resultant conservation of energy stores more rapidly than could be accomplished through changes in the total circulating T_4 pool. Hence, circulating T_3 levels are low in uremia as in other chronic illnesses. Levels of reverse T_3 in uremia are variable. Weissel et al. (5) reported low rT_3 in 14 hemodialysis patients with no shift in the ratio of T_3 to rT_3. This suggests that deiodination of T_4, whether to T_3 or rT_3, is depressed. Other authors, however, have found increased ratios of rT_3 to T_3 (6, 7). T_3 metabolism is not accelerated in renal disease, and, after development of uremia, serum T_3 concentration is not further reduced by nephrectomy. T_4 conversion to T_3 is markedly reduced, but the total disposal of T_4 is similar to normals. It can be inferred that reverse T_3 concentrations are elevated because of stereospecific monoiodination of the inner aromatic ring of T_4 similar to findings in other chronic illnesses.

The mechanism responsible for low circulating T_4 levels in uremia is controversial. In some patients with heavy proteinuria, loss of thyroid binding globulin (TBG) in the urine has been postulated, but this is probably not an adequate explanation. It is more likely that there is a change in total body economy of thyroxine in chronic uremia, such that levels of the total metabolically active fraction of T_4, which is not bound to protein (so-called free T_4), remains within normal limits. Reliable estimates of circulating free T_4 probably provide the best laboratory index of thyroid function in uremia. The technique used for determination of free T_4 is critical. When the free T_4 is calculated from (a) total T_4 levels and (b) the "T_3 resin uptake," i.e., the binding of tracer thyroid hormone to resin in the presence of the patient's serum (the so-called free T_4 index), values are obtained in uremic patients which are often in the hypothyroid range (8). On the other hand, when free thyroxine is measured directly by equilibrium dialysis methods, values are almost invariably normal. In one series free T_4 was normal in all but 2 of 87 uremic patients examined (9). It was postulated that the aberrant relationship between the T_3 resin uptake and the free T_4, as measured by equilibrium dialysis results from (a) some unknown substance competing with thyroxine for binding to TBG or (b) changes in binding affinity secondary to the increased ionic strength of uremic serum. It is of interest that Chopra *et al.* (*3, 4*) showed that severely ill patients with no known thyroid or renal disease may have low or borderline-low total T_4 levels. They usually have low free T_4 as calculated from the T_3 resin uptake, but almost always have normal free T_4 by equilibrium dialysis. Similar results are seen in uremia. The accuracy of eight commercially available free T_4 kits was compared with measurements of free T_4 determined by equilibrium dialysis in distinguishing true hypothyroidism from the "low T_4, low T_3 syndrome" due to unusual protein binding (*9*). With six of the eight commercial methods tested, free T_4 estimates did not distinguish patients with nonthyroid illness from hypothyroidal subjects. The two most successful were the gamma coat ^{125}I Free T_4 RIA by Clinical Assays and the Free T_4 Index from Abbott Laboratories.

Thyrotropin (TSH) levels in uremic subjects are usually not elevated (*10–12*). The response of TSH to a bolus of thyrotropin releasing hormone (TRH) is quite variable. Some subjects show a blunted response; in others, the response is delayed and may be prolonged. The significance of these observations is unclear. As we shall describe later uremia distorts the pattern of pituitary responsiveness with respect to growth hormone, prolactin, and the gonadotropins, as well as to TSH.

The heterogeneity of laboratory findings in uremia is well illustrated by the findings of Spector *et al.* (*13*). They studied 30 patients on hemodialysis and found that mean levels of total T_4, free T_4 and TBG were normal. Half the group had T_3 levels that were in the hypothyroid range. Despite this, only one subject had a TSH value greater than 10 $\mu U/ml$. Spector *et al.* studied seven metabolic indices of thyroid function by evaluating results of basal metabolic rate (BMR), Achilles tendon half relaxation time, serum cholesterol, serum creatine phosphokinase (CPK) and the Q-Kd interval (elapsed time between the QRS complex of the electrocardiogram and the diastolic Korotkoff sound). They established that 43% of their subjects had low circulating T_3 concentrations despite normal circulating T_4 levels. They grouped subjects into normal T_3 and low T_3 categories and compared the metabolic parameters. There was no difference in clinical scoring of hypothyroidism, Q-Kd interval, Achilles relaxation time, or BMR between these two groups. Serum CPK was lower in the low T_3 group, and serum cholesterol was higher in the normal T_3 group, results that are inconsistent with low T_3 values as indicators of hypothyroidism. The lack of correlation between symptoms and laboratory indices of hypothyroidism supports the conclusion that hypothyroidism is not the usual metabolic situation in uremia.

There has only been one therapeutic trial of thyroxine supplementation in uremic subjects on chronic dialysis. In 1973 Silverberg *et al.* (*14*) noted cold intolerance, skin dryness, sluggishness, sallow complexion, and other symptoms suggestive of hypothyroidism in 54 hemodialyzed subjects. They documented decreased T_4, T_3 resin uptake, and TSH levels. Only one had a significant goiter, and this was present prior to the onset of renal disease. Five subjects were selected because of low T_4 levels and an abnormal free thyroxine index and were treated with L-thyroxine in daily doses of 100 μg. Patients demonstrated reduced fatigue and improved cold tolerance within a few weeks. When the dosage was increased to 200 μg daily, further reduction in fatigue was noted in two, but symptomatic hyperthyroidism appeared in three.

Attention has been drawn to abnormalities in thyroid function which may be consequent to dialysis therapy. Although most centers have not found goiter to be a common problem in the dialysis population, some geographic areas have reported goiter incidence as high as 58% among dialysis subjects (15). In this study, ^{131}I uptake was low at 2 and 6 hr, but normal at 24 hr. T_4 levels were low; T_3 resin uptake was normal in the majority of patients; T_3 and TSH levels were normal; and there was no evidence of autoimmune thyroid disease as detected by antithyroglobulin and antithyroid microsomal antibody. In this population, iodide deficiencies were highly unlikely, and a contaminant, possibly a water pollutant, was thought responsible for the presence of goiter. Fluoride has been suggested as a dialysis goitrogen (13). Supporting the notion that an abnormality in thyroid gland metabolism results in the reported dialysis-induced goiter are (1) subnormal thyroid response to injected TSH; and (2) the finding that mean TSH concentration is statistically elevated (although still in the normal range). Gelfand et al. (16, 17) and others have described the HHH syndrome (heparin-associated hemodialysis hyperthyroidism). They have found a significant blunting of TSH response to TRH as seen in physiological hyperthyroidism. These authors demonstrated that the regional and systemic heparinization used in most hemodialysis centers produced no change in the total T_4, but that the free T_4 can double with systemic heparinization and may rise significantly with only regional use of heparin. TRH tests after heparin use were significantly more blunted than when performed at the initiation of dialysis and prior to heparin administration.

In summary, there is evidence of changes in thyroid hormone economy in patients with ESRD. These include (a) a possible intrathyroid abnormality; (b) variable pituitary TSH response to TRH; (c) low circulating thyroxine levels; (d) subnormal peripheral generation of T_3; (e) changes in the binding affinity of transport proteins exposed to the uremic milieu; (f) possible transient hyperthyroidism induced by the displacement of T_4 from its binding protein by the heparin used in dialysis; and (g) goiter secondary to a postulated goitrogen present in the dialysate. Nevertheless, there is little objective evidence of independent hypothyroidism in chronic uremia.

III. GLUCOSE AND INSULIN METABOLISM IN UREMIA

Under normal circumstances, man controls the concentration of blood glucose with rather small fluctuations after meals and during food-free intervals. Following the ingestion of glucose, insulin secretion is increased manyfold which, in turn, enhances the clearance of the sugar from the blood-stream. During food-free intervals, insulin secretion declines. The chief source of blood glucose is the liver via breakdown of stored glycogen (glycogenolysis) and the formation of glucose from amino acids (gluco-neogenesis). The very different metabolic milieus occurring during post-prandial and postabsorptive periods are delicately integrated such that euglycemia is maintained (*18*). Patients with ESRD generally display an abnormal response to challenge with either oral or intravenous glucose. However, fasting blood glucose levels usually remain within normal limits. Occasional patients exhibit frank hyperglycemia and rarely may become hypoglycemic under conditions of food deprivation. Hypoglycemia may be more of a problem in patients with malnutrition or liver disease, patients who dialyze against no glucose, or who receive β-blocking medications. It is noteworthy that, despite the severe metabolic derangements which ac-company uremia, control of glucose is so well maintained. The abnormalities following glucose challenge in the uremic patient have nevertheless been the subject of intense investigation. Clearance of glucose from the plasma is slowed, and there are abnormalities in insulin secretion and subresponsive-ness of peripheral tissues to the actions of both endogenous and exogenous insulin (*19–21*).

The insulin response to glucose is heterogeneous. Interpretation of such data is complicated by the fact that ESRD is associated with delayed clear-ance of insulin from the plasma (*22*). This probably reflects the important role played by the normal kidney in degrading circulating insulin. Hypocal-cemia or hypokalemia accompanying uremia may adversely influence the ability of the pancreatic β cell to secrete insulin appropriately after glucose challenge (*23, 24*).

A second abnormality seen in uremia is subresponsiveness of peripheral tissues to the action of insulin. Westervelt infused insulin directly into the brachial artery of patients with uremia and examined the changes in forearm metabolism (*25*). He observed that the insulin-induced glucose uptake was only one-fourth of that noted in normal subjects.

DeFronzo *et al.* (*21*) have studied patients with uremia using the "glucose and insulin clamp" techniques, in which sufficient insulin is infused to maintain concentrations which are 100 $\mu U/ml$ above basal levels. Glucose is simultaneously infused at a variable rate such that euglycemia is main-tained. The amount of glucose infused is a measure of the individual's sensitivity to exogenous insulin. A second technique employs the infusion of glucose only with the infusion rate modified so as to maintain an ambient glucose concentration of 125 mg/dl. Plasma insulin levels are measured at frequent intervals. This procedure provides an index of the endogenous insulin response to the challenge of hyperglycemia. Furthermore, the amount of glucose infused is a measure of the body's responsiveness to the endogenous insulin. From such studies DeFronzo *et al.* have concluded that there is peripheral resistance to both endogenous and exogenous insulin in the patient with ESRD. As in other studies, patterns of endogenous insulin secretion were heterogeneous both before and after dialysis.

The basis of the subresponsiveness to insulin in uremia remains uncertain. Elevated levels of glucagon and growth hormone have been reported (*26, 27*). Sherwin *et al.* (*28*) noted elevations in basal and in alanine-stimulated glucagon concentrations in uremia. Furthermore, the clearance of glucagon was depressed, and exogenous glucagon produced significantly greater hyperglycemia in ESRD than in controls. Others have described increased gluconeogenesis in uremia which could be accounted for by an increase in glucagon (*29*). The conclusion that hyperglucagonemia is found in uremia is complicated by recent findings that circulating immunoreactive glucagon is heterogeneous (*30*). Three peaks of activity are detectable by separation on a Biogel P-30 column: peak A elutes in the void volume, peak B has a molecular weight of about 9000 daltons, and peak C corresponds to true pancreatic glucagon with a molecular weight of 3500 daltons. Peaks A and B are thought to represent possible precursors of peak C and have reduced bioactivity. In uremia an increase in peak A accounts for much of the increase in total glucagon immunoreactivity (*31*). Therefore, the finding of increased circulating glucagon in uremia does not imply a corresponding increase in glucagon bioactivity. Other workers have suggested that there may be changes in glucagon receptors in experimental uremia (*32*). While the metabolic picture in uremia corresponds in part to that elicited by exogenous glucagon, there is no firm evidence that glucagon hypersecretion can be incriminated in the glucose abnormalities of ESRD.

In summary, most patients with uremia maintain euglycemia. Abnormalities in insulin secretion and peripheral resistance to endogenous and exogenous insulin have been demonstrated. In general, these abnormalities are not clinically significant, although they may play a role in the pathogenesis of hyperlipidemia which is discussed later in this chapter.

The Diabetic Patient with End-Stage Renal Disease

The kidney is estimated to be the site of degradation of approximately 7 units of insulin per day (*33*). The renal clearance of insulin, and perhaps also hepatic clearance, is significantly diminished in the presence of uremia. The clearance of insulin from plasma is therefore reduced, i.e., insulin remains in the serum longer than in normal individuals, and this may increase its bioactivity in the whole organism. In addition, patients with ESRD may have a decrease in body mass, decrease in caloric intake, hemodialytic loss of glucose, decrease in metabolic rate and decrease in energy expenditure, all of which contribute to a precipitous decline in insulin requirements. As glomerular filtration declines, insulin dosage should be concomitantly decreased. Subjects who are treated with oral sulfonylurea agents, some of which are metabolized by the kidney, also require dosage adjustments to avoid hypoglycemia as renal function declines. Most authorities believe that peritoneal dialysis is the preferable treatment in the insulin-dependent uremic subject (see Chapter 8). Experience is also being obtained on (a) the use of multiple daily subcutaneous injections of insulin combined with home glucose monitoring, (b) continuous intravenous or subcutaneous insulin infusion by portable pump, and (c) the addition of insulin to the peritoneal dialysate (34, 35). It is hoped that these techniques will reduce the accelerated atherosclerosis, neuropathy, and retinopathy of the uremic diabetic. Pancreatic or islet cell transplantation and closed loop insulin infusion devices are still in experimental stages.

IV. THE HYPERLIPIDEMIAS

Hyperlipidemia, an abnormal elevation of serum triglyceride and/or cholesterol, is noted in at least one-third of patients with ESRD. This is true irrespective of whether the patients are being treated conservatively or are on maintenance dialysis. Patients with ESRD have a very high prevalence of coronary atherosclerosis and of peripheral vascular disease (36). Hyperlipidemia has been implicated as an important etiological factor in atherosclerosis, and it has been suggested that abnormalities in lipid metabolism in ESRD account for the extensive atherosclerosis observed (37). We shall consider first some aspects of the normal transport of lipids and then examine the possible etiological factors accounting for the hyperlipidemia of uremia. When fats are ingested, dietary triglyceride is assembled into a large particle containing both lipid and protein, the chylomicron. Chylomicrons traverse the thoracic duct from which they enter the bloodstream. The enzyme lipoprotein lipase (LPL) clears triglyceride from the circulation by hydrolyzing the molecule into free fatty acid and glycerol which are then taken up by peripheral organs, particularly adipose tissue. LPL requires the apoprotein C-II for activation. Insulin also appears important for full activity of the enzyme. Endogenous triglycerides, chiefly synthesized in the liver, are assembled into a lipid–protein molecule known as very low density lipoprotein (VLDL) which enters the circulation from which it is cleared by LPL. Cholesterol is chiefly transported to the periphery in low density lipoprotein (LDL). The latter is taken up by peripheral tissues through a specific membrane receptor. Excess cholesterol is transported from the periphery on the molecule, high density lipoprotein (HDL), which also serves as a source for apoprotein C-II, the activator of LPL. Hence, HDL is thought to have a protective effect on the atherosclerotic process.

The commonest form of hyperlipidemia encountered in end-stage renal disease is Type IV, i.e., elevation of VLDL and of circulating triglycerides (38). Total serum cholesterol is usually normal, but HDL cholesterol may be reduced (39). In the absence of uremia, Type IV hyperlipidemia is characteristically observed in states of hyperinsulinism and insulin resistance, such as obesity and Type II diabetes mellitus. However, Type IV hyperlipidemia is frequently observed in uremic subjects who are neither obese nor diabetic. Furthermore, there is evidence that the clearance of exogenous fat administered intravenously as Intralipid is decreased in subjects with ESRD (40). This may be secondary to LPL abnormalities occurring in these patients (41). One index of the action of LPL is the measurement of lipolytic activity present in plasma after the injection of heparin. Heparin is believed to release lipases from hepatic and peripheral endothelial surfaces. Hence, the measurement of postheparin lipolytic activity (PHLA) represents a combination of peripheral and hepatic lipase activity. Recent studies have established that PHLA is decreased in uremia (42). Apoprotein C-II, the activator of LPL, is also depressed in patients with ESRD (43). The insulin resistance that accompanies uremia may also contribute to decreased LPL activity. The evidence, although incomplete, tends to support a defect in VLDL clearance as the major pathogenetic mechanism for type IV hyperlipidemia in ESRD. Epidemiologically, atherosclerosis is more tightly coupled to hypercholesterolemia than to hypertriglyceridemia. We have stated previously that total cholesterol levels are normal in uremia. However, HDL cholesterol is reduced, as is the enzyme lecithin cholesterol acyltransferase (LCAT), which facilitates transfer of cholesterol to HDL (44). Thus, qualitative abnormalities of cholesterol metabolism may play a role in the pathogenesis of atherosclerosis in ESRD.

Frank et al. (45) have shown a correlation between the duration of dialysis and the prevalence of hyperlipidemia. In their study, patients maintained on dialysis for more than 5 years were more likely to have normal lipid patterns than those who had been dialyzed for less than 5 years. It is unclear whether this observation represents a beneficial effect of hemodialysis or the effect of chronic heparin administration on lipid metabolism, or alternatively, early death of the hyperlipidemic group of dialysis subjects. Most uremic patients receive a variety of medications, such as androgens and propranolol, which may aggravate hyperlipidemia.

Lipid Metabolism following Renal Transplantation

Neither peritoneal dialysis nor hemodialysis corrects the abnormalities described in fat metabolism in ESRD. It has become apparent that successful renal transplantation is also accompanied by accelerated atherosclerosis and a high prevalence of death from cardiovascular disease. Whereas hypertriglyceridemia is most common in ESRD treated conservatively or with dialysis, hypercholesterolemia is recorded in up to 50% of subjects after renal transplantation (46). The hyperlipidemia corresponds to type IIA (an increase in LDL and in cholesterol), but type IIB (an increase in VLDL, LDL, cholesterol, and triglycerides) is also seen. Glucocorticoids and immunosuppressive therapy are thought to account for these abnormalities (47). These medications are said to enhance VLDL production by the liver. The clearance of VLDL improves after renal transplantation, but the remnants of the VLDL molecule are converted to LDL, the concentration of which rises excessively.

V. GROWTH HORMONE AND SOMATOMEDIN METABOLISM IN UREMIA

Under normal conditions growth hormone secretion is increased by starvation and in the presence of hypoglycemia. Conversely, growth hormone output is blunted by oral or intravenous glucose administration. There are profound changes in the control of growth hormone secretion in uremia. Fasting levels are often elevated and fail to suppress following glucose loading (48). Furthermore, growth hormone release is not enhanced by hypoglycemia but responds to the administration of TRH. This releasing hormone is ineffective in normal persons as a growth hormone secretogogue, but can initiate growth hormone release in acromegalics and patients with anorexia nervosa. It has been suggested that the pattern of growth hormone release in uremia resembles that seen in states of protein–calorie malnutrition. Growth hormone initiates the formation of a group of growth factors, the somatomedins, which exert important anabolic bioeffects. In protein–calorie malnutrition, growth hormone levels are elevated, whereas somatomedin concentrations are subnormal. The latter has classically been assayed by examining the capacity of serum to enhance radioactive sulfate incorporation into excised cartilage. Elevations in serum sulfate concentrations in uremia have complicated measurements of somatomedin activity (49). Somatomedin levels in uremia have disparately been reported as increased or decreased (50). Newer immunoassays for somatomedin may clarify the present confusion. The role, if any, of growth hormone hypersecretion in uremia remains uncertain. There is no correlation between the severity of glucose intolerance in uremia and growth hormone hypersecretion. Nevertheless, the findings suggest a generalized disturbance in hypothalamic–pituitary function involving growth hormone, prolactin, and possibly TSH and the gonadotropins.

VI. PITUITARY ADRENOCORTICAL FUNCTION IN UREMIA

There is a diurnal rhythm for ACTH and cortisol. Levels are usually maximal in the early morning and fall during the day to a nadir around midnight. Release of ACTH and subsequently of cortisol is also initiated in response to stress including fever and acute induction of hypoglycemia. Acute lowering of ambient cortisol levels (e.g., by administration of metyrapone) triggers ACTH release, whereas cortisol and synthetic glucocorticoids inhibit ACTH secretion.

In the circulation, cortisol is tightly bound to cortisol binding globulin (CBG). The free fraction of circulating cortisol available for metabolism is relatively small unless total cortisol levels are raised to greater than approximately 20 μg/dl, above which CBG approaches saturation. Metabolic clearance of cortisol involves hepatic inactivation by reduction to tetrahydro-reduced derivatives and conjugation to form water-soluble glucuronides, which are then available for urinary excretion as urinary 17-hydroxy-corticosteroids. With diminishing renal function, 17-hydroxysteroid conjugates accumulate in plasma (51). The presence of steroid metabolites in subjects with renal failure has hampered investigations of pituitary–adrenal dynamics. A recent evaluation of four commonly used, commercially available cortisol radioimmunoassays (RIA) showed that all four gave erroneously high plasma cortisol estimations in uremic serum, unless dichloromethane extraction and/or chromatography was performed to remove cross-reacting material (52). It was noted that a substance that interfered with accuracy of one RIA procedure may have no effect on another. These technical factors may explain the previous discrepancy in plasma cortisol determinations among uremic subjects.

Early studies reported normal fasting plasma cortisol levels and a normal adrenal response to exogenous ACTH in patients with ESRD. More recent studies point to abnormalities in cortisol secretion in these patients. Cortisol secretion remains pulsatile, and the diurnal rhythm is retained, although it may be distorted by dialysis which can cause stress-induced ACTH secretion (53, 54). Plasma cortisol levels measured at 8 AM and 4 PM have been reported as normal or somewhat elevated. When cortisol was sampled every 20 min for 24 hr, mean cortisol levels in uremic subjects were twice normal (55). Both insulin-induced hypoglycemia and metyrapone administration failed to initiate a normal ACTH and cortisol response (56, 57). A more recent report found normal suppression of plasma cortisol following a large dose of metyrapone (3G) given at midnight (58). Further evidence of the partial autonomy of ACTH secretion in uremia is provided by the finding of inadequate suppression of cortisol by dexamethasone. In one study, 9 of 10 patients had abnormal suppression after 1 mg of oral dexamethasone; 6 of 10 failed to suppress normally with 2 mg of dexamethasone for 2 days; 1 of 10 failed to suppress with 8 mg of dexamethasone a day for 2 days. When free plasma cortisol was measured, mean values in uremic subjects after suppression by 8 mg of dexamethasone were greater than in normal subjects who received only a single 1 mg dose (55). Intravenous dexamethasone was more effective than oral in suppressing cortisol in uremic subjects. Nevertheless, the suppression of IV dexamethasone was less complete than in normals (59). Ramirez et al. (58) were able to achieve suppression of morning cortisol concentrations in uremic subjects who were given 3 mg of dexamethasone at midnight. They noted the plasma levels of dexamethasone following an oral 1 mg loading dose were significantly lower in uremic subjects than in controls. The rate of disappearance of an intravenous bolus of dexamethasone was similar in control and uremic subjects. There may therefore be a defect in the absorption of dexamethasone and possibly metyrapone in uremia. It is unlikely, however, that the abnormalities in pituitary adrenal function observed in uremia are entirely due to a gastrointestinal cause. We have noted that hypoglycemia is ineffective in initiating ACTH and cortisol release in uremia (58). We suggest that ACTH secretion in uremia resembles that of growth hormone and prolactin in being partially autonomous. Uremia appears to share with syndromes of protein–calorie malnutrition, an acquired defect in the normal negative feedback mechanism controlling ACTH secretion. These abnormalities may be of more than academic interest if a state of true hypercortisolism exists in uremia. This may be implicated in the muscle wasting, hyperlipidemia, accelerated atherosclerosis, and overall catabolic state.

The dialysis process exerts an influence on pituitary–adrenal metabolism. The multiple stresses can initiate a rise in ACTH secretion. Circulating free cortisol is dialyzable, whereas cortisol bound to CBG is not. Approximately 0.5 mg of cortisol is thought to be lost during each dialysis, a quantity that is insignificant compared to the daily production rate of 20–30 mg (60).

Nevertheless, total plasma 17-hydroxycorticosteroid levels drop pre-cipitously during dialysis and rise again within 3 hr after discontinuation of dialysis. Clearance of plasma cortisol rises 30–60% during dialysis (61). This is not consequent to loss of cortisol into the dialysate but appears to indicate increased hepatic clearance. This interesting finding has been explained by postulating that between dialysis treatments there is inhibition of hepatic conjugation of cortisol by circulating steroid conjugates. When the conju-gates are removed by dialysis, hepatic steroid metabolism returns to normal as reflected by the enhanced hepatic clearance.

Aldosterone and Renin

Aldosterone secretion is stimulated by three factors in normal man: the renin–angiotensin system, ACTH secretion, and the plasma potassium concentration. In a study of eight normokalemic subjects with advanced chronic renal insufficiency (mean creatinine clearance 14.3 ml/min), Berl and colleagues (62) reached three conclusions: (a) many patients were in a state of hyperaldosteronism; (b) aldosterone production could be further stim-ulated by a change in posture or by hypovolemia; and (c) aldosterone contributed to the maintenance of plasma potassium level and was anti-natriuretic in the subjects since spironolactone therapy resulted in both an increase in sodium excretion and in plasma potassium concentration. The syndrome of hyporeninemic hypoaldosteronism should be considered in patients with creatinine clearances of 10–50 ml/min who display inappro-priate hyperkalemia (63). Typically, diabetes mellitus and a hyperchloremic metabolic acidosis will also be present. In most patients hypoaldosteronism can be explained by inadequate renin secretion. Control of acidosis and of hyperkalemia can usually be achieved with a mineralocorticoid supplement.

Investigations of the renin–angiotensin–aldosterone system in patients whose renal function has deteriorated sufficiently so as to require chronic dialysis have been in general agreement. First, elevations of the plasma potassium concentration will still increase plasma aldosterone levels (64). These alterations also occur in surgically anephric patients who have no plasma renin activity (PRA) (60). Second, baseline plasma aldosterone levels are quite variable depending on several factors including the surgical anephric state. Hyperaldosteronism is commonly found and does not change over the course of 26 months of chronic hemodialysis (65). Also, PRA is unaltered over the same period. Patients with a history of accelerated hyper-tension often have the highest PRA and aldosterone values. Third, volume depletion by isolated ultrafiltration without dialysis in nephric subjects acutely increases both plasma aldosterone and PRA (66). Conventional hemodialysis can increase, decrease (aldosterone is dialyzable), or leave plasma aldosterone unchanged depending on the interplay of extracellular fluid volume, heparin, plasma potassium level, and dialysis losses of the hormone (60, 66). Fourth, when surgically anephric patients were compared to normal controls, there was no diurnal fluctuation in plasma aldosterone in the anephric patients, all of whom had undetectable PRA (67). In this same study plasma cortisol demonstrated a diurnal variation in both groups. It may be concluded that ACTH plays little role in the diurnal variation in plasma aldosterone and that PRA is the probable regulator of this phenomenon.

Renal transplantation is frequently accompanied by hyperreninemic hyperaldosteronism and hypertension. This state may originate in the recipient's own kidneys, from chronic allograft rejection, or not infrequently from stenosis of the transplanted renal artery (68). Therapy is usually directed toward control of hypertension by medical means. Occasionally, repair of transplant renal artery stenosis or surgical extirpation of the recipient's own kidneys will be beneficial.

VII. PITUITARY–GONADAL AXIS

With the development of progressive renal failure and its attendant systemic symptoms, there is a loss of fertility and interest in sexual activity. When dialysis treatment is started, most subjects experience an increase in their sense of well-being, but the disturbances of gonadal function commonly associated with renal failure generally persist. In males decreased libido, gynecomastia, impotence, and hypogonadism with sterility due to oligospermia or azoospermia are virtually consistent findings, and may be among the most psychologically and socially disabling aspects of the illness (69–72). With occasional exceptions, these abnormalities in sexual function are not corrected by adequate dialysis, but may be reversed by successful renal transplantation (73–75). Women have severe disturbances in gonadal and sexual function which are not corrected and may be worsened by dialysis (76–79). Amenorrhea may develop in 50% of women. In the group that continues to have menstrual activity, the anticoagulants used during hemodialysis may cause severe hemorrhage, which may necessitate oophorectomy or hysterectomy in another 25% of patients.

A. Gonadal Function in Men with End-Stage Renal Disease

Impotence has been reported in between 28 to 80% of males with ESRD. A recent study examined nocturnal penile tumescence (NPT) in patients with

ESRD and in chronically ill subjects with normal renal function (79). Forty percent of the former and 18% of the latter group complained of erectile dysfunction. Objective evidence of depression was found in 43% of uremic subjects and 27% of the chronically ill group. There was, however, no correlation between the presence of depression and the frequency of successful intercourse. Abnormalities of NPT were recorded in about half of the uremic subjects studied. The pathogenesis of impotence in uremia is complex. Many patients have vascular insufficiency and/or autonomic neuropathy. Furthermore, most patients are receiving drugs that can adversely influence sexual function, such as antihypertensive medications and psychotropic drugs. Some authors have proposed that the elevated parathyroid hormone and prolactin levels commonly encountered in ESRD may adversely affect gonadal function (80–82). Zinc deficiency, possibly secondary to dialysis, has been postulated as a cause of the decreased libido and potentia (83). There are usually objective abnormalities of testicular function present in males with ESRD. The majority of male patients with uremia have oligo- or azoospermia and low serum levels of total testosterone and of free testosterone (i.e., not bound to protein) (71). Production rates of testosterone are low and the level of testosterone binding globulins is variable and appears to correlate with the nutritional status of the patient. Histological examination of the testis reveals differing degrees of impairment of spermatogenesis which can be so severe as to resemble germinal cell aplasia. These abnormalities may be the consequence of direct testicular damage or may be secondary to reduced secretion of the gonadotropins, follicle stimulating hormone (FSH), and luteinizing hormone (LH) (72). When large series of subjects have been studied, the results have been heterogeneous, although most authors have concluded that serum LH levels are usually elevated in uremia (84). For example, in one recent series, LH levels were above the 95th percentile of normal in 78% of patients, and FSH was above the 95th percentile in 31% of patients with ESRD. These studies suggest that there is primary testicular damage in uremia. This conclusion is supported by the generally subnormal response of serum testosterone to exogenous human chorionic gonadotropin (hCG) in uremia. hCG appears to have bioactivity very similar to that of LH. There is, however, one important study that incriminates hypogonadotropism in the etiology of the hypogonadism of uremia. Lim and Fang (70) noted normal serum gonadotropin levels in approximately half of their patients despite universally low testosterone levels. Furthermore, they reported that clomiphene citrate therapy produced striking increases in FSH, LH, and testosterone levels, and corresponding improvement in potentia and libido in five men treated for up to 12 months (85). The pituitary gonadotroph was stimulated by clomiphene and by exogenous luteinizing hormone releasing hormone (LHRH). Thus, they established the integrity of the hypothalamic pituitary unit and suggested that this had been inappropriately inhibited by the uremic state. Serum prolactin levels were normal in their patients. This is important because hyperprolactinemia is not uncommon in uremia and can independently depress gonadotropin secretion (80, 86). Thus, euprolactinemic hypogonadotropic hypogonadism has been observed in a subset of patients with uremia and should be diligently sought since it is eminently treatable. We have studied a relatively small group of male subjects with ESRD (87). Since the heterogeneity previously reported may have reflected the influence of medications, none of the patients whom we examined were receiving medication known to have any influence on the pituitary–gonadal axis. Results from this study are shown in Fig. 1. Serum testosterone levels were subnormal and serum LH and FSH levels were clearly elevated. LH and FSH responses to exogenous LHRH were either normal or supranormal. The response of serum testosterone to exogenous hCG administration (4000 Units IM daily for 4 days) was subnormal. Serum prolactin levels were not elevated. These data are consistent with primary testicular disease, i.e., hypergonadotropic hypogonadism. We did not find evidence of increased circulating 17-hydroxy-progesterone. Thus, the data did not support a block in testosterone synthesis secondary to inhibition of the enzyme 17,20-desmolase.

Hyperprolactinemia has been suggested as an etiological factor in the hypogonadism of uremia. Gomez *et al.* (*88*) reported that 73% of women and 25% of men with ESRD, none of whom were receiving interfering drugs, had prolactin levels outside the normal range. Prolactin secretion in uremia is relatively autonomous. Oral L-dopa and intravenous dopamine fail to

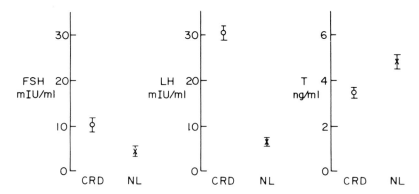

Fig. 1.   Serum LH, FSH, and testosterone levels in normal male subjects and in a group of individuals with end-stage renal disease. (Unpublished data of G. McLean, W. Stone, and D. Rabin, 1981. Reprinted from D. Rabin and T. J. McKenna, "Endocrinology and Metabolism: Principles and Practice." Grune & Stratton, New York, 1982.)

suppress prolactin, while the stimulatory effect of TRH is blunted (*81*, *86*). By contrast, the dopaminergic agonist bromocriptine will suppress prolactin if given in sufficient dosage over a prolonged period (*89*). While prolactin clearance is decreased in uremia, this alone does not account for the hyperprolactinemia, i.e., there is a significantly increased secretion rate of prolactin. We have stated that hypogonadism may be seen despite euprolactinemia, and in our personal series, hyperprolactinemia was very rare. There is evidence, however, that abnormalities of prolactin secretion may contribute to the hypogonadism of uremia in a subgroup of patients. Gomez *et al.* (*88*) reported that all males with prolactin levels greater than 39 ng/ml were impotent. Therapy with bromocriptine 3.75–5 mg/day suppressed prolactin consistently, but no increase in potency or libido was noted. Three of 10 women with amenorrhea similarly treated had menstrual bleeding after 6 weeks of therapy. Bohnet *et al.* (*90*) reported that eight of 15 uremic subjects were unable to continue therapy with bromocriptine because of hypotension occurring within 1 hr of receiving the drug. A fall in serum prolactin, increased libido, penile erections, and frequency of intercourse were reported in those patients who were able to continue with the therapy. Since the study was not conducted in a double-blind method, the results should be interpreted with caution. We have experienced great difficulty in administering L-dopa to patients with uremia. We have observed acute hypotension, angina, and psychosis, and we believe that dopaminergic agonists should be used with great caution in uremia.

In summary, male hypogonadism is a common concomitant of ESRD. There appear to be three mechanisms which play a role: hypogonadotropism, hyperprolactinemia, and primary testicular damage. The first two mechanisms are rare, but should be assiduously sought since successful treatment with clomiphene citrate and bromocriptine, respectively, has been reported. Primary testicular damage is by far the most common syndrome which we have encountered. In this situation improvement may occur after renal transplantation (see below). In some males, impotence associated with subnormal serum testosterone levels may be ameliorated by the use of exogenous androgen therapy. Testosterone enanthate, 200 mg i.m. at 2-week intervals, is the safest regimen. For those patients who do not tolerate injections, synthetic androgens such as methyltestosterone, 25–50 mg daily, or fluoxymesterone, 2–4 mg daily, may be prescribed. These compounds are not free of side effects including hepatotoxicity.

B. Effect of Renal Transplantation on Gonadal Function

Successful renal transplantation restores libido and fertility in some patients (*91–93*). Improvement of potentia is observed in 50–70% of male patients receiving a kidney transplant. In part, this can be attributed to an improvement in general health and sense of well-being. There is usually objective improvement in laboratory indices of gonadal function, although evaluation is complicated by the immunosuppressive and glucocorticoid medications that these patients are receiving. Serum prolactin levels fall, and sensitivity to the inhibitory effects of dopamine is restored (86). Holdsworth et al. (74) reported a rise in serum testosterone levels and a fall in LH levels, which indicate an improvement in Leydig cell function. There is evidence for persisting gonadal dysfunction despite transplantation: gonadotropin levels remain statistically elevated, the response to LHRH is exaggerated, and hCG-stimulated testosterone secretion may be subnormal. Abnormalities in sperm count persist in over half of the patients undergoing transplantation. The role of immunosuppressants (azathioprine, cyclophosphamide) in oligospermia is probably important. Normal sperm density and fertility have, however, been reported in some patients. It is important to recall that impotence may persist or even become worse in a minority of subjects undergoing renal transplantation (94). Manipulation of the epigastric artery during transplant surgery may adversely affect penile blood flow, since objective abnormalities in erectile function were observed in 13 of 15 posttransplant patients who were impotent.

C.   Gonadal Function in Women with End-Stage Renal Disease

Ninety percent of females with ESRD have disturbances in menstrual function and about half develop amenorrhea (76–78). Hemodialysis does not ameliorate this and may bring on menorrhagia secondary to chronic heparin use. Galactorrhea is common among females receiving dialysis. LH and prolactin levels are usually elevated. FSH levels are variable, and serum estradiol and progesterone levels are usually low. The LH and FSH response to LHRH is normal or prolonged. In some patients, there is primary ovarian pathology; in others, hyperprolactinemia may underlie the gonadal suppression. Some women treated with bromocriptine have resumed cyclical ovulatory menstruation; others have displayed an increase in gonadotropin levels without a return of ovarian function (88). Conception may occur after successful renal transplantation.

VIII.   GASTROINTESTINAL HORMONES

Elevations in serum gastrin, cholecystokinin, gastric inhibitory peptide, glucagon and vasoactive intestinal peptide have been reported in patients with ESRD (57, 95–97). Serum gastrin immunoreactivity is heterogeneous and comprised of at least three molecular forms: big big gastrin, big gastrin (known as G34 because it is composed of 34 amino acids), and gastrin (known as G17). Ingestion of food is a powerful stimulus for gastrin release in normal subjects. Gastrin, in turn, stimulates acid secretion from the stomach which is important in the normal process of digestion. Gastrin levels are elevated in uremia and the rise correlates with elevations in serum creatinine (96). Food ingestion fails to bring about an elevation in G17 in uremic patients, but levels of G34 rise within 2 hr of eating. Gastric acid secretion is either normal or increased in patients with ESRD, and peptic ulcer disease may be more frequent. No clear relationship has been found between ulcer disease and circulating total gastrin immunoreactivity in serum. It is likely that much of the gastrin measured in uremic serum represents the accumulation of biologically inactive hormone, which is usually metabolized by the healthy kidney. This is probably true, at least in part, for many of the other hormones of gastrointestinal origin.

IX. SYNTHESIS

We have described the changes in endocrine function which accompany chronic ESRD. Elevations of many hormones are observed, partly due to inadequate inactivation by the diseased kidney and partly due to increased secretion. The polypeptide hormones measured in uremic serum are comprised of multiple molecular species, and a varying percentage of total immunoreactivity measured represents hormone fragments that have escaped destruction. Similarly, water-soluble products of steroid degradation and conjugation accumulate in uremic serum. The abnormalities in laboratory endocrine indices may be clinically silent or may profoundly influence morbidity and mortality. There is often intolerance to glucose loading in uremia accompanied by changes in insulin secretion. The departures from normal in glucose metabolism do not appear to have clinical sequelae. On the other hand, the disturbances in insulin metabolism have been implicated in the pathogenesis of the hyperlipidemias, which may contribute to accelerated atherosclerosis. ESRD is accompanied by a lowering of the metabolic rate, and some indices of thyroid function (e.g., total thyroxine and triiodothyronine) are subnormal. It is likely that these changes are secondary to chronic illness and do not represent accompanying independent hypothyroidism. This conclusion is supported by the finding of normal free thyroxine levels in serum when measured by equilibrium dialysis. Conventional measurements of free thyroxine using indirect methods may yield erroneous results in uremia, and the possible incorrect prescription of exogenous thyroxine. There is partial autonomy of the hypothalamic pituitary axis in uremia. Examples of this include (a) failure to suppress growth hormone secretion by glucose loading, (b) failure to suppress prolactin secretion with dopamine or to stimulate it with TRH, and (c) inadequate suppression of ACTH by dexamethasone. Hyperprolactinemia may play a role in suppressing gonadal function in uremic subjects. The question of whether true hypercortisolism is present in uremia and contributes to the overall catabolism remains controversial. Most subjects with failing renal function display overactivity of the renin–angiotensin–aldosterone system manifest clinically as difficult to control hypertension. Hyporeninemic hypoaldosteronism is occasionally observed in ESRD, particularly in diabetic glomerulosclerosis. This often leads to profound and life-threatening hyperkalemia and requires therapy with synthetic mineralocorticoids. There are extensive changes in gonadal function among males and females with ESRD. Loss of libido and potency and oligo- or azoospermia occur frequently. In most male patients, testosterone levels are depressed and gonadotropin levels are elevated. These findings are consistent with primary testicular damage. In some patients, the hypogonadism is secondary to hyperprolactinemia or to hypogonadotropism. Male gonadal function is usually not improved by dialysis, but can be restored following renal transplantation. Under such circumstances, testosterone levels may return to normal, but improvement in sperm density is more variable. Among females there may be primary ovarian disease, but elevated prolactin concentrations can play an important role in suppression of ovarian activity. The changes in endocrine function noted after transplantation are not uniform. We contrast the improvement often observed in gonadal function with the persistence of hyperlipidemia and accelerated atherosclerosis.

GENERAL REFERENCE

Emmanouel, D. S., Lindheimer, H. D., and Katz, A. I. Pathogenesis of endocrine abnormalities in uremia. *Endocr. Rev.* **1,** 28–44 (1980).

REFERENCES

1. Leiter, L. Observations on the relation of urea to uremia. *Arch. Intern. Med.* **28,** 331–354 (1921).
2. Knochel, J. P., and Seldin, D. W. The pathophysiology of uremia. *In* "The Kidney" (B. M. Brenner and F. C. Rector, eds.), 2nd ed., pp. 21–37. Saunders, Philadelphia, Pennsylvania, 1981.
3. Chopra, I., Solomon, D. H., Hepner, G. W. *et al.* Misleadingly low free thyroxine index and usefulness of reverse triiodothyronine measurement in nonthyroidal illnesses. *Ann. Intern. Med.* **90,** 905–912 (1979).

4. Chopra, I. J., Chopra, U., Smith, S. R. *et al.* Reciprocal changes in serum concentrations of 3,3'5'-triiodothyronine (reverse T_3) and 3,3'5-triiodothyronine (T_3) in systemic illnesses. *J. Clin. Endocrinol. Metab.* **41,** 1043–1049 (1975).

5. Weissel, M., Stummvoll, H. K., Wolf, A. *et al.* Thyroid hormones in chronic renal failure. *Ann. Intern. Med.* **86,** 664–665 (1977).

6. Lim, V. S., Fang, V. S., Katz, A. I. *et al.* Thyroid dysfunction in chronic renal failure—a study of the pituitary thyroid axis and peripheral turnover kinetics of thyroxine and triiodothyronine. *J. Clin. Invest.* **60,** 522–534 (1977).

7. Ramirez, G., O'Neill, W., Jubiz, W. *et al.* Thyroid dysfunction in uremia: Evidence for thyroid and hypophyseal abnormalities. *Ann. Intern. Med.* **84,** 672–676 (1976).

8. Joasoo, A., Murray, I., Parkin, J. *et al.* Abnormalities of in vitro thyroid function tests in renal disease. *Q. J. Med.* **43,** 245–261 (1974).

9. Kaptein, E. M., Macintyre, S. S., Weiner, J. M. *et al.* Free thyroxine estimates in nonthyroidal illness: Comparison of eight methods. *J. Clin. Endocrinol. Metab.* **52,** 1073–1077 (1981).

10. Pokroy, N., Epstein, S., Hendricks, S. *et al.* Thyrotropin response to intravenous thyrotropin releasing hormone in patients with hepatic and renal disease. *Horm. Metab. Res.* **6,** 132–136 (1974).

11. Gonzalez-Barcena, D., Kastin, A. J., Schalch, D. S. *et al.* Responses to thyrotropin-releasing hormone in patients with renal failure and after infusion in normal men. *J. Clin. Endocrinol. Metab.* **36,** 117–120 (1973).

12. Gomez-Pan, A., Alvarez-Ude, F., Yeo, P. P. B. *et al.* Function of the hypothalamo-hypophysial thyroid axis in chronic renal failure. *Clin. Endocrinol. (Oxford)* **11,** 567–574 (1979).

13. Spector, D. A., Davis, P. J., Helderman, J. H. *et al.* Thyroid function and metabolic state in chronic renal failure. *Ann. Intern. Med.* **85,** 724–730 (1976).

14. Silverberg, D. S., Ulan, R. A., Fawcett, D. M. *et al.* Effects of chronic hemodialysis on thyroid function in chronic renal failure. *Can. Med. Assoc. J.* **109,** 282–286 (1973).

15. Ramirez, G., Jubiz, W., Gutch, C. F. *et al.* Thyroid abnormalities of chronic renal failure. A study of 53 patients on chronic hemodialysis. *Ann. Intern. Med.* **79,** 500–504 (1973).

16. Gelfand, M. C., Rodelas, R., McAnally, J. F. *et al.* Heparin associated hemodialysis hyperthyroidism (HHH): A physiologically significant phenomenon. *Proc. Clin. Dial. Transplant Forum* **8,** 255–259 (1978).

17. Schatz, D. L., Sheppard, R. H., Steiner, G. *et al.* Influence of heparin on serum free thyroxine. *J. Clin. Endocrinol. Metab.* **29,** 1015–1022 (1969).

18. Porte, D., and Halter, J. B. The endocrine pancreas and diabetes mellitus. *In* "Textbook of Endocrinology" (R. H. Williams, ed.), 6th ed., p. 716. Saunders, Philadelphia, Pennsylvania, 1981.

19. Bagdade, J. D. Disorders of glucose metabolism in uremia. *Adv. Nephrol.* **8,** 87–100 (1979).

20. DeFronzo, R. A., Andres, R., Edgar, P. *et al.* Carbohydrate metabolism in uremia: A review. *Medicine (Baltimore)* **52,** 469–481 (1973).

21. DeFronzo, R. A., Tobin, J. D., Rowe, J. W. *et al.* Glucose intolerance in uremia. Quantification of pancreatic beta cell sensitivity to glucose and tissue sensitivity to insulin. *J. Clin. Invest.* **62,** 425–435 (1978).

22. Chamberlain, M. J., and Stimmler, I. The renal handling of insulin. *J. Clin. Invest.* **46,** 911–919 (1967).

23. Witzel, D. A., and Littledike, E. T. Suppression of insulin secretion during hypocalcemia. *Endocrinology* **93,** 761–766 (1973).

24. Spergel, G., Bleicher, S. J., Goldberg, M. *et al.* Effect of potassium on the impaired glucose tolerance in chronic uremia. *Metab., Clin. Exp.* **16,** 581–585 (1967).

25. Westervelt, F. B. Insulin effect in uremia. *J. Lab. Clin. Med.* **74,** 79–84 (1969).
26. Bilbrey, G. L., Faloona, G. R., White, M. G. *et al.* Hyperglucagonemia of renal failure. *J. Clin. Invest.* **53,** 841–847 (1974).
27. Samaan, N., and Freeman, R. M. Growth hormone levels in severe renal failure. *Metab., Clin. Exp.* **19,** 102–113 (1970).
28. Sherwin, R. S., Bastl, C., Finkelstein, F. O. *et al.* Influence of uremia and hemodialysis on the turnover and metabolic effects of glucagon. *J. Clin. Invest.* **57,** 722–731 (1976).
29. Rubenfeld, S., and Garber, A. J. Abnormal carbohydrate metabolism in chronic renal failure. The potential role of accelerated glucose production, increased gluconeogenesis, and impaired glucose disposal. *J. Clin. Invest.* **62,** 20–28 (1978).
30. Emmanouel, D. S., Jaspan, J. B., Kuku, S. F. *et al.* Pathogenesis and characterization of hyperglucagonemia in the uremic rat. *J. Clin. Invest.* **58,** 1266–1272 (1976).
31. Kuku, S. F., Zeidler, A., Emmanouel, D. S. *et al.* Heterogeneity of plasma glucagon: Patterns in patients with chronic renal failure and diabetes. *J. Clin. Endocrinol. Metab.* **42,** 173–176 (1976).
32. Soman, V., and Felig, P. Glucagon and insulin binding to liver membranes in a partially nephrectomized uremic rat model. *J. Clin. Invest.* **60,** 224–232 (1977).
33. Rabkin, R., Simon, N. M., Steiner, S. *et al.* Effect of renal disease on renal uptake and excretion of insulin in man. *N. Engl. J. Med.* **282,** 182–187 (1970).
34. Flynn, C. T., and Nanson, J. A. Intraperitoneal insulin with CAPD—An artificial pancreas. *Trans. Am. Soc. Artif. Intern. Organs* **25,** 114–117 (1979).
35. Zimmerman, A. L., Cohn, J. I., Ranieri, R. *et al.* Continuous low dose insulin infusion in diabetics receiving peritoneal dialysis. *Trans. Am. Soc. Artif. Intern. Organs* **24,** 490–497 (1978).
36. Scharf, S., Wexler, J., Longnecker, R. E. *et al.* Cardiovascular disease in patients on chronic hemodialytic therapy. *Prog. Cardiovasc. Dis.* **22,** 343–356 (1980).
37. Lindner, A., Charra, B., Sherrard, D. *et al.* Accelerated atherosclerosis in prolonged maintenance hemodialysis. *N. Engl. J. Med.* **290,** 697–701 (1974).
38. Bagdade, J. D., Porte, D., and Bierman, E. L. Hypertriglyceridemiae. A metabolic consequence of chronic renal failure. *N. Engl. J. Med.* **279,** 181–185 (1968).
39. Rapoport, J., Aviram, M., Chaimovitz, C. *et al.* Defective high density lipoprotein composition in patients on chronic hemodialysis. *N. Engl. J. Med.* **299,** 1326–1329 (1979).
40. Chan, M. K., Varghese, Z., Persaud, J. W. *et al.* Fat clearance before and after heparin in chronic renal failure—Hemodialysis reduces post-heparin fractional clearance rate of intralipid. *Clin. Chim. Acta* **108,** 95 (1980).
41. Mordasini, F., Frey, F., Flury, W. *et al.* Selective deficiency of hepatic triglyceride lipase in uremic patients. *N. Engl. J. Med.* **297,** 1362–1366 (1977).
42. Appelbaum-Bowden, D., Goldberg, A. P., Hazzard, W. R. *et al.* Postheparin plasma triglyceride lipase in chronic hemodialysis: Evidence for a role for hepatic lipase in lipoprotein metabolism. *Metab., Clin. Exp.* **28,** 917–924 (1979).
43. Chan, M. K., Varghese, Z., and Moorehead, J. F. Lipid abnormalities in uremia, dialysis, and transplantation. *Kidney Int.* **19,** 625–637 (1981).
44. Guarnieri, G. F., Moracchiello, M., Campanacci, L. *et al.* Lecithin-cholesterol acyltransferase (LCAT) activity in chronic uremia. *Kidney Int.* **13,** S26 (1978).
45. Frank, W., Rao, T. K. S., Manis, T. *et al.* Uremic hyperlipoproteinemia: Correlation with residual renal function and duration of maintenance hemodialysis. *Trans. Am. Soc. Artif. Intern. Organs* **23,** 59–64 (1977).
46. Ponticelli, C., Barbi, G. L., Cantalupi, A. *et al.* Lipid disorders in renal transplant recipients. *Nephron* **20,** 189–195 (1978).

47. Chan, M. K., Varghese, Z., Persaud, J. W. *et al.* The role of multiple pharmacotherapy in the pathogenesis of hyperlipidemia after renal transplantation. *Clin. Nephrol.* **15**, 309–313 (1981).

48. Ramirez, G., O'Neill, W. M., Bloomer, H. A. *et al.* Abnormalities in the regulation of growth hormone in chronic renal failure. *Arch. Intern. Med.* **138**, 267–271 (1978).

49. Phillips, L. S., Pennisi, A. J., Belosky, D. C. *et al.* Somatomedin activity and inorganic sulfate in children undergoing hemodialysis. *J. Clin. Endocrinol. Metab.* **46**, 165–168 (1978).

50. Takano, K., Hall, K., Kastrup, K. W. *et al.* Serum somatomedin-A in chronic renal failure. *J. Clin. Endocrinol. Metab.* **48**, 371–376 (1979.

51. Engelerte, E., Brown, H., Willardson, D. G. *et al.* Metabolism of free and conjugated 17-hydroxycorticosteroids in subjects with uremia. *J. Clin. Endocrinol. Metab.* **18**, 36–48 (1958).

52. Nolan, G. E., Smith, J. B., Chavre, V. J. *et al.* Spurious overestimation of plasma cortisol in patients with chronic renal failure. *J. Clin. Endocrinol. Metab.* **52**, 1242–1245 (1981).

53. Mishkin, M. S., Hsu, T., Walker, W. G. *et al.* Studies on the episodic secretion of cortisol in uremic patients on hemodialysis. *Johns Hopkins Med. J.* **131**, 160–164 (1972).

54. Akmal, M., and Manzler, A. D. Simplified assessment of pituitary adrenal axis in a stable group of chronic hemodialysis patients. *Trans. Am. Soc. Artif. Intern. Organs* **23**, 703–706 (1977).

55. Wallace, E. Z., Rosman, P., Toshav, N. *et al.* Pituitary adrenocortical function in chronic renal failure: Studies of episodic secretion of cortisol and dexamethasone suppressibility. *J. Clin. Endocrinol. Metab.* **50**, 46–51 (1980).

56. McDonald, W. J., Golper, T. A., and Mass, R. D. Adrenocorticotropin-cortisol axis abnormalities in hemodialysis patients. *J. Clin. Endocrinol. Metab.* **48**, 92–95 (1979).

57. Drueke, T. Endocrine disorders in chronic hemodialysis patients (with the exclusion of hyperparathyroidism). *Adv. Nephrol.* **10**, 351–382 (1981).

58. Ramirez, G., Gomez-Sanchez, C., Meikle, W. A., and Jubiz, W. Evaluation of the hypothalamic hypophyseal adrenal axis in patients receiving long-term hemodialysis. *Arch. Intern. Med.* **142**, 1448–1452 (1982).

59. Rosman, P. M., Farag, A., Peckham, R. *et al.* Pituitary-adrenocortical function in chronic renal failure: Blunted suppression and early escape of cortisol levels after intravenous dexamethasone. *J. Clin. Endocrinol. Metab.* **44**, 528–533 (1982).

60. Feldman, H. A., and Singer, I. Endocrinology and metabolism in uremia. A clinical review. *Medicine (Baltimore)* **54**, 345–376 (1974).

61. Deck, K. A., Fischer, B., and Hiollen, H. Studies on cortisol metabolism during hemodialysis in man. *Eur. J. Clin. Invest.* **9**, 203–208 (1979).

62. Berl, T., Katz, F. H., Henrich, W. L. *et al.* Role of aldosterone in the control of sodium excretion in patients with advanced chronic renal failure. *Kidney Int.* **14**, 228–235 (1978).

63. Schambelan, M., Sebastian, A., and Biglieri, E. G. Prevalence, pathogenesis, and functional significance of aldosterone deficiency in hyperkalemic patients with chronic renal insufficiency. *Kidney Int.* **17**, 89–101 (1980).

64. Sterns, R. H., Feig, P. U., Pring, M. *et al.* Disposition of intravenous potassium in anuric man: A kinetic analysis. *Kidney Int.* **15**, 651–660 (1979).

65. Studer, A., Zaruba, K., Grimm, J. *et al.* Control of plasma aldosterone during chronic hemodialysis. *Clin. Nephrol.* **13**, 172–176 (1980).

66. Farinelli, A., Squerzanti, R., De Paoli, V. E. *et al.* Response of plasma aldosterone to sequential ultrafiltration, dialysis, and conventional hemodialysis. *Nephron* **26**, 274–279 (1980).

67. Cooke, C. R., Whelton, P. K., Moore, M. A. *et al.* Dissociation of the diurnal variation of aldosterone and cortisol in anephric subjects. *Kidney Int.* **15,** 669–675 (1979).

68. Pollini, J., Guttmann, R. D., Beaudoin, J. G. *et al.* Late hypertension following renal allotransplantation. *Clin. Nephrol.* **11,** 202–212 (1979).

69. de Kretser, D. M., Atkins, R. C., and Scott, D. F. Disordered spermatogenesis in patients with chronic renal failure on maintenance hemodialysis. *Aust. N. Z. J. Med.* **4,** 178–181 (1974).

70. Lim, V. S., and Fang, V. S. Gonadal dysfunction in uremic men. A study of the hypo-thalamo-pituitary-testicular axis before and after renal transplantation. *Am. J. Med.* **58,** 655–662 (1975).

71. Chen, J. C., Vidt, D. G., Zorn, E. M. *et al.* Pituitary-leydig cell function in uremic males. *J. Clin. Endocrinol. Metab.* **31,** 14–17 (1970).

72. Holdsworth, S., Atkins, R. C., and de Kretser, D. M. The pituitary-testicular axis in men with chronic renal failure. *N. Engl. J. Med.* **296,** 1245–1249 (1977).

73. Morley, J. E., Distiller, L. A., Unterhalter, S. *et al.* Effect of renal transplantation on pituitary gonadal function. *Metab., Clin. Exp.* **27,** 781–785 (1978).

74. Holdsworth, S. R., de Kretser, D. M., and Atkins, R. C. A comparison of hemodialysis and transplantation in reversing the uremic disturbance of male reproductive function. *Clin. Nephrol.* **10,** 146–150 (1978).

75. Phadke, A. G., MacKinnon, K. J., and Dossetor, J. B. Male infertility in uremia: A restoration by renal allografts. *Can. Med. Assoc. J.* **102,** 607–608 (1970).

76. Lim, V. S., Henriquez, C., Sievertsen, G. *et al.* Ovarian function in chronic renal failure: Evidence suggesting hypothalamic anovulation. *Ann. Intern. Med.* **93,** 21–27 (1980).

77. Swamy, A. P., Woolf, P. D., and Cestero, R. V. M. Hypothalamic-pituitary-ovarian axis in uremic women. *J. Lab. Clin. Med.* **93,** 1066–1072 (1979).

78. Morley, J. E., Distiller, L. A., Epstein, S. *et al.* Menstrual disturbances in chronic renal failure. *Horm. Metab. Res.* **11,** 68–72 (1979).

79. Procci, W. R., Goldstein, D. A., Adelstein, J. *et al.* Sexual dysfunction in the male patient with uremia: A reappraisal. *Kidney Int.* **19,** 317–323 (1981).

80. Cowden, E. A., Ratcliffe, W. A., Ratcliffe, J. G. *et al.* Hyperprolactinemia in renal disease. *Clin. Endocrinol.* **77,** 15P–16P (1978).

81. Ramirez, G., O'Neill, W. M., Bloomer, H. A. *et al.* Abnormalities in the regulation of prolactin in patients with chronic renal failure. *J. Clin. Endocrinol. Metab.* **45,** 658–661 (1977).

82. Massry, S. G., Goldstein, D. A., Procci, W. R. *et al.* Impotence in patients with uremia: A possible role for parathyroid hormone. *Nephron* **19,** 305–310 (1977).

83. Atkin-Thor, E., Goddard, B. W., O'Nion, J. *et al.* Hypogeusia and zinc depletion in chronic dialysis patients. *Am. J. Clin. Nutr.* **31,** 1948–1951 (1978).

84. Blackman, M. R., Weintraub, B. D., Kourides, I. A. *et al.* Discordant elevation of common alpha subunit of the glycoprotein hormones compared to beta subunits in serum of uremic patients. *J. Clin. Endocrinol. Metab.* **53,** 39–48 (1981).

85. Lim, V. S., and Fang, V. S. Restoration of plasma testosterone levels in uremic men with clomiphene citrate. *J. Clin. Endocrinol. Metab.* **43,** 1370–1377 (1976).

86. Lim, V. S., Kathpalia, S. C., and Frohman, L. A. Hyperprolactinemia and impaired pituitary response to suppression and stimulation in chronic renal failure: Reversal after transplantation. *J. Clin. Endocrinol. Metab.* **48,** 101–107 (1979).

87. McLean, G. W., Stone, W. J., and Rabin, D. Unpublished observations.

88. Gomez, F., de la Cueva, R., Wauters, J. *et al.* Endocrine abnormalities in patients under-going long term hemodialysis. The role of prolactin. *Am. J. Med.* **68,** 522–530 (1980).

89. Sievertsen, G. D., Lim, V. S., Kathpalia, S. *et al.* Hyperprolactinemia in chronic renal failure: Altered lactotroph response to dopaminergic suppression. *Clin. Res.* **26,** 495A (1978).

90. Bohnet, H. G., Dahlen, H. G., Wutte, W. *et al.* Hyperprolactinemic anovulatory syndrome. *J. Clin. Endocrinol. Metab.* **42,** 132–143 (1976).

91. Chopp, R. T., and Mendez, R. Sexual function and hormonal abnormalities in uremic men on chronic dialysis and after renal transplantation. *Fertil. Steril.* **29,** 661–666 (1978).

92. Mies, R., Baeyer, H., Figge, H. *et al.* Investigation of pituitary and leydig cell function in chronic hemodialysis and after renal transplantation. *Klin. Wochenschr.* **53,** 611–615 (1975).

93. Sherman, F. P. Impotence in patients with chronic renal failure on dialysis: Its frequency and etiology. *Fertil. Steril.* **26,** 221–223 (1975).

94. Brannen, G. E., Peters, T. G., Hambidge, K. M. *et al.* Impotence after kidney transplantation. *Urology* **15,** 138–146 (1980).

95. Hansky, J. Effect of renal failure on gastrointestinal hormones. *World J. Surg.* **3,** 463–467 (1979).

96. Korman, M. G. Laver, M. C., and Hansky, J. Hypergastrinemia in chronic renal failure. *Br. Med. J.* **1,** 209–210 (1972).

97. O'Doriso, T. M., Sirinek, K. R., Mazzaferri, E. L. *et al.* Renal effects on serum gastric inhibitory polypeptide (GIP). *Metab., Clin. Exp.* **26,** 651–656 (1977).

5

Psychiatric Aspects
of End-Stage Renal Disease:
Diagnosis and Management

◆

PAULINE L. RABIN

111

Copyright © 1983 by Academic Press, Inc.
All rights of reproduction in any form reserved.
ISBN 0-12-672280-3

END-STAGE RENAL DISEASE

I. PERSONALITY CHANGES IN END-STAGE RENAL DISEASE

The following features characterize the psychological responses of patients with end-stage renal disease (ESRD).

A. Responses to Multiple Losses (*1, 2*)

1. Loss of Health—Implications and Reactions

A perceptible feeling of loss invariably accompanies chronic debilitating disease, with the realization that one can no longer enjoy good health. The uremic syndrome is characterized by weakness, malaise, lethargy, and debilitation. In addition, the patient has difficulty in concentration, and his memory may be impaired. Loss of libido and impotence secondary to organic changes in gonadal function not infrequently accompany chronic renal disease. These problems may only present after the initiation of dialysis and be blamed on "the machine." A similar constellation of symptoms is also observed in the depressed patient. It is important to distinguish the role that depression plays in the patient's symptomatology. The differential diagnosis will be discussed later.

2. Loss of Work, Loss of Economic Stability,
    and Financial Independence

Many patients cannot return to their previous employment, especially if it entails physical labor. Patients in white collar jobs or in professions tend to find it easier to return to work. However, some employers prefer not to employ the chronically ill. Thus, most patients with ESRD face an uncertain work future. This, in turn, threatens economic stability and exaggerates feelings of anxiety and depression. In male patients, in particular, the loss of the dominant role as the chief family breadwinner is a cause of chronic dissatisfaction. In addition, the wife may have to assume many responsibilities previously undertaken by her husband. The reversal of roles and loss of previous status creates further insecurity for the patient. The same dilemma faces women with ESRD who have had active careers. Some women, however, have less difficulty accepting the "passive sick" role and may make a better adjustment to chronic illness.

3. Loss of Mobility and Flexibility

Any form of dialysis must be carried out regularly. Center dialysis patients are required to report at a given hour two or three times a week. This imposes restrictions on the patient and his family. There is a loss of flexibility. Family schedules must be rigidly planned around the dialysis program. Patients on home hemodialysis or home peritoneal dialysis have a greater measure of freedom in planning their treatment. They can dialyze in hotel rooms, in campers, or at the homes of their friends. This is particularly true of patients on CAPD. Nevertheless, these time-consuming procedures always restrict mobility to some degree.

4. Loss of Freedom concerning Diet and Fluid Intake

The dialysis patient must consistently restrict and monitor his fluid intake. In addition, he must adhere to a rigid diet, particularly in regard to potassium. This is especially difficult during the summer months when fresh fruits and vegetables are in abundant supply. The patient cannot eat or drink freely at a party or picnic.

5. The Syndrome of Impending Loss

Even when the patient is stabilized on a dialysis program, the future is fraught with the dangers of multiple medical complications, hospitalizations with separation from family and friends, and a shortened life expectancy. In addition, drastic changes in the patient's state of health may pose a threat to the marriage. This has been observed more frequently in younger individuals who cannot tolerate the new and unexpected stresses attendant on chronic illness in a spouse.

6. Loss of a Kidney Transplant

The patient who opts for kidney transplantation inevitably faces a loss of that kidney. The average best survival time is approximately 8 years, and many transplanted kidneys will be rejected sooner. Rejection will be accompanied by some feelings of depression despite use of denial by the patients. They try to minimize the loss by saying, "Well, I knew I only had a fighting chance," or "I took a gamble and lost." These patients will, nevertheless, be mourning the loss and may experience the emotional and/or the physiological symptoms of depression.

Implications of the Losses

The universal response to loss is to grieve. The grief reaction is a normal and expected response. Clinically, the patient will describe sadness or feeling blue. He may even be tearful. He may express hopelessness about his future and have a negative outlook. Feelings of self-reproach or guilt are common. Behavior may become withdrawn or more dependent and clinging. There is loss of interest in usually stimulating activities together with feelings of fatigue, loss of energy, and anhedonia. Preoccupation with thoughts of death may be present. Certain physiological or vegetative symptoms are often seen:

1. Sleep disturbance: this is usually characterized by early morning awakening and is accompanied by a tired feeling all day. A vast array of other sleep disturbances are encountered, including excessive daytime sleepiness and restless night sleep.

2. Loss of appetite: this may be accompanied by weight loss. Some patients, however, lose their enjoyment of food, but eat nonetheless and may even eat excessively. Uremia may dull both taste and smell sensations which further reduce appetite.

3. Loss of libido: patients usually have little or no desire for sexual intercourse. Males may complain of impotence; females of anorgasmia.

4. Somatic symptoms: somatic symptoms encountered are (a) gastrointestinal complaints, and (b) pain, usually vague but persistent. Headache is common, but chest and low back pain are also found.

5. Addiction to drugs: narcotics and sedatives may be prescribed by physicians to relieve pain and suffering, while the underlying grief reaction may not have been recognized. Depressed patients may abuse these drugs in an attempt to alleviate symptoms of depression.

6. Noncompliance with diet and/or prescribed medications: This is often an expression of feelings of hopelessness experienced by the patient.

The grief reaction is a normal response to loss. Although the signs and symptoms are extensive and affect mood, they are usually not sufficiently pervasive as to impair the individual's ability to function. Intensification of the signs and symptoms of the grief reaction or persistence for more than 2–3 months may herald the onset of frank depression. The signs of depression include psychomotor retardation or an overt agitation with wringing of the hands and tense pacing. The patient's attention span is limited, and this will be manifested by an inability to sustain concentration when performing relatively simple tasks. The patient may ruminate excessively about his symptoms, which will be described with hopeless resignation. Self-worthlessness and pessimism will color the patient's perspective. Addiction to drugs and alcohol may occur secondary to depression. In the presence of the characteristic features of depression, one should not, however, be misled by the "smiling depression," the patient who conceals his mood behind a mask of smiles.

Depressed patients should always alert one to the danger of suicide. The physician should ask specifically about suicidal ideation, intention, or plans if the patient appears depressed. Patients are usually relieved to have the opportunity to talk about their self-destructive impulses. A frank discussion about the patient's depression can provide an avenue for therapeutic intervention. Overt suicide has been documented when patients refuse to continue dialysis, tamper with their shunt, allow themselves to exsanguinate from a shunt, or deliberately overdose on medications. Abram et al. (3) in 1971 reported that suicide was 100–400 times as frequent in the dialysis population as in the general population in the United States. A similar study repeated in 1979 in Europe revealed the suicide rate among patients on chronic dialysis to be 10 times that of the general population (4). Our own experience during the past 5 years is more in keeping with the findings in the latter study. This may be due to the fact that the physical demands of dialysis have been decreased considerably by reducing time on the machine. In the past few years, the introduction of more efficient dialyzers has decreased the usual time on dialysis from 30 to 12 hr per week. It may also reflect the patient's recognition that people are living a decade or longer on dialysis and that alternative modes of therapy such as transplantation are available.

Noncompliance with the medical regimen may lead to intractable complications which can be life threatening. As one example, excessive fluid and salt intake can lead to pulmonary edema. Patients may resent adherence to the restrictive diet and feel they have lost control over their lives. They may act out their anger by refusing to comply with medical instructions or deny that their behavior can influence their medical status (5). Other patients may knowingly opt for a more flexible life-style, despite the knowledge that this will shorten their life-span. They choose quality of life rather than quantity of life.

There is a striking and perplexing overlap in the signs and symptoms of depression with those of uremia. Depressed patients may not be treated because the signs and symptoms are attributed to the underlying disease process. Physicians may consider depression an "appropriate" response to severe medical illness and do not attempt to treat it. Furthermore, independent and potentially treatable psychological causes may be overlooked and inadequately explored.

Treatment of the Depressed Patient

The untreated uremic patient may exhibit a depressed affect in association with an acute organic brain syndrome. We stress that it is often impossible to distinguish whether the component of depression is primarily attributable to ESRD or is secondary to independent causes. Therefore, the disordered biochemical picture accompanying uremia (i.e., elevated BUN, acidemia, electrolyte disturbances including hyperkalemia, and disordered calcium metabolism) should first be vigorously corrected and the patient's mood reassessed thereafter.

When evaluating any patient with depression, and especially ESRD patients who are often on a host of medications, one must consider that the depression may be drug induced. The antihypertensive medications as a group are the most common cause of drug-induced depression; reserpine, methyldopa and the β blockers are frequently implicated. Steroids, barbiturates, cimetidine, and benzodiazepines may also cause depression. Discontinuing a drug is the simplest way to test its role in producing mood changes. It may be dangerous to discontinue a drug precipitously. The drug should be tapered and the clinical response observed. Substitution of one antihypertensive for another may be effective in alleviating the depression.

When depressive symptoms persist, especially for more than 2 months, are severe, or are marked by feelings of hopelessness, negative attitudes and suicidal ideation, the diagnosis of depression can be confidently made and warrants treatment. Psychological tests can be helpful in obtaining a more objective evaluation of the patient's mental status. The physician must then explore the origins of these feelings and actively treat the depression. One should never assume that the depression is necessarily secondary to the renal disease. For example, a 55-year-old man who had been on dialysis for 5 years became increasingly depressed and threatened to stop dialysis. When a psychiatric evaluation was made, the patient was encouraged to speak about his personal life. It was learned that he was very disturbed by a letter he had received from his 19-year-old son stationed in Korea. The young man wrote that he was marrying a Korean girl whom he had met 2 months previously. The father was overwrought that the son was taking on a responsibility in an impulsive, immature way, and he was sad that he would not be able to attend his only child's wedding.

Supportive psychotherapy with discriminating use of antidepressant medication is the suggested therapeutic approach to the depressed patient. The tricyclic antidepressant drugs, particularly doxepin HCl and imipramine HCl, are safe and effective. These are rapidly absorbed, rapidly concentrated in the tissues and tightly bound to plasma protein (6). Because of this, renal dialysis probably has little effect on reducing levels in the plasma. This group of drugs is metabolized almost entirely by the liver, and only small quantities of unchanged drug are found in the urine (7). A major dose modification in renal patients is therefore not required (8). During tricyclic therapy, problems with blood pressure maintenance on dialysis have rarely been encountered in our experience. The cardiotoxic and anticholinergic side effects of antidepressants must be kept in mind. The therapeutic dose recommended ranges from 150 to 250 mg daily, usually given in one dose at bedtime. Initially, one will start with 50 mg h.s. and gradually increase the dose over the next 10 days. A clinical response will only be observed after a minimum of 2–3 weeks. It is important to remember that the antihypertensive effect of guanethidine can be blocked by antidepressant medication. However, guanethidine has not been a useful drug in our ESRD population due to its propensity to cause sudden, severe hypotension during dialysis.

Involvement of the family is essential in treating the depressed patient. Problems that the family are facing may be projected or "blamed" on the patient, or the patient may experience guilt feelings because he cannot participate more actively in their solution. The active participation of a social worker is often critical in successfully coping with the problems facing the family.

Loss of Sexual Potency: Differential Diagnosis (9–11)

Patients often refrain from discussing sexual problems with their doctor. However, over one-half of uremic men and one-third of uremic women experience severe sexual disorders. Women report a marked decrease in desire for intercourse and frequency of orgasm, and most men consider themselves partially or totally impotent (9). Prescribed drugs (particularly antihypertensives) and psychogenic factors (depression, denial, or interpersonal difficulties) may play major roles in sexual dysfunction. The differentiation of psychogenic from organic impotence can usually be made in men by measurements of nocturnal penile tumescence. Patients with organic impotence do not have nocturnal erections. Those with psychogenic impotence exhibit nocturnal penile tumescence, usually in association with REM sleep.

TREATMENT.   The therapeutic approach is dictated by the etiology of the impotence. An unequivocal definition of the cause of impotence may help patients and their partners in their adaptation to chronic illness. If antihypertensive medication is implicated, changing the regimen is sometimes useful. When serum testosterone levels are found to be very low, exogenous testosterone therapy can restore potency in some but not all uremic patients. Parenteral testosterone enanthate is recommended. Impotence consequent to depression is amenable to treatment. The use of antidepressant medications in conjunction with psychotherapy usually yields the best results. Marital counseling is indicated for those couples who are having interpersonal problems. Sex therapy is helpful to encourage couples to consider alternate ways of expressing affection and intimacy. Implantation of a penile prosthesis may be considered for male patients who are refractory to other therapy.

B.   Responses to Potential Gains

The introduction of dialysis has made it possible to extend life for the patient with ESRD. When renal disease has progressed so that dialysis is necessary, a crisis or turning point occurs in the life of the patient. As with every crisis, there is both danger and opportunity. The danger is that of death from uremia or other complications. This contrasts with the opportunity to translate the extension of life by the artificial kidney into meaningful existence. We have observed patients who have made determined efforts and succeeded in introducing new dimensions to their lives. This extension of life-span has enabled some to raise their families, help in the completion of their children's education, and see their children married. For other patients, the crisis has been an opportunity to face up to and resolve intrapersonal conflicts and interpersonal relationships. Some patients have sought and completed vocational rehabilitation in areas that would allow them to become independent while continuing on dialysis. In others, the crisis has catalyzed previously dormant initiative, and they have flourished in independent business enterprises, juggling their schedules to meet the demands of the dialysis. Exceptional patients whose employers were amenable have continued to work full-time in demanding jobs and have dialyzed at home in the evenings.

Despite the catalogue of losses described, the gains for many patients make dialysis treatment worthwhile and can enhance not only the length, but also the quality, of life.

C.   Behavioral Changes Accompanying Chronic Disease

1.   Dependency, Regression, and the Behavioral Manifestations of Denial and Displacement of Affect (11–15)

In general, the mentally and physically healthy individual strives to maintain independence. When confronted with real physical illness and accompanying limitations, it is necessary to accept help. Ideally, the patient should come to terms with the fact that he is dependent on others, but can maintain some independence in areas not affected by his illness. Only then can he engage productively in work, family activities, and other pursuits within the limitations of his illness and his treatment (1). In practice, many patients exhibit a more global *regression* and become dependent on their families in more ways than can be explained by their illness and its treatment. This is often expressed by failure to participate actively in family undertakings, from household chores to financial decision making.

Denial is a widely used defense mechanism whereby a person avoids awareness of an emotionally painful aspect of reality. Denial is useful when it provides a respite from anxiety and fear attendant on all severe chronic disease. It is destructive when it prompts behavior that is inimical to the patient's therapeutic regimen. At one extreme this may lead the patient to discontinue regular dialysis treatments in the mistaken belief that he only requires infrequent dialysis. Denial can also lead to dietary indiscretion and abuse of liquids. Medications may be discontinued or erratically taken. For example, the immediate benefit of phosphate binders is not apparent to the patient and thus are often disregarded. However, having to be hemodialyzed three times a week serves as a persistent reminder of the illness and counteracts significantly the patient's denial mechanisms. Even when the patient is not undergoing dialysis, the presence of the shunt and the accompanying hum are a constant reminder to the patient of the reality of his illness. Yet, despite the ravages of the disease and the restrictions imposed by treatment, the average dialysis patient may look and feel relatively well especially on the day following dialysis. This may reinforce the patient's denial of illness. For some patients there is a dilemma of whether to assume the sick role or the healthy role. It is our conclusion that patients need assistance in accepting and living with both of these roles.

Younger patients (under 50 years) are often considered transplant candidates. The perception of this alternative as a "cure" increases frustration and intolerance with dialysis as a treatment modality and may foster denial of the possible difficulties associated with transplantation. If the transplant fails, an excessive feeling of loss may result.

2. Exaggeration of Preexistent Neurosis

All adult persons have developed a set of defense mechanisms with which they cope with any threat to their self-integrity. The neuroses develop when these defense mechanisms become a dominant feature in life-style causing interference with effective functioning. Stress, such as chronic illness, will trigger the use of defense mechanisms and may make an underlying neurosis overt or exaggerate a preexisting neurosis.

For example, a 50-year-old man with an obsessive personality trait utilized his defenses to structure his life on dialysis in a very regimented manner. He was considered an ideal patient by the treatment team, but his marriage and family life were jeopardized because of his extreme rigidity and need to control the entire household.

Another example of the emergence of a full-blown neurosis is the case of a well-educated 48-year-old married woman with a 25-year history of chronic renal disease. When hemodialysis was eventually required, she resented being "tied down on a machine" and threatened to refuse further treatment. During her third hospital dialysis, she revealed a strong belief in her ability to communicate with God via automatic writing. Psychiatric consultation was obtained. By this time, she contended that God urged her to choose life and that meant acceptance of the dialysis program. She did not exhibit any other psychotic features. The team was advised to ignore this delusion because it provided the patient with a rationale for continuing dialysis, which heretofore she had considered unacceptable and had almost rejected. She has maintained this fixed delusion for 3 years, functioning effectively as a housewife and mother.

In approaching behavioral changes, the underlying feelings that patients are experiencing must first be explored. The potentially harmful defense mechanisms like denial must be understood by the patient, and healthy new coping skills encouraged by the physician. Fear of losing control of one's life and the implicit fear of death often underlie abuse of diet and fluid intake. The patient should be helped to realize the origins of behavior and to utilize the controls that he does have in order to manage and favorably modify the course of his disease.

D. Responses to Dependency on a Machine

Patients suffering from chronic renal disease in our society anticipate prolongation of life by one or another form of dialysis treatment. Although they do not look forward to this and many disclaim intention of participation, few refuse to start this treatment. The survival instinct predominates over the fears and revulsion of machine dependency. Conflicts persist and patients exhibit different phases in their adaptation to dialysis. Three stages have been classically described by Reichsman and Levy (16): honeymoon, disenchantment and discouragement, and long-term adaptation. The *honeymoon period* is characterized by marked emotional and physical improvement of which the patient has clear and conscious awareness. This generally begins 1–3 weeks after the patient's first dialysis treatment and usually lasts from 6 weeks to 6 months. There are feelings of hope, confidence, joy, and, at times, euphoria. The patients tend to minimize the inconvenience of the illness and its treatment and accept their marked dependency on the machine with phrases such as "It's not so bad. What's all the fuss about?" Because dialysis as a treatment modality is readily available in the United States, patients now tend to come for treatment earlier. Nephrologists, in general, tend to start dialysis sooner than they did two decades ago, i.e., before the patient develops a full-blown uremic syndrome. In consequence, we do not see so floridly "the honeymoon period" described by writers such as Reichsman and Levy (*16*) and Abram (*17*). The phase of *disenchantment and discouragement* may begin either abruptly or quite gradually and lasts from 3 to 12 months. In Reichsman and Levy's series, 12 or 16 patients displayed a decrease and even disappearance of feelings of contentment, confidence and hope. These authors found a strong temporal relationship between the onset of this period and the planning or resumption of an active role in the family and at work. In our experience, the end of the honeymoon is generally triggered by an intercurrent complication, either social or medical, for example, news that application for a financial loan has been refused; disturbing family problems such as the patient who learned that his un-married daughter was pregnant; or a medical setback such as pneumonia or the loss of a dialysis access site. Confrontation with one's illness or with one's inability to influence events exposes a patient's vulnerabilities and re-focuses his attention on the intractability of his chronic illness.

The third phase, *long-term adaptation*, begins when the patient comes to terms, to a greater or lesser degree, with his physical limitations and with the shortcomings of the treatment. The adaptation will be an expression of the patient's personality and the defense mechanisms he usually employs.

1. Anxieties while on the Machine (18, 19)

There are significant stresses which inevitably accompany the hemodial-ysis procedure. The venipunctures, followed by observation of one's hepa-rinized blood being continually pumped through a machine with nurses and paramedical personnel in attendance, all contribute to an increased aware-ness of one's illness. Muscle cramping and a sense of general discomfort may accompany the procedure. In addition, being on the machine reinforces a sense of dependency (the "sick" role) and the fact that the patient is not in control. The heightened anxiety thus produced is defended by a variety of behavioral responses. Patients may complain incessantly or may make excessive demands on the nursing staff. Having the undivided attention of the nurse or dialysis assistant for some patients restores a sense of security. Some patients masturbate while dialyzing. Masturbation is an anxiety relieving mechanism, which symbolically restores a male patient's sense of manhood. The same explanation pertains to the overtly sexual overtures made by male patients to female staff. Female patients may be flirtatious or seductive to male attendants or physicians in an effort to deny their illness and assert their femininity. Methods for handling these behaviors are dis-cussed in Section V.

Some patients dramatically regress while on the machine. A 45-year-old diabetic male who, until he started dialysis, was actively employed as a welder exhibited very disturbing behavior during hemodialysis. He would curl up in a fetal position and literally moan from beginning to end of every dialysis treatment. Group pressure, by way of a petition from other patients who shared the center facility, and structured support by the nurses eventually had some impact in reversing this behavior.

Reviewing the long-term adjustment of our patients on hemodialysis, we have made similar observations to those of Anderson (*20*). He described two patient populations, an assertive independent group and a more passive dependent group. The patients with independent personality traits will suffer the greatest difficulties initially when they feel they are losing control over their lives, but usually make a more successful adjustment when they are well enough to resume their previous active role in society. The dependent group generally can more easily accept the sick role, but their attempts at professional and social rehabilitation are usually fraught with difficulties. This group should be encouraged to dialyze at home and accept responsibility for their own medical care. This will improve their self-esteem and general sense of well-being. For those patients who are unable to dialyze at home, structured recreational programs allowing the individual to participate in group activities may counterbalance their passivity.

2.   Misperceptions of Being "On the Machine"

Not uncommonly, there are unrecognized deleterious effects of the jargon used by personnel at the renal clinic and dialysis center on patients before their first dialysis. Repetitive use of the term "on the machine" may be seriously misperceived by patients who have not been educated about, or have avoided acquainting themselves with, dialysis procedures. The following case is a striking example (*21*). A 55-year-old man had been followed for some years in a renal clinic with a diagnosis of polycystic kidney disease. He had previously worked on an assembly line in a bicycle factory. When told that his medical condition warranted dialysis "on the kidney machine," he resisted opportunities to learn about the procedure and repeatedly postponed hospitalization arranged for the construction of the shunt. The psychiatrist was able to establish rapport with the patient and learned that he fantasized "being on the machine" as a process similar to the one with which he was familiar in the bicycle factory. "I thought I would be strapped down on the machine and the nurses and doctors would subject me to a variety of different procedures just the way we put together a bicycle." These ideas frightened him, but he kept them to himself and denied troublesome symptoms in an effort to postpone dialysis. He was relieved and surprised by what actually constituted the hemodialysis procedure.

This patient exemplifies many of the unspoken fears and misperceptions that patients have of the new and more sophisticated medical techniques (*22, 23*). Fear may lead to denial of symptoms and self-destructive behavior, in that timely initiation of maintenance hemodialysis may be delayed. This example emphasizes the importance of a continuing education program for patients with pre-ESRD.

II. EDUCATION FOR PATIENTS WITH PRE-END-STAGE AND END-STAGE RENAL DISEASE

As a result of our experience with the patient described above and others, we initiated formal visits to the dialysis center for all patients with progressive kidney disease. Second, we instituted an ongoing weekly session of "Kidney Talk." These 1 hr sessions, held each renal clinic day, review all aspects of kidney disease and its treatment. The "Kidney Talk" sessions are open to renal patients and their families. Areas related to living with chronic renal disease including hemodialysis, peritoneal dialysis, and renal transplantation are covered. The goals of "Kidney Talk" are two-fold, patient education and supportive group therapy.

A. Patient Education

On alternate weeks a minilecture is presented by a member of the staff of the hemodialysis and transplant teams, which includes the nephrologist, renal transplant surgeon, psychiatrist, social worker, clinical nurse specialist, and dietitian. These lectures are informal and range from the history of dialysis, aspects of renal physiology, and understanding of shunt construction, to the signs and symptoms of depression. In addition to lectures, we have used movies, slides, and posters to demonstrate important principles and ideas. The lecturers encourage questions during and after their presentation, and other staff members in the audience generally stimulate discussion by the patients and their families.

B. Supportive Group Therapy

Alternate weeks are devoted to open discussion, with a staff member serving as the group leader. By creating a forum for patients to meet with one another and with members of the staff, patients share some of their problems and receive support from other patients. Topics include ways to cope with diet restrictions at holiday times, interesting hobbies that can be converted to satisfying full-time occupations, techniques for shunt care, and how to budget on a fixed income.

Patients are often afraid to ask "silly questions" of their busy doctors. In the relaxed atmosphere of "Kidney Talk," they feel free to question any member of the staff and receive satisfactory explanations to their queries.

Many myths and misperceptions have been clarified in these sessions. We encourage the combined attendance of patients with chronic renal disease, patients on hemodialysis or peritoneal dialysis, and patients who have received a kidney transplant. This allows transmittal of firsthand information from persons who have experienced a treatment with which others are unfamiliar. One of the most dramatic effects which we have observed from this program is the support and encouragement that patients on hemodialysis are able to give those who are imminent dialysis candidates. No anxiolytic agent is as effective or as long-lasting. From close contact with nephrology patients attending "Kidney Talk," I have observed that almost every patient with chronic renal illness harbors the hope that he will be the virtually unique exception to avoid ESRD and the medical and therapeutic consequences. Patients may have confidence in their physician but nevertheless believe he may have erred in judgement and clinical assessment in their particular case. From our work with patients attending a renal clinic, we have been able to describe three discrete types of responses (21): Compliers (Group 1), Partial Deniers (Group 2), and Total Deniers (Group 3).

Among Group 1 are individuals who accept their doctor's advice, adhere to their medical regimen closely, and follow through with therapeutic recommendations. On review of their psychiatric histories, Group 1 individuals are usually law-abiding, disciplined citizens who have been raised in an environment dominated by the presence of an authority figure. These patients pay attention to advice from physicians and dietitians, make an adequate adjustment to dialysis, and are regarded by their physicians as ideal or "good" patients.

Group 2 patients characteristically do not believe that their condition is as serious as their doctor has stated. Feelings of anger seem to make up a large component of the patients' conscious reaction to their illness. They have a need to test the doctor in an attempt to disprove his diagnosis, which they do by ignoring instructions, abusing their diet or mismanaging their medication schedules. They are apt to follow the medical regimen for a few days prior to their clinic visit in order to placate their physicians, perhaps out of a sense of guilt or as a result of real fear that they are unable to repress, a fear that the doctor may indeed be right. Such patients convey an attitude of playing games and arouse intense frustration in the treatment team.

Group 3 patients may be divided into two subsets. Some deny the significance of many of their chronic symptoms and often present acutely requiring emergency hemodialysis. The second subgroup attend the outpatient renal clinic erratically, follow medical instructions poorly, and assiduously avoid visiting a dialysis center. They decline any opportunity to familiarize themselves with the kidney machine. This reaction can be explained on the basis of fear and denial that they may require dialysis. This denial is perpetuated by magical thinking of which the following represent examples: "If I never see the machine, perhaps I may never even need one," or "Other people need the machine and it saves their lives, but I don't need it, so why should I upset myself by seeing the whole thing," or "It's all too complicated for me—I'm no doctor—if and when I need to be on the machine I'm sure my doctor will give me all the information necessary."

III. PSYCHOLOGICAL FACTORS INFLUENCING THE CHOICE OF ALTERNATE METHODS OF TREATMENT

The patient with pre-ESRD has a choice of several modalities of therapy: hemodialysis in center, home hemodialysis, peritoneal dialysis, continuous ambulatory peritoneal dialysis, or kidney transplantation. The nephrologist will make a recommendation based on medical considerations. For example, the diabetic patient with ESRD almost invariably has attendant diabetic retinopathy. The dangers of retinal or preretinal bleeding are exaggerated by the frequent use of heparin necessary in the hemodialysis technique. Consequently, an alternative therapeutic approach is recommended, usually peritoneal dialysis. The medical indications which determine therapeutic modalities are discussed in Chapter 8. The availability of an assistant and the proximity to a dialysis center are nonmedical factors that may influence the type of dialysis treatment adopted. We confine our discussion to the psychological factors that affect a patient's choice when all modes of therapy remain viable options. Several patients have expressed their personal choices articulately (*24. 25*).

A. Hemodialysis

This is the most commonly recommended dialysis treatment. The individuals that adapt best to this form of treatment are (a) well organized and able to use the time on the machine in a constructive manner, e.g., reading, watching television, or making phone calls; and (b) those persons who are realistic about the demands of the illness and the loss of time that must necessarily be spent on the machine. We concur with Levy and Wynbrandt (*2*) who noted that dialysis adversely affected the quality of life in persons whose equanimity relied heavily on employment and physical activity.

Hemodialysis may be psychologically more salutary than renal transplantation for those patients who cannot tolerate the unknown. Transplantation is colored with uncertainty: Will the transplant take? Will side effects from the medications develop? Will there be any rejection episodes? Some patients prefer the routine of dialysis to the uncharted territory accompanying transplant. A support system is present at dialysis centers where social workers, nurses, doctors, and dietitians are regularly present and available for encouragement and advice (26). For chronically ill patients, the dialysis center may provide a pivotal segment of their social life which they would lose after transplantation.

B. Home Hemodialysis (27–29)

Distance from a center and flexibility of schedule are usually the dominant factors in persuading patients and their families to train for home hemodialysis. Absolutely essential is an available dialysis assistant, usually a spouse or family member. We have trained patients and assistants from every social and educational background. In our opinion, the decisive factor determining success in training is the degree of motivation in both the patient and the assistant. Highly motivated couples with meager formal education can master the intricacies of hemodialysis. However, home dialysis introduces a stressful situation in a family where one member treats another in a life-saving, yet potentially life-threatening, way. An evaluation of the emotional status of the patient and the dialysis assistant is essential before a home training program is undertaken. Psychological support for the patient, the assistant, or for the couple may be vital to assure successful performance of home dialysis. Patients on home dialysis tend to do very well. This may well be a consequence of selection: the more severely ill patients with multiple medical complications tend to be treated in center dialysis programs. On the other hand, the high degree of motivation, the acceptance of responsibility for their medical care, and maintenance of a degree of control among the home dialysis patients undoubtedly contribute to a better outcome in this group.

An inherent part of the home dialysis program is the active involvement of the patient in the entire procedure. Patients must be thoroughly knowledgeable about the workings of the machine, and they are responsible for setting up and cleaning the apparatus. This active role prevents the dependency and regression so commonly seen in center dialysis patients.

C. Intermittent Peritoneal Dialysis (CIPD)

The advantages of this mode of treatment are (1) a dialysis assistant is not always necessary; (2) the patient can sleep through part of the procedure; (3) less muscle cramping is experienced although some abdominal cramping is inevitable; and (4) there is none of the anxiety associated with the sight of one's blood being pumped through a kidney machine. The disadvantages include (1) fear of infection; (2) claustrophobic feelings; (3) general abdominal discomfort; (4) dissatisfaction concerning long hours on dialysis; and (5) protrusion of a plastic cannula through the skin. In addition, some patients have real concern about the abdominal penetration that they consider life threatening.

D. Continuous Abdominal Peritoneal Dialysis (CAPD)

This relatively new treatment approach offers a striking advantage. The patient is not tied down to a machine, and he does not usually require any assistance. He can be absolutely mobile, can travel freely, and work a full week. The patient who opts for CAPD predictably is the independent, highly motivated, careerist individual. The disadvantages are that the procedure is time consuming and bags must be changed with great attention to sterility. During travel the sheer weight and number of bags required can be a burden. Patients complain that they never have "a day off." The dangers of this treatment are infection and a subtle encouragement of denial of illness.

E. Factors Associated with a Decision to Discontinue Dialysis

Patients may actively make a decision to discontinue dialysis and be allowed to die. This generally occurs in a setting where the quality of life has deteriorated to such an extent that the suffering is constant and obvious to family and medical staff. Physicians, however, are usually very reluctant to be involved in such decisions and request a psychiatric evaluation of the patient's competence to make such a decision. When psychiatric evaluation reveals a depressed patient in contact with reality and expressing appropriate hopelessness about his grim prognosis, the treatment team should give consideration to the request to discontinue dialysis.

A 37-year-old blind diabetic patient with polyneuropathy was satisfactorily maintained on home peritoneal dialysis for 8 months. He rather suddenly developed generalized seizures, which heralded the onset of the syndrome of dialysis dementia including dysarthria, muscle twitchings, and typical EEG changes. After 2 weeks of vigorous therapy, including hemodialysis, he questioned his physicians about the prognosis. They were unable to give him any hope of a cure, but expressed certainty that they could control the seizures. The patient could not accept the suffering he endured on hemodialysis with the knowledge that dialysis dementia was a progressive condition. He made the decision to stop dialysis while he was in full control of his faculties.

Many patients do not come to this active and declared decision, but instead adopt a passive, aggressive stance. Patients on peritoneal dialysis may become careless in their catheter management. Patients on hemodialysis may abuse diet and fluid restrictions. When confronted, these patients deny a wish to die, but express a loss of desire to live. They are usually depressed, hopeless, and tired of the whole dialysis routine (22). Usually family support has ebbed. The patient has lost a meaningful role in society, has no outside interests, and considers himself a burden. These patients have given up and are usually resistant to psychotherapy and often refuse antidepressant medication.

F. Transplantation (30–33)

Successful renal transplantation is regarded by some patients as a "permanent cure." Under the appropriate medical conditions, this choice becomes particularly desirable for those patients who (a) cannot abide the rigid schedule of dialysis, the lack of mobility, or the limitations imposed by diet and fluid restriction; (b) are not doing well medically on dialysis; or (c) are young, desire to "return to normalcy," and are considered good transplant candidates.

It is incorrect to view transplantation as a cure. Since rejection episodes are very common, patients who receive a renal transplant require long-term and continued surveillance. In addition, the complications from the immunosuppressant drugs prescribed for all transplant patients are multiple and are often overlooked by the patient eagerly seeking a "magical cure."

A survey was taken of our dialysis population to determine the factors that influence patients to choose a renal transplant. All these patients had participated in education programs and had received information pertaining to the advantages and disadvantages of renal transplantation. This notwithstanding, the majority of patients did not reach their decision on the basis of a rational examination of the facts; rather, theirs was a "gut" decision. Specifically, the patients who opted for a renal transplant did so mainly because of their dissatisfaction with life on the dialysis machine. Their comments included, "I can't stand the machine," "This is not living—I'd rather die," "I want to give transplant a chance—what do I have to lose?" When confronted about the possible complications, patients indicated a willingness to gamble on escaping these hazards. "At least with transplant there is a chance that I may be well. On this machine I'm going downhill all the time." One element that dissuaded patients was a clear signal from their doctor that he had definite reservations about the procedure. The opposite also holds true, namely, the patient may concur with a recommendation for transplantation because he feels vulnerable, dependent, and wishes to please the staff and/or his family. In the latter situation, a patient's decision may be guided by the hope that he will be less of a burden on his family. Those patients considered good transplant candidates but who refused to be on the "active list" for future transplantation expressed preference for the treatment they knew rather than face the uncertainty attendant with transplantation. As one patient said, "Rather the devil I know than the devil I don't know."

G. Counseling Patients Who Are Considering Renal Transplantation

It should be the patient's decision whether or not to have a renal transplant. An informed decision is desirable. The information should be relayed in an unbiased manner with the intention of neither persuading nor dissuading the patient. To this end, the counseling is preferably given by a member of the nephrology team who is not identified explicitly with dialysis or with transplant. Our approach has been to have an experienced nurse impart the information, and, in a pretransplant interview, the psychiatrist will try to evaluate the patient's understanding of the information. Many of the patients whom I have evaluated have retained only that information that is nonthreatening. Too many look on transplantation as a cure and express surprise at the long-term, postoperative treatment that is a vital part of the maintenance of the transplanted kidney.

The psychiatrist's role is to ensure that the patient is aware of at least some of the drawbacks and difficulties that will occur even with the most optimal surgical results. In my experience, an element of repression of all the dangers and complications must be present to allow a patient to go through with the procedure. On the other hand, global denial of these problems is a prominent factor in the causation of postoperative depression and failure to cooperate with the medical regimen. The following principles are useful for both the nephrology nurse and the psychiatrist in preoperative counseling.

1. Transplantation is a treatment modality, not a cure. Unless this is understood, the patient is allowed to develop unreal expectations, which may be betrayed by the posttransplantation complications. He may then feel cheated and unable to cope with any setback, however minor.

2. The patient should have a good understanding of the surgical procedure, its possible complications and the immediate postoperative course, including the use of mask isolation, input–output chartings, and change in diet.

3. The patient must be knowledgeable about the medical treatment. He must be told the reasons for the use of steroids and other immunosuppressants and the side effects of these medications. Two side effects that are not

serious medically, but must be given due consideration in view of psychological sequelae, are moon facies and acne. Several patients, in our experience, have been so devastated by the change in their appearance that they have deliberately discontinued the medication. "At least on dialysis I don't look strange and disfigured to others."

4. Transplant rejection phenomena and their treatment must be understood. The patient must realize that it is dangerous to deny early rejection symptoms because this may delay initiation of appropriate treatment and result in loss of the graft.

5. There are specific considerations relating to the use of a cadaver kidney as opposed to a live donor kidney. In the former, the patient knows that a healthy person must die so that he can receive a kidney. For some, this provokes anxiety and guilt. They must be reassured that their need for a kidney in no way influences accidents and other deaths. The donor being dead and unknown allows free reign for fantasy. The patient needs to be able to speak about his thoughts and feelings concerning the origin of the transplanted kidney and also about his own ideas regarding death and dying. One white patient learned a new respect for the brotherhood of man. Upon accidentally learning that his kidney transplant had come from a black donor, he resigned from the Ku Klux Klan.

6. Patients who will be the recipients of live donor kidneys from one of their relatives must have an opportunity to examine their feelings about accepting such a gift. Many patients reject the idea because they feel they cannot deal with the attendant obligation it could arouse. Some patients fear that, as a result of the donation, the donor may in some way jeopardize his own health. An unresolved conflict between the recipient and the donor regarding the transplant may adversely affect the outcome of the procedure. We have observed this in several adolescents who received transplants from their parents and then failed to comply with the medical management postoperatively. Unresolved, rebellious feelings or anger were consistent features in these patients. When parental donors are involved, one must be alert to past and present dependency conflicts in the parent–child relationship. These may be magnified by the actual dependency imposed on the child recipient in the transplant situation irrespective of his age (31).

Complexities are also seen in sibling donor–recipient situations. In some cases, the siblings become closer, while in others there is resentment by the recipient because he feels an obligation to the donor. Some siblings become concerned that they will develop characteristics of the donor which they find undesirable. such as homosexual behavior.

The complex emotions experienced by the designated donor relative are often overlooked. Despite all precautions to preserve strict confidentiality regarding HLA typing among relatives, the family will inevitably learn who are the most desirable donors. Family pressure may subtly be brought to bear on a relative who demonstrated a good match with the patient. The prospective donor may have intense ambivalence regarding the loss of one of his kidneys. The kidney team has an obligation to the mental health of the donor. It is always possible to find a face-saving formula that relieves the donor of his perceived obligation without incurring guilt and the displeasure of his family, including the patient.

Postoperatively, donors may react to the pain and discomfort that inevitably follow major abdominal surgery. Some donors may become very angry and feel that they have experienced a very traumatic event (*33*). One donor called up his brother recipient on an intrahospital phone and demanded that the recipient "take good care of my kidney." The recipient became very agitated and obsessed with his "numbers" and was found studying his record in a very bizarre manner. He later became acutely psychotic. This was followed by rejection of the kidney and a severe depressive reaction. It is not possible to prove that psychological factors influence rejection; nevertheless, the association between intense, interpersonal conflicts and the phenomena of rejection is impressive.

We do not understand the many complex factors that influence compliance with a rigorous medical regimen following transplantation. Patient motivation here, as in dialysis therapy, is the overriding factor. A clear understanding of the process whereby medications influence successful functioning of the transplant will often increase patient cooperation. The patient should be encouraged to take responsibility for his behavior and become an active partner in the treatment program.

IV. NEUROPSYCHIATRIC MANIFESTATIONS ASSOCIATED WITH END-STAGE RENAL DISEASE

Patients who have suffered from chronic illness with manifest psychotic episodes may continue to display such symptoms either chronically or episodically after starting on a dialysis program. These patients are usually difficult to manage and do not comply with medications for their renal or for their psychiatric illness. Psychosis is an uncommon response to the stress of hemodialysis, but psychosis may develop *de novo* in patients on dialysis. In most cases, functional psychiatric syndromes begin in patients under the age of 40. Any patient over the age of 40 presenting for the first time with psychiatric complaints merits careful scrutiny of his general medical condition that may account for the new symptomatology. Delirium and dementia presenting in a patient on dialysis require a similar diligent approach.

Patients with ESRD who display behavior that is decidedly unusual for them may be clinically subdivided into two categories, acute and chronic.

A. Acute Onset of Disturbed Behavior

1. Delirium

Delirium most often is due to a problem whose primary focus lies outside of the central nervous system and produces diffuse cellular metabolic dysfunction involving the whole brain (34). Variability of its clinical manifestations is a hallmark of delirium. Patients present with clouding of consciousness, disorientation, hallucinations (usually visual), and paranoid ideation. These symptoms may be accompanied by clinical signs of sympathetic or parasympathetic hyperactivity. Various forms of tremor are frequently present. Bilateral asterixis and multifocal myoclonus are virtually pathognomonic of delirium. Neurological signs other than the abnormal movements are not common. It is most desirable to identify delirium during its prodrome when the patient may complain of trouble thinking, restlessness, irritability, insomnia, or vivid, frightening dreams. A brief mental status examination focusing on arousal level, attention span, short-term memory, and orientation should be done.

Any intercurrent infection can produce delirium. The delirium may also be precipitated by a drug reaction. In addition, the acute onset of disturbed behavior is often seen secondary to endocrine or electrolyte imbalance. Hypercalcemia, hypocalcemia, hypo-, or hypernatremia can produce profound psychiatric disturbances in a setting of ESRD. There is often no parallel between the degree of behavioral change and the quantitative alterations in serum chemistry.

It should be a rule to consider and definitively exclude a cerebrovascular insult or a subdural hematoma in any patient with ESRD presenting with an acute or subacute onset of change in behavior or mentation, even in the absence of any objective neurological deficits. This is one area where the use of the CT scan has been of inestimable value. Because of the chronic intermittent use of heparin, the patient receiving hemodialysis is prone to the development of subdural hematoma. This can present relatively acutely with disturbances of mentation and vague complaints by the patient of feeling "under par" or being disinterested in life. This picture could be mistaken for depression, but on close questioning the patient will not manifest the mood changes of depression. It is important to stress that there may be no focal neurological findings and no history of head trauma in dialysis patients who have developed subdural hematomas.

2. Steroid Psychosis (35)

The use of steroids in large doses is universal after kidney transplantation. There are no reliable predictors of the type of psychiatric response to massive doses of the glucocorticoid hormones. Steroids induce marked fluctuations in mood, either euphoria or dysphoria and depression. These mood fluctuations may or may not progress to a full-blown psychosis. The steroid psychosis usually presents during the first weeks following initiation of steroid hormone therapy and is characterized by visual hallucinations and paranoid ideation. These paranoid ideas often reflect the patients' concern about the safety and success of their transplant. They are usually anxious and irritable, but remain oriented to place and person. Some disturbance of the passage of time is common, "time is rushing by." Easily distracted by noise and unable to screen out extraneous sounds, they lose attention span and ability to concentrate on a task. They often appreciate that visual hallucinations are not real but may act out in response to them. For example, one teenaged patient receiving large doses of steroids vividly described a passing parade of her favorite cartoon characters in the street 10 floors below. While this might have been viewed as fantasy and wish fulfillment, the danger was that she was tempted to lean out of the window to see if, perhaps, they were real.

The following are characteristics of steroid psychoses (36):

1. The psychosis may occur at any point during steroid therapy without obvious precipitating factors.
2. The psychosis is commonly affective in nature.
3. The psychosis occurs in approximately 5% of patients receiving steroid therapy.
4. Delusional and hallucinating behavior is a frequent feature of the psychotic process.
5. The occurrence of the psychosis is not predictable from the premorbid personality.
6. Suicide is a significant problem with this psychotic process.

Treatment of Acute Behavioral Disturbances

Treatment should be directed at correcting the underlying cause. This, however, may not be immediately feasible (e.g., steroid psychosis). Therefore, it may be important to treat the behavioral disturbance symptomatically for a period of time. Haloperidol has been the drug of choice in these circumstances. The liquid concentrate preparation is easily absorbed. If a more rapid response is necessary, this medication can be given by intramuscular injection. A test dose of 2 mg is given initially. If necessary, this can be followed by a 5 mg dose after 30 min. Thereafter, one can titrate the dose according to the response elicited. An acute dystonic reaction may be observed as a side effect subsequent to the use of haloperidol. This usually responds well to an antihistamine such as diphenhydramine hydrochloride, 50 mg IM or IV.

Steroid psychosis responds dramatically to haloperidol. The psychiatrist and nephrologist should work together in reducing the steroid dose when possible, while adjusting the amount of neuroleptic necessary to control the disturbed behavior. Supportive measures are often very valuable in decreasing the anxiety and agitation that are common features of steroid psychosis. Moving patients into a quieter atmosphere in the presence of a close family member whom they know and trust is often beneficial.

Another cause of an acute psychiatric disturbance is a postoperative delirium. The patient described below illustrates that the syndrome responds very well to small doses of a neuroleptic medication and supportive measures (37).

A 37-year-old married woman received a transplanted kidney from her younger sister. She became acutely agitated and hostile while in the recovery room, accusing the staff there of trying to "dope her up." She was hyperalert and overtly suspicious of everyone and accused the staff of trying to tamper with her new kidney. We decided to move her into a private room and made provisions for her husband to stay overnight in the same room. Haloperidol, 2 mg IM, was given, followed 1 hr later by 5 mg IM. This achieved sedation, and she fell into a peaceful sleep. She subsequently required 2 mg t.i.d. for 3 days, and this was then tapered and discontinued after 1 week. The dosage of prednisone, 60 mg daily, was not altered. The transplanted kidney continued to function optimally, and her posthospital course was unremarkable.

B.   Chronic Onset of Disturbed Behavior

The insidious onset of disturbances in behavior suggests the following differential diagnosis.

1.   Psychiatric Illnesses

a.   Pseudo-dementia, i.e., a clinical picture that can resemble and partially mimic dementia, but is a reflection of an underlying psychiatric disorder, usually depression (38). Patients with pseudo-dementia characteristically complain repeatedly of their memory loss, and often family members can date the onset to a specific event or time. The cognitive difficulties are erratic, as are the disturbances in attention and concentration. Memory loss is generalized with no sparing of remote memory, unlike truly demented patients. Patients with pseudo-dementia often have a history of previous psychiatric difficulties. Depression is a treatable condition; hence, the importance of delineating this diagnosis and instituting vigorous therapy.

b. Other psychiatric disorders. These usually present prior to the onset of the ESRD, but can develop later, e.g., affective disorders and schizophrenia.

2. *Causes Related to Dialysis or Other Therapy*
   for End-Stage Renal Disease

a. DIALYSIS DEMENTIA. This can be defined as an encephalopathy presenting with the symptom complex of dementia, dysarthria, muscle twitchings, seizures, and specific EEG changes (*39*). This may begin weeks to years after the initiation of dialysis and occurs in patients of all ages. The course is usually rapid and can be fatal within weeks or months. While the presentation is usually subacute or chronic we have seen several patients who presented acutely with the onset of seizures or dysarthria. We have also seen two patients in whom the presenting symptoms were primarily psychiatric. The EEG tracings, however, were unequivocally abnormal and led us to suspect dialysis dementia. Only much later in the course of the illness did neuromuscular, speech and cognitive decline become manifest. Psychiatric presentations reported in dialysis dementia include depression, euphoria, irritability, paranoid delusions, auditory, and visual hallucinations (*40–45*). Abnormal EEG tracings provide the only method of suspecting dialysis dementia in patients presenting with psychiatric symptoms. The etiology is not well understood although aluminum intoxication has been postulated. There is no specific treatment but the withholding of aluminum containing medications has ameliorated the course of the illness in some cases (Chapter 3). Neuroleptic medication such as haloperidol has been used for behavioral modification in patients with delusions, hallucinations, and manic symptomatology. Antidepressants have been effective in alleviating depressive symptoms which may or may not be secondary to the dementia. Transplantation has produced remission in some patients with dialysis dementia.

b. COMPLICATIONS FROM LONG-TERM USE OF STEROID THERAPY. We and other centers have seen a variety of unusual meningeal and cerebral infections in patients on long-term steroid therapy. Often these are fungal in origin, and the symptoms of infection are masked by the steroids. The patients present with behavioral disturbances with or without neurological deficits. The importance of a lumbar puncture in establishing the diagnosis is emphasized. CT scan of the cranium may reveal an unexpected abscess and is equally important.

c. DEMENTIA THAT MAY BE DRUG INDUCED. Patients with chronic ESRD are often on numerous medications, which may be the cause of a dementia-like syndrome. The most common drugs causing this are the benzodiazepines and the barbiturates, both of which are excreted by the kidneys. Decreasing a dose or altering the type of drug may ameliorate the disturbed behavior. Medications which raise seizure threshold should not be stopped precipitously because of the danger of inducing seizure activity. Drug interactions, chronic alcoholism, and abuse of prescribed sedatives and tranquilizers should not be overlooked in the workup of dementia.

3. *Causes of Dementia Unrelated to Psychiatric or Renal Disease*

Dementia usually represents an insidious, destructive process primarily involving the cortex (*46*). Deficits in the higher cortical functions are the most prominent manifestations of dementia, and changes in arousal or attention are unusual until the terminal phase. Clinically, one will detect impairment of orientation, memory, and judgment with deterioration of all intellectual functions such as comprehension, calculation, and learning. There is associated lability and shallowness of mood. Patients with ESRD are susceptible to the multiple pathogenic factors that can underlie any chronic brain syndrome. There are five clinical subtypes of organic brain syndromes, each characterized by the most striking presenting feature: amnesia, delusions, hallucinations, mood alterations, and changes in personality. The most frequent cause of dementia is Alzheimer's disease, accounting for more than 50% of cases and for which there is no definitive treatment. However, approximately 15% of patients who meet criteria for dementia have potentially reversible disorders (*46*). It is important not to overlook treatable causes such as anemia, vitamin deficiencies, endocrinopathies, normal pressure hydrocephalus, chronic infections, and primary or secondary brain tumors. Hemodialysis can cause thiamine deficiency, and this can produce damage to the mammillary bodies. Clinically, thiamine deficiency can present as a Wernicke–Korsakoff psychosis characterized by confabulation in an attempt to fill vast memory gaps.

When dementia is suspected, the following studies on initial evaluation will help to identify the patients with treatable causes: complete hematological evaluation, serological test for syphilis, standard metabolic screening tests (for example, sequential multiple analyzer computer), serum thyroxine by column, serum B_{12} and folate levels, computerized cranial tomography, and chest X-ray. Appropriate vitamin supplements should be given, and other indicated treatment initiated.

4. Disturbed Behavior Due to Multiple Causes

DEPRESSION SECONDARY TO DEMENTIA. Some patients developing manifestations of dementia may be aware of the decrease in their cognitive abilities and may subsequently react by becoming severely depressed. The features of depression may dominate the clinical picture, and the underlying dementia may be overlooked. Thus, while depression may present as pseudodementia, dementia and depression may occur together as illustrated by the following case.

The patient, a 50-year-old airline pilot, had been on dialysis for 5 years. He was regarded as the best adjusted patient in the renal clinic. His wife had gradually become aware that his memory was unreliable, so he was admitted for evaluation. The patient was very tearful, cried frequently, and expressed pessimistic concerns about his health. He was very distressed by his inability to recall recent events, and he admitted that he was very forgetful. He was oriented for time, place, and person, but he had some difficulty estimating the passage of time. He thought he had been in the hospital for 1 week when, in fact, he had been there for only 2 days. His attention span was short, and his ability to concentrate was markedly diminished. His performance of recent memory tests was poorer than tests of remote memory. The diagnosis made at that time was one of depression, with probable underlying organic brain damage. Several features of his clinical presentation were more indicative of dementia rather than pseudo-dementia. These include the insidious onset, the absence of previous psychiatric difficulties, poor attention and concentration, and the severe loss of recent memory. Psychological tests confirmed the presence of organic brain damage. The EEG was diagnostic of an encephalopathy, but CT scan was negative. During the ensuing weeks, the patient deteriorated rapidly, developing dysarthria, muscular twitchings, and the unambiguous clinical picture of dialysis dementia.

V. REACTIONS OF STAFF IN A DIALYSIS CENTER

Since the introduction of chronic hemodialysis for patients with ESRD, a large literature has developed on the psychological adjustments of patients undergoing this treatment. Less attention has been given to the stressful influences of this regimen on the nursing staff. Stress may be defined as the cause or trigger of disturbances in the body's equilibrium which result in a characteristic group of symptoms. These symptoms can include increased muscular tension, headaches, irritability, and gastrointestinal discomfort.

A. Factors Contributing to Stress in the Dialysis Nurse

We will consider these factors under the following headings:

1. The unique features of the dialysis treatment program
2. Patient behavior
3. The specialized role of the nurse in a dialysis center
4. Tension resulting from interpersonal staff relationships
5. Off-duty stress

1. The Unique Features of a Dialysis Treatment Program

In a center dialysis program, treatment schedules are rigid, three times a week for each patient, every week, and the nurse is in a vitally responsible position. Because of the frequency and regularity of the treatments, the relationship between the nurse and the patient can become quite intense. Cramond *et al.* (*47*) have stressed that it is a new and heavy burden for members of the team to give emotional support over periods of months or years to patients and their families. This may be a rewarding experience when the patient is doing well, but is more difficult when complications occur or when patients become reproachful and hostile.

During the interval between treatments, patients often express their independence by deviating from their dietary and medical program. Thus, they can seemingly "undo" the beneficial effects painstakingly achieved by the nurse while they are "on the machine." In this way, patients can destroy the expectations the nurses hold for them, thereby provoking frustration and tension.

2. Patient Behavior

We have emphasized that some patients have problems in adjusting to a chronic illness which is both demanding and restricting. Chronic illness engenders a sense of dependency. This dependency is exaggerated for the dialysis patient by virtue of the treatment regimen. An intense conflict arises between the patient's desire for independence and his very real dependency needs. As the struggle to survive becomes more difficult, the patient will become more anxious and will develop defensive maneuvers to assist him in lowering anxiety levels. These may take the form of acting out anger while on the machine, becoming overly demanding, frankly rebellious, or openly flirtatious (*48*). Staff stress increases when patients are considered to be uncooperative, or when the patient's behavior makes the nurse feel unappreciated or worthless.

a. COMMON PATTERNS OF BEHAVIOR OBSERVED. i. The Rebellious Patient. The patient pursues behavior that he has specifically been told to avoid. He ignores dietary restrictions and arrives for dialysis having gained excessive amounts of weight. This provokes feelings of frustration in the nurse who recognizes that the patient is contributing to his own deterioration. When this happens, it is imperative that the patient become more involved in his own care which should decrease his denial of illness. A useful approach is to involve the patient as a part of the treatment team, so that he can take responsibility for monitoring his own weight and blood pressure. In addition, he should be given an opportunity to help other patients, for example, by working for the Kidney Foundation. However, most patients in this category refuse to be helped.

ii. The Passive Demanding Patient. Early on in dialysis, these patients are more passive and generate a favorable reaction in the nursing staff. The nurses feel needed, and initially the patient is very responsive to nursing attention. Gradually, however, the patient's demands increase as he continues to regress, and he is eventually unwilling to do anything for himself. The nurse cannot meet the new demands and begins to feel increasingly tense. The nurse should provide appropriate attention, but at designated times which the patient can come to expect, and to which he can look forward. This is therapeutically more effective than attention given on demand only. Self-care programs can also be beneficial in encouraging responsible behavior.

iii. The Flirtatious Patient. Among the most troublesome and embarrassing patients are those who are flirtatious or seductive. The nurse may feel threatened and uncomfortable by these advances, and will often respond by totally ignoring the patient except to attend to the most essential duties. The patient's passive dependent role on dialysis can threaten his masculinity, and he may have a need to prove his manliness to himself and to others, for example, by masturbating and/or exposing himself. While recognizing that this is a means of relieving tension, it should only be tolerated when carried out in a discreet manner.

The nurse should respond to the above situations by reminding the patient of their professional relationship. She should also set clear limits regarding what is acceptable behavior. Nurses themselves should be aware that some casual remarks may be perceived as encouraging sexual advances by the patient.

b. OTHER FACTORS THAT COMPLICATE THE PATIENT–NURSE RELATIONSHIP

1. Many patients have serious economic and social problems; some are able to continue to work, but the majority cannot. Nurses will be troubled by this, will feel quite helpless, and may become anxious and depressed

themselves. Referring the patient for consultation with a social worker may alleviate the nurse of this burden.

2.   Families of patients, while usually concerned, often do not know how to cope with the situation. They may become overprotective and make inappropriate demands of the nurses, requesting unreasonable favors for their relative. The social worker is adept at working with families, and nurses should be encouraged to use their expertise.

3.   Patients are not spared intercurrent life stresses and are subject to disappointments, losses, separations, and other problems that invariably occur during any person's life. Patients' anxieties are transmitted to those who treat them. Lefebvre *et al.* (*49*) have succinctly described "depressive currents" circulating between patients and staff.

4.   Medical complications occur during the course of chronic hemodialysis. The nurse will be a participant observer in the patient's deterioration, and this can engender extreme feelings of helplessness and hopelessness.

5.   Death and dying are frequent events in a dialysis center. Few patients actually die while they are at the center on the machine, but many die while in the hospital or between dialysis treatments. News of a patient's death is always disturbing to the dialysis nurse.

3.   The Specialized Role of the Nurse in a Dialysis Unit

The dialysis nurse has serious nursing responsibilities. She monitors patients on dialysis and is required to make decisions that can determine very directly the moment-to-moment survival of the patient on the machine. The stress associated with the intensity of these nursing responsibilities is obvious. It is only by experiencing satisfaction and gratification from her work that the nurse can contend with these stresses.

4.   Tension Resulting from Interpersonal Staff Relationships

Interstaff relations between nurse and nurse, nurse and technician, nurse and social worker, nurse and administrator, and nurse and physician cannot always be smooth. Nurses are encouraged to talk through these problems openly with their peers and with other involved parties. While they usually manage this well with most personnel, they often have difficulty working through problems with physicians who are viewed as authority figures not to be challenged.

The nurse who spends many hours with a patient as a trained observer should have the opportunity of conveying her impressions to the attending physician. Frank discussions of a problem with the physician will improve patient care and will consolidate the nurse's value as a member of the treatment team.

5. Off-Duty Stress

Nurses have their own private lives and must contend with inevitable intercurrent problems. The dialysis nurse is not immune from marital problems, stressful family situations, financial strains, and losses. While the personal problems of the nurse may appear relatively insignificant in comparison to those of their patients, this should not preclude nurses from seeking help for themselves.

B. Techniques for Decreasing or Alleviating Staff Stress

Experience with four separate groups of center dialysis nurses has led to an appreciation that certain factors, separately or together, can substantially alleviate staff stress.

1. General Considerations

An attractive physical plant generally has a salutary effect on staff as well as on patient morale. Also important is a flexible work schedule that can meet the needs of an individual nurse. The nurse's education in medical and psychological areas should be ongoing, so that she can develop a clear understanding of her patients' problems. Opportunities to attend conferences away from the clinic will stimulate interest and create situations for nurses to interact with others who are similarly employed. Exercise and relaxation are both effective methods of decreasing anxiety levels and dispersing aggression.

2. The Role of the Psychiatrist

For some years, I have met on a regular basis with four separate groups of center dialysis nurses in the Nashville area (*50*). These meetings usually last from 60 to 90 min, have a flexible structure, and, when indicated, will include social workers, dietitians, technicians, secretarial staff, and occasionally physicians. These group sessions have proved to be an effective vehicle for alleviation of stress, enhancement of morale, and improvement of the self-esteem of the dialysis nurse.

During a session, a member of the team may present a difficult problem with which the nurse is currently contending. The medical, psychologic and social aspects of the patient's problem will be reviewed. The psychiatrist acts as the group leader and encourages participation by all present. Alternatively, the psychiatrist will present a problem for which a consultation had been requested. The group will explore avenues for management of the problem and of improving staff attitudes. A common example is masked depression in a patient either diagnosed as having organic brain damage by some staff members, or seen as "merely an irritable, demanding patient" by others. The diagnosis often emerges when the various staff members who have close contact with the patient come together and review their observations.

A recurring theme is the inability of the nursing personnel to understand the rationale of a physician's approach to a particular patient. During the course of discussion, the staff may come to understand the physician's strategy. Not infrequently, however, there is no consensus, and the group may reach a decision to invite the physician to explain to them his treatment approach.

When the dialysis nurse is confronted by a difficult interaction, usually with a manipulative patient, we have found that role playing in the group is a very effective technique to help the nurse consider various approaches to the patient. Inclinations to reject a manipulative patient by a nurse engenders guilt. A supportive group can help the nurse to recognize this pattern of behavior and can explore its origins. With this new found awareness, a nurse can be encouraged to alter his/her approach to the problem patient.

We have also utilized educational movies which cover subjects such as patients' rights, death and dying, and the decision-making process. These are followed by open discussions. On occasion, we have invited the hospital chaplain to participate. These settings provide an opportunity for the dialysis nurse to express the conflict between professional responsibilities, which result in the prolongation of a patient's life, and the visceral feeling that therapeutic intervention serves to increase the agony for the patient and his family. The interactions through group discussion allow the nurse to comprehend a very wide range of standards compatible with life, some of which, while at variance with a personal credo, are acceptable to others.

Frequently requested topics for group discussion include suicidal behavior, depression, organic brain syndrome, and anxiety reactions. These talks have helped nurses to identify problematic patterns of behavior in their patients. This enhanced understanding increases their tolerance and effectiveness which, in turn, fosters self-confidence and decreases stress.

Group meetings can be very supportive when the staff is feeling despondent. The group is the ideal place to grieve. Instead of each nurse harboring the loss on her own, nurses can legitimately share the pain of death and dying in the group. Grieving is a normal response to loss. Many nurses try to deny the significance of the loss of a patient, thinking that it is not professional. The long association with many patients intensifies the relationship and a bond develops between patient and nurse. Recognition of the depth of the lost relationship must be worked through in the grieving process.

The effectiveness of the group sessions in alleviating staff tension can be attributed to several elements. Self-esteem is increased by the fact that the clinic has arranged for a consultant psychiatrist to meet with the staff on a regular basis. The opinions and observations of the dialysis nurse are actively sought and encouraged and do not go unheeded. The group leader actively directs the group to define problem areas and seek solutions in which the nurse will participate. Other authors (51) have also commented on the usefulness of regular contact between a consultant psychiatrist and the dialysis staff.

Although physician–patient contact is not as intense as that of the nurse–patient relationship, physicians are not immune to the stresses of working with patients on long-term dialysis. The same bonds that develop between nurse and patient are also encountered between doctor and patient. The decline in a patient's mental and physical condition inevitably has an impact on the physician. Physicians seem to cope with this in a constructive way by developing study and research interests that will improve the treatment they can offer their patients. Unfortunately, as their patients become more incapacitated, some physicians tend to withdraw emotionally from them and tend to concentrate on the technologic aspects of treatment.

VI. THE ROLE OF THE PSYCHIATRIST AS A TEAM MEMBER OF A NEPHROLOGY UNIT

A clear understanding of the psychological factors accompanying ESRD and the superimposed neuropsychiatric complications is vital to the physician who is providing primary care to the patient (52). In every case, it is essential that the patient be heard by his physician, i.e., be given the time to discuss his problems. Many patients think their doctor is too busy to hear about sexual problems or social and economic difficulties. Some patients turn to the nurse, who should bring these problems to the attention of the physician. Dietitians may be aware of problems in the family long before the social worker, nurse, or doctor. If there is no coordination, the patient will receive conflicting information from the various disciplines. Hence, a team approach is essential in the integration of any treatment plan.

The most effective psychiatric input occurs when the psychiatrist is accepted by the staff and the patients as an integral member of the nephrology treatment team. Under these circumstances, a psychiatric consultation does not provoke excessive anxiety, and patients accept it as a part of comprehensive treatment. In our program the psychiatrist is introduced to all the patients by participation at the weekly "Kidney Talk" program described earlier. The psychiatrist may be consulted for acute situations and diagnostic problems. Interventions should be crisis oriented and should concentrate on practical solutions to the immediate problem without creating further dependency for the patient. The most common diagnostic problems for which I am consulted are the masked depressions, drug abuse, the unexplained and occasionally unrecognized delirium, and the challenging protean manifestations of the dementias or chronic organic brain syndromes.

As a member of the treatment team and with knowledge of the patient's personality and family constellation, the psychiatrist can be of help in formulating a specific treatment approach for the patient. Since depression, in its many and varied forms, seems to be the most common psychiatric problem in patients with ESRD, the psychiatrist can be of help in determining the etiology and in treatment of this disorder. Whenever the competence and/or the cooperation for home dialysis is in question, the psychiatrist should evaluate the patient and the potential assistant.

A psychiatric evaluation may be medicolegally necessary when a patient requests to discontinue dialysis treatment. The competence of the patient needs to be documented. The patient may want to talk over his decision with a physician other than the nephrologist, preferring not to disappoint the doctor who has saved his life. An opportunity to talk to a psychiatrist who can appreciate his predicament and will also listen to an expression of the painful feelings associated with death and dying is often beneficial to the patient. This may lead to a reevaluation or a confirmation of the decision.

The psychiatrist should be available for all living kidney donors. That is not to say that everyone must see a psychiatrist, but they should know that a psychiatrist is available and that it is considered an acceptable and recommended practice. Every patient considering transplant should, likewise, be offered an opportunity to discuss any concerns regarding this decision with the psychiatrist.

The psychiatrist should be a resource person for the entire team. The consultation model is a useful one for the physician, the social worker, the dietitian, and the nurse; i.e., patients and problem situations are discussed with the psychiatrist who may have suggestions or insights to add, without himself getting involved with the patient directly. The psychiatrist's role as group discussant with the dialysis nurses has been described above.

VIII. SUMMARY

In this chapter we have reviewed psychiatric aspects of chronic renal disease, emphasizing the following features:

1. The dynamic changes in personality consequent upon chronic debilitating disease and the features unique to ESRD and living "on a machine."
2. Psychological factors which influence the modality of therapy with special consideration to kidney transplantation.
3. Diagnostic considerations in the approach to neuropsychiatric problems in ESRD.
4. Reactions of the dialysis nurses.
5. The team approach to the care of patients with ESRD and the role of the psychiatrist in the rehabilitation of patients with ESRD.

ACKNOWLEDGMENTS

I wish to thank Dr. C. E. Wells for his helpful suggestions and Ms. Bettye Ridley and Deborah Petty for their untiring secretarial assistance.

GENERAL REFERENCES

Castelnuovo-Tedesco, P., ed. "Psychiatric Aspects of Organ Transplantation." Grune & Stratton. New York, 1971.
Czaczkes, J. W., and Kaplan De-Nour, A. "Chronic Hemodialysis As a Way of Life." Brunner/ Mazel, New York, 1978.
Levy, N. B. "Living or Dying: Adaptation to Hemodialysis." Thomas, Springfield, Illinois, 1974.
Levy, N. B., ed. "Psychonephrology." Plenum, New York, 1981.
U.S. Department of Health, Education and Welfare. "Living with End-Stage Renal Disease: A Book for Patients," DHEW Publ. No. 76-3001, Stock #017-026-00043-7. U.S. Govt. Printing Office, Washington, D. C., 1973.

REFERENCES

1. Abram, H. S. Psychological responses to illness and hospitalization. *Psychosomatics* **10,** 218–224 (1969).
2. Levy, N. B., and Wynbrandt, G. D. The quality of life on maintenance hemodialysis. *Lancet* **1,** 1328–1330 (1975).
3. Abram, H. S., Moore, G. L., and Westervelt, F. B. Suicidal behavior in chronic dialysis patients. *Am. J. Psychiatry* **127,** 1199–1204 (1971).
4. Haenel, T. H., Brunner, F., and Battegay, R. Renal dialysis and suicide: Occurrence in Switzerland and in Europe. *Compr. Psychiatry*, **21,** 140–145 (1980).
5. Goldstein, A. M., and Reznikoff, M. Suicide in chronic hemodialysis patients from an external locus of control framework. *Am. J. Psychiatry*, **127,** 1204–1207 (1971).
6. Maher, J. G., and Schreiner, G. E. Current status of dialysis of poisons and drugs. *Trans. Am. Soc. Artif. Intern. Organs* **15,** 461–477 (1969).

7.   Abram, H. S. Repetitive dialysis. *In* "Massachusetts General Hospital Handbook of General Hospital Psychiatry" (T. P. Hackett and N. H. Cassem, eds.), pp. 342–364. Mosby, St. Louis, Missouri, 1978.

8.   Haffke, E. A., Somasundaram, R., and Egan, J. Dialysis, depression and antidepressants. *J. Clin. Psychiatry* **39,** 759–760 (1978).

9.   Levy, N. B. Sexual adjustment to maintenance hemodialysis and renal transplantation: National survey by questionnaire: Preliminary report. *Trans. Am. Soc. Artif. Intern. Organs* **19,** 138–143 (1973).

10. Karacan, I., Dervent, A., Cunningham, G., Moore, C. A., Weinman, E. J., Cleveland, S. E., Salis, P. A., Williams, R. L., and Kopel, K. Assessment of nocturnal penile tumescence as an objective method for evaluating sexual functioning in ESRD patients. *Dial. Transplant.* **7,** 872–876 (1978).

11. Procci, W. R., Goldstein, D. A., Adelstein, J., and Massry, S. G. Sexual dysfunction in the male patient with uremia: a reappraisal. *Kidney Int.* **19,** 317–323 (1981).

12. Steele, T. E., Finkelstein, S. H., and Finkelstein, F. O. Hemodialysis patients and spouses. Marital discord, sexual problems and depression. *J. Nerv. Ment. Dis.* **162,** 225–237 (1976).

13. Kaplan De-Nour, A., Shaltiel, J., and Czaczkes, J. W. Emotional reactions of patients on chronic hemodialysis. *Psychosom. Med.* **30,** 521–533 (1968).

14. Shea, E. J., Bogdan, D. F., Freeman, R. B., and Schreiner, G. E. Hemodialysis for chronic renal failure. IV. Psychological considerations. *Ann. Intern. Med.* **62,** 558–563 (1965).

15. Abram, H. S. Survival by machine: The psychological stress of chronic hemodialysis. *Psychiatry Med.* **1,** 37–50 (1970).

16. Reichsman, F., and Levy, N. B. Problems in adaptation to maintenance hemodialysis. *Arch. Intern. Med.* **130,** 859–865 (1972).

17. Abram, H. S. The psychiatrist, the treatment of chronic renal failure and the prolongation of life. II. *Am. J. Psychiatry* **126,** 157–167 (1969).

18. Kemph, J. P. Renal failure, artificial kidney and kidney transplant. *Am. J. Psychiatry* **122,** 1270–1274 (1966).

19. Wright, R. G., Sand, P., and Livingston, G. Psychological stress during hemodialysis for chronic renal failure. *Ann. Intern. Med.* **64,** 611–620 (1966).

20. Anderson, K. The psychological aspects of chronic hemodialysis. *Can. Psychiatr. Assoc. J.* **20,** 385–391 (1975).

21. Rabin, P. L. Misperception of hemodialysis. *Psychosomatics* **23,** 549–553 (1982).

22. Beard, B. H. Fear of death and fear of life. *Arch. Gen. Psychiatry* **21,** 373–380 (1969).

23. Menzies, I. C., and Stewart, W. K. Psychiatric observations on patients receiving regular dialysis treatment. *Br. Med. J.* **1,** 544–547 (1968).

24. Eady, R. A. J. Why I have not had a kidney transplant after nine and one half years as a hemodialysis patient. *Transplant. Proc.* **5,** 1115–1117 (1973).

25. Coene, R. E. Dialysis or transplant: One patient's choice. *Hastings Cent. Rep.* **8,** 5–7 (1978).

26. Basch, S. H. Emotional dehiscence after successful renal transplantation. *Kidney Int.* **17,** 388–396 (1980).

27. Gross, J. B., Keane, W. F., and McDonald, A. K. Survival and rehabilitation of patients on home hemodialysis. Five years experience. *Ann. Intern. Med.* **78,** 341–346 (1973).

28. Streltzer, J., Finkelstein, F., Feigenbaum, H., Kitsen, J., and Cohn, G. L. The spouse's role in home hemodialysis. *Arch. Gen. Psychiatry* **33,** 55–58 (1976).

29. Shambaugh, P. W., Hampers, C. L., Bailey, G. L., Snyder, D., and Merrill, J. P. Hemodialysis in the home—emotional impact on the spouse. *Trans. Am. Soc. Artif. Intern. Organs.* **13,** 41–45 (1967).

30. Abram, H. S., and Buchanan, D. C. The gift of life: A review of the psychological aspects of kidney transplantation. *Int. J. Psychiatry Med.* **7**, 153–164 (1976–1977).
31. Basch, S. H. The intrapsychic integration of a new organ. A clinical study of kidney transplantation. *Psychoanal. Q.* **42**, 364–384 (1973).
32. Burns, S., and Johnson, H. K. Rehabilitation potential of a dialysis versus a transplant population. *Dial. Transplant.* **5**, 54–56 (1976).
33. Kemph, J. P. Psychotherapy with patients receiving kidney transplant. *Am. J. Psychiatry* **124**, 623–629 (1967).
34. Wells, C. E., and Duncan, G. W. "Neurology for Psychiatrists," pp. 45–64. Davis, Philadelphia, Pennsylvania, 1980.
35. Ling, M. H. M., Perry, P. J., and Tsuang, M. T. Side effects of corticosteroid therapy. Psychiatric aspects. *Arch. Gen. Psychiatry* **38**, 471–477 (1981).
36. Blazer, D. G., Petrie, W. M., and Wilson, W. P. Affective psychoses following renal transplant. *Dis. Nerv. Syst.* **37**, 663–669 (1976).
37. Abram, H. S. Psychological aspects of the intensive care unit. *Hosp. Med.* **5**, 94–95 (1969).
38. Wells, C. E. Pseudodementia. *Am. J. Psychiatry* **136**, 895–900 (1979).
39. Poisson, M., Mashaly, R., and Lafforgue, B. Progressive dialysis encephalopathy. *Ann. Neurol.* **6**, 88 (1979).
40. Chokroverty, S., Bruetman, M. E., Berger, V., and Reyes, M. G. Progressive dialysis encephalopathy. *J. Neurol. Neurosurg. Psych.* **39**, 411–419 (1976).
41. Barratt, L. J., and Lawrence, J. R. Dialysis-associated dementia. *Aust. N. Z. J. Med.* **5**, 62–65 (1975).
42. Scheiber, S. C., and Ziesat, H. Dementia dialytica: a new psychotic organic brain syndrome. *Compr. Psych.* **17**, 781–785 (1976).
43. Burks, J. S., Alfrey, A. C., Huddlestone, J., Norenberg, M. D., and Lewin, E. A fatal encephalopathy in chronic hemodialysis patients. *Lancet* **1**(7963), 764–768 (1976).
44. Nadel, A. M., and Wilson W. P. Dialysis encephalopathy: a possible seizure disorder. *Neurology* **26**, 1130–1134 (1976).
45. Jack, R. A., Rabin, P. L., and Rivers-Bulkeley, N. T. Secondary mania as a presentation of progressive dialysis encephalopathy. *J. Nerv. Ment. Dis.* (in press).
46. Wells, C. E. Diagnosis of dementia. *Psychosomatics* **20**, 517–522 (1979).
47. Cramond, W. A., Knight, P. R., and Lawrence, J. R. The psychiatric contribution to a renal unit undertaking chronic hemodialysis and renal homotransplantation. *Br. J. Psychiatry* **113**, 1201–1212 (1967).
48. Abram, H. S. "The Nurse and the Chronic Dialysis Patient," A dialysis Symposium for Nurses, pp. 3–5. U.S. Dept. of Health, Education and Welfare, Washington, D.C., 1968.
49. Lefebvre, P., Nobert, A., and Crombez, J. C. Psychological and psychopathological reactions in relation to chronic hemodialysis. *Can. Psychiatr. Assoc. J.* **17**, SS9–SS13 (1972).
50. Rabin, P. L. Stress and the dialysis nurse. *Dial. Transplant.* **11**, 536–554 (1982).
51. Kaye, R., Leigh, H., and Strauch, B. The role of the liaison psychiatrist in a hemodialysis program: A case study. *Psychiatry Med.* **4**, 313–321 (1973).
52. Abram, H. S. Psychiatric reflections on adaptation to repetitive dialysis. *Kidney Int.* **6**, 67–72 (1974).

6

Social Work
with Renal Failure Patients:
Roles of the Social Worker

ELINOR MOORES

I. INTRODUCTION

Social work with renal failure patients begins with a thorough assessment of the patient in his total environment. In any medical setting it is especially important to come to an understanding of aspects of the patient's social situation that affect his medical condition and are, therefore, relevant to clinical medical practice (1).

The information gathered by the social worker encompasses all aspects pertinent to social functioning; personal, interpersonal and practical. These

149

components of social functioning were found by Doremus (*1*) to combine four factors that provide a comprehensive understanding of the patient and his difficulties: an assessment of the patient's social *roles*, his emotional *reactions*, his interpersonal *relationships*, and his practical *resources*. The assessment of these factors which Doremus calls "the four R's of medical-social diagnosis" provides the basis for devising effective social work intervention.

II. ROLES OF THE SOCIAL WORKER

In essence, the relationship between social worker and patient is an explicit or implied contractual one in which the worker's efforts are designed to help the patient in the achievement of certain jointly established goals. In the broadest general terms, the goal with renal failure patients is to help the patient and/or his family or a patient group in making the best possible adjustment to the altered life imposed by this medical condition. Intermediate objectives toward achievement of that broad goal may cover the spectrum of intra- or interpersonal or purely practical issues generated by the illness, with the specific problem being addressed at any given time determining the role the social worker will assume in this joint undertaking with the patient.

Although the social worker is by no means limited to these, probably the five most commonly assumed direct service roles are those of *enabler*, *teacher*, *mediator*, *advocate*, and *social broker*. In addition, the social worker's role may extend beyond the direct worker/patient relationship to a more indirect service role in the community to develop and promote additional resources, or to lobby for more favorable legislation on behalf of an entire population of patients.

A. The Social Worker as Enabler

When acting as an enabler, the social worker's intervention is chiefly supportive in nature, geared toward assisting patients to develop coping strengths and inner resources to produce desired changes in themselves, their interpersonal relationships, and their environment.

Many of the emotional reactions and disturbances of interpersonal relationships that renal failure patients experience stem from the inevitable distortions of their usual social roles imposed by their disease. There is a profound relationship between social roles and human identity: the concept of person is inseparable from that of role (2). Thus, loss of even a single, highly valued role central to the self-image can be a devastating event in human experience.

Sustained ambiguity is not easily tolerated by anyone. Yet role ambiguity becomes an inescapable fact of life for patients undergoing chronic maintenance dialysis. Society has made allowance for the fact that from time to time people become ill and are rendered incapable of meeting their usual responsibilities. No censure attaches to the patient's need to be cared for by others, his regression, his ill temper, or display of behaviors that would not otherwise be tolerated, *provided* that he tacitly acknowledges the temporariness of the privileges accorded him and does all in his power to get well as soon as possible.

In contrast, life-extending technological advances have created a departure from the classic "role of the sick" for the renal failure patient. Except for periods when the patient becomes acutely ill and requires hospitalization, he may appear and feel relatively well, but he is never free from the demanding medical regimen or the limitations on his functioning imposed by his disease. Basic human drives such as for food and water must be closely monitored. Energy is diminished, so that he may have the capacity for moderate recreational activities but lack the strength and endurance to work regularly. Sexual functioning is generally impaired. In short, his inability to conform to societal norms held for the well person sets him apart in a new kind of deviance in the eyes of his contemporaries.

While emphasizing that no facet of the renal failure patient's life escapes the impact of persistent role ambiguity, many patients experience the most distress in relation to family and employment.

It is obvious that the serious illness of a family member will require a reallocation of duties and responsibilities. Performance expectations and emotional responsiveness are quite different for sick compared to well family members. A mother, for example, who is not acutely sick but never truly well strains the adaptive capacity of the best integrated family. With the onset of illness, many patients' families are willing to promise to do *anything* if only the patient's life can be saved, and they are quite sincere in their intention. The initial joy and relief at what seems truly a return from the dead diminish for a while the burden of the radical adjustments they are called on to make. Sooner or later, however, the distortion of family roles, reallocation of responsibilities, sacrifices of personal dreams and ambitions, recurring crises, and the uncertainty of what to expect from day to day take their toll. And sooner or later, it may occur to some of the family members that the way out of the dilemma is for the patient to die. Although these thoughts may never be openly expressed, the mere knowledge that they were entertained, however briefly, can create a crushing guilt to add to other existing strains on family relationships.

Case 1: Miss N., a 28-year-old blind diabetic woman, entered the hospital to begin chronic peritoneal dialysis. While she was there, her mother suffered a stroke and died. This double tragedy made it necessary for Miss N's younger brother to drop out of college to help maintain the home, while her father continued to try to keep the family farm productive. Both the father and the brother assumed many tasks formerly performed by the mother in addition to carrying out the lengthy dialysis routine. After a long and complicated course of illness punctuated by many hospitalizations, Miss N. died. Her weeping brother acknowledged that he was unable to know if his tears were prompted by grief at the loss of his sister or by joy "at getting my life back."

The importance of employment, not only as a means of providing the necessities of daily living, but also as a component of social status, self-image, and self-esteem cannot be overestimated. In an achievement-oriented society such as ours, occupation offers the principal opportunity for persons to achieve a rise in rank. Inevitably, the high or low status of the job becomes the status of the person in the job.

Aside from status, it is the norm for people to perform work. Only the independently wealthy and those who are incapacitated in some way are exempted. While most people must work to provide for the necessities of life, work for its own sake is highly valued. Even those who do not "need" to work are held in higher regard if they make some contribution of useful service.

Society may provide for persons who are legitimately unable to provide for themselves, but such consideration is not without cost to the self-esteem. Recipients of the public dole are expected to be aware of their humble estate; to refrain from any but the most frugal living; to be grateful for the favors bestowed on them; and, hopefully, to resume gainful employment at the earliest possible moment. Internalized values and societal expectations can exert enormous pressures even on persons legitimately disabled as the result of accident or illness. Almost everyone has known of some severely disabled person who overcame immense obstacles to regain independence, then went on to overachieve in the effort to compensate for the severe damage sustained by his sense of personal worth. Society applauds and rewards such efforts. The more severely disabled the person, the more approval he wins for his extraordinary achievement, although few would be willing to change places with him.

End-stage renal disease (ESRD) patients are acutely aware of both silent and spoken pressures on them to become rehabilitated in the specific sense of returning to gainful employment. There is also a growing awareness that the failure of sufficient numbers of them to do so may ultimately jeopardize the enormously expensive governmental programs that fund their life-extending treatments. Ironically, based on promising evidence of rehabilitative potential among early, handpicked patient populations, maintenance dialysis was made generally available. This general availability of maintenance dialysis has produced patient populations who are older, more debilitated, possibly less motivated, and who, consequently, have less rehabilitative potential. Despite this contradiction, occupational rehabilitation remains the primary criterion on which the success of the patient and the program is judged.

An extremely important factor, as far as maintenance dialysis patients are concerned, is that they often do not appear obviously disabled to the casual observer. Many such patients who have been unable to find employment report that "people" regard them as malingerers, especially if they engage in recreational activities as they are encouraged to do by their physicians. This is both a projection of the patient's own discomfort with his uncertain state and a true perception of fact. As a member of society, the patient shares societal values, which condemn his exempted state without visible justification.

Whether or not a dialysis patient can rejoin the work force is much more than the simple matter of sufficient physical restoration to permit him to work. For in-center patients, the dialysis schedule alone can present an insurmountable obstacle in some cases. Other patients find employers unwilling to hire them because of doubts about the amount or regularity of work they can perform, or because hiring a chronically ill person can adversely affect insurance rates. Still others lack the stamina to resume their former physically demanding jobs, and lack the skills that would enable them to qualify for more sedentary work. Another group of patients may find themselves forced to choose between the witch and the devil: whether to continue to exist on Social Security Disability benefits (a sure thing), as opposed to reentering gainful employment (a not-so-sure thing). Moreover, such employment often produces less income than the disability benefits because of the limited amount of time available for the patient to work.

When a provider is no longer able to contribute his usual share to family income, or when a patient dependent on a provider perceives himself as causing a disproportionate drain on family resources, self-esteem can be seriously eroded. Other members of the family, struggling to cope with a reduced standard of living, may have little capacity or inclination to offer reassurance; in fact, they may feel an irrational resentment toward the patient for causing their deprivation.

Many of the social ramifications which can be produced by embarking on a course of chronic maintenance dialysis are clearly illustrated in the following case:

Case 2: Mr. B., a 46-year-old married man, was a construction worker prior to becoming ill and beginning a course of maintenance dialysis. Mrs. B. took pride in her ability as a homemaker and had never aspired to any other career. Following his initial adjustment to the dialysis regimen, Mr. B. usually felt quite well, but was unable to resume his physically demanding job. Financial pressures forced Mrs. B. to seek employment for the first time in her life. Fortunately, she developed an aptitude for selling real estate and was soon producing an adequate income. However, she never ceased to resent having to make such a drastic change in her life-style and complained bitterly about how unhappy the change had made her. Mr. B. blamed himself for his wife's unhappiness and felt obliged to make things up to her by becoming as meticulous a housekeeper as she had been despite the fact that he was already diminished in his own eyes by the loss of his preferred masculine pursuits. No matter how he cooked and cleaned, ironed the curtains, and mopped the floors, the housework he performed never came up to Mrs. B's standards. She would frequently stay up late at night redoing some task "properly." To make matters worse, Mr. B. had accepted the dialysis treatments against the teachings of his religion, and the thrice weekly sessions on the kidney machine were a constant reminder of his "lack of faith." He was, in his own eyes and his wife's, a failure as a husband, as a "wife," and as a church member.

Whenever the strains imposed by the "not sick" dimension of his role became too much for this chronically depressed man, he would bake a chocolate cake and eat most of it. An overdose of chocolate invariably won him admission to the hospital where he was safely congruent with societal expectations for a sick person. Once there, his depressed affect promptly diminished. He gained a respite from an intolerable home situation in this manner. This was so important to him that it was extremely difficult for Mr. B. to "remember" the potentially deadly consequences of consuming high potassium foods, such as chocolate.

Fortunately, many families avoid the extremes of maladaptive behavior exemplified by this couple. Nevertheless, the B's situation is not an uncommon one; the effects of serious family and occupational role disturbances and the accompanying emotional responses differ only in degree.

The task of the enabling social worker in such situations is to assist the patient and his family in identifying and strengthening inner resources, in developing more effective coping mechanisms, and in making practical changes in their environment to make life more tolerable. Intervention in the case of the B's would undoubtedly have been more effective had it been possible to involve Mrs. B. However, she remained inaccessible, partly because of the demands of her job, and partly because of her religious beliefs, which were opposed to medical intervention of any kind. The worker's efforts, therefore, concentrated on Mr. B., helping him to rebuild his severely damaged sense of personal worth, encouraging him to resume contact with his male friends and share recreational activities with them as he had once done; and especially, helping him to find alternatives to hospitalization when things became too much for him to bear at home.

B. The Social Worker as Teacher

This is an educative role in which the social worker provides the patient with new information necessary for dealing with the problem situation.

The majority of patients and their families, faced with the onset of maintenance dialysis, know little beyond the fact that a thing called a kidney machine exists. Most of what they do know has been gained from television and popular publications, and much of it is based on misconception. Even those who know (or know of) someone receiving this treatment are little better off as far as realizing what to expect. The phrase in common parlance "going *on* the kidney machine," for example, frequently causes patients to envision a frightening thing that must be mounted. Many have only rudimentary knowledge of the operation of their own bodies, much less the sophisticated apparatus encountered in a medical setting. Thus, the new renal patient and his family can be likened to a modern day Rip van Winkle awakening in a changed world with familiar landmarks swept away. The patient's body no longer works as it once did. He barely speaks the language. Financial security may be replaced with the prospect of financial ruin. The present is uncertain and the future incomprehensible.

In the midst of all this, with anxiety at a peak, the patient and his family are called on to master a bewildering array of new information. High anxiety levels and the effects of uremia on mental functioning impede the patient's ability to comprehend. Effective teaching in such a climate demands a high degree of skill and patience from the social work and nursing staff.

The social worker's educational role begins with the first contact with the patient and is usually a part of every contact thereafter. Teaching may be a discrete function through which the social worker acquaints patient and family with facts relevant to their new situation, and helps them anticipate stresses brought about by the patient's illness and formulate plans for dealing with these problems. Teaching is also an aspect of all other roles the social worker may assume. While acting on behalf of the patient in various capacities as the need arises, the social worker's ultimate objective is to equip the patient through instruction, encouragement, and effective role modeling to resume responsibility for himself to the extent that he is able.

The social worker strives to put patients and their families at ease and to create an atmosphere in which the lack of understanding of medical matters can be revealed without embarrassment. This presents an excellent opportunity for the worker to reinforce and perhaps clarify information previously given by other team members, as well as providing a gauge of how much understanding the patient has achieved. The worker must, of course, exercise discretion in deciding which questions he can address and which must be referred back to other team members.

By making other professionals aware of gaps in the patient's comprehension, and by sharing with them an understanding of elements in the patient's social situation which will serve to promote or impede his compliance with the medical regime, the social worker complements the efforts of other team members in devising a plan of effective medical management.

C.   The Social Worker as Mediator

This is an essentially neutral role in which the social worker acts as liaison between the patient and other elements of his environment to improve communication, promote better understanding and cooperation, and to work toward conflict resolution. Here the relationship between the patient and the medical community comes under scrutiny.

The need to consult a physician constitutes an acknowledgement of the patient's helplessness to improve his own situation. The awareness of helplessness is extremely uncomfortable for some people to tolerate. While the patient must, sooner or later, call on the special knowledge and skill of a doctor if he is to get better, his need to turn to someone else for help may (logically or not) make him feel diminished in his own eyes. Further, most patients have no means of judging for themselves the qualifications of doctors. They must take it on faith that the doctor is well trained in his field and that he is a conscientious and ethical person to whom they can safely entrust their lives. For some, such trust does not come easily.

At least in the beginning, the doctor is a stranger to the patient. But if the doctor is to be able to help him, the patient must cooperate by revealing the most intimate information about his behavior and his body, information often so secret in nature that it may not have been shared with anyone else. The patient is, literally and figuratively, revealed naked before the doctor and is thus rendered very vulnerable. These special properties of the relationship between doctor and patient require that the interaction between them be strictly limited to the area of concern; i.e., the physical well-being of the patient.

Differences in perspective can create problems. Physicians may know that factors in the private life of the patient have tremendous influence on his willingness or ability to follow medical instructions and stay well. However, doctors sometimes do not probe into delicate areas of the patient's life because of a personal reluctance to intrude, or on the assumption that if problems exist the patient will reveal them. Patients, on the other hand, may not appreciate the relevance of personal matters to the medical situation, or they may simply regard their private affairs as none of the doctor's business.

It must be stressed that it is not so much the physician's personal characteristics as the patient's perception of the physician *in his professional role* which constrains communication. However much the doctor may strive to present himself to patients as being kind, interested, and approachable may prove to be beside the point. The patient, although he may be gratefully aware of his doctor's benevolent attitude, may nevertheless be subject to his own vulnerability at the hands of the doctor. As he sees it, it behooves him to cultivate the good will of the doctor toward him; he cannot risk losing that benevolent regard by "pestering" the doctor with questions, or by burdening him with matters that the patient sees as his own personal problems.

Consciously or unconsciously, doctors convey the idea to patients that they are very busy and pressed for time. Consequently, patients may conclude that the doctor will be annoyed if demands on his time are excessive. In addition, communication may be further inhibited by the patient's fear that he will be revealed as ignorant if he asks questions. It is not uncommon for a patient to accept the doctor's explanation of his condition with a knowing nod when, in truth, he does not understand at all; or to preface the few questions he does ask with a shamefaced, "I hope you won't think I'm stupid, but. . . ."

The educational background and frame of reference of doctor and patient may be so different that even very careful explanations do not bridge the gap. The doctor's familiarity with complex medical knowledge can make it difficult for him to recall how little he once knew about the operation of the human body, and it can cause him to assume more knowledge of basic physical facts on the part of the patient than the patient actually possesses.

Paradoxically, as time goes by the opposite of this situation may evolve. Renal failure patients are encouraged to take an active part in the management of their illness. They are taught to understand the significance of their laboratory values and the effects of medication and diet on their bodies. They are made responsible for managing their medicines and sometimes for adjusting the dosage as needed. They are expected to resist having blood samples taken from the shunt arm, and they often administer their own dialysis treatments at home. In short, it is not unusual for renal patients to become to some extent experts on kidney disease. While the development of expertise and active participation are strongly promoted within the renal failure community, these traits are not always welcomed by medical professionals in other settings who are more accustomed to the classic passive stance of "the good patient."

It is generally recognized that physicians, nurses, and technicians involved in the direct physical care of patients must, for their own and the patients' protection, stand outside the reciprocities of ordinary social intercourse in their dealings with patients. The differences between these functionally specific complementary roles and familial or friendly relationships constitute important levers that permit their necessary transactions to take place.

Nevertheless, society continues to pay homage to the belief, one might say the mythology, that a magical thing called "the doctor–patient relationship" exists which somehow automatically creates communication and instant understanding. While some physicians may possess the ability to establish such rapport with relative ease, others do not. In this day of rapid technological advances, doctors are trained to be expert in their areas of specialization, and demands on them for their special knowledge are enormous. They may not have the training, the inclination, or the time to devote to building the type of relationships that promote understanding their patients as human beings. Thus, there is a need for an ally, someone who can bridge the gap between the doctor with his knowledge of treatments and diseases on the one hand, and the patient, the person with the disease, with all its social, emotional, and environmental ramifications on the other.

The social worker has the training and the inclination, and takes the time to understand the patient as a person, along with the practical and interpersonal aspects of his particular situation. He understands the ramifications of the medical condition while remaining outside any direct involvement with the patient's physical care, or the responsibility for making life or death decisions. By virtue of these factors, the social worker is in a unique position to act as intermediary between patient and medical community in the gathering, assessment, and exchange of information.

D.   The Social Worker as Advocate

In acting as an advocate for the patient the social worker assumes a partisan stance in which he may argue, bargain, debate, negotiate, and manipulate the environment on behalf of the patient.

Effective advocacy requires that the social worker have a working knowledge of the persons, systems, institutions, or agencies with which he must deal, and the skill and sensitivity to employ the techniques most likely to achieve the ends he hopes to attain for his patient. He selects from the information available to him the data most likely to influence a favorable decision for the patient, according to the orientation of the person who will make the decision. The social worker may choose to assume the advocacy role on behalf of an inexperienced or incapacitated patient, or he may use it as a role model and teaching tool to prepare the patient to act on his own behalf at a later time.

Acting as advocate for a hospitalized patient whose income had ceased when his illness began, a social worker contacted the patient's creditors and arranged for postponement of payments until alternate income could be established. Another case involved the research and presentation of information (couched in terms of advantage to the granting agency) that was successful in securing an exception to state policy to obtain a needed service for a patient. On another occasion information presented by a social worker resulted in a change of state policy to the benefit of a number of patients as well as considerable savings to the state. Social workers may negotiate with agencies to secure housing or other services, with the courts to arrange for the release of jailed dialysis patients, and with charitable organizations to obtain relief for patients in financial emergencies.

E.   The Social Worker as Social Broker

The social worker as social broker is the resource person who understands the intricacies and limitations of available community resources that can be brought to bear on the patient's problems, and provides the linkage between the patient and community sources of help.

An understanding of the stunning impact of ESRD on social *roles*, interpersonal *relationships*, and emotional *reactions* is incomplete without consideration being given to the fourth "R," the practical *resources*. The matter of resources is not an independent factor, but one that is closely interwoven with the other three. The management of funds can damage or cement relationships, and often evokes very intense emotional reactions. The giving or receiving of money or goods is a traditional aspect of certain social roles and, as such, has great symbolic importance to the self-concept.

Whether as the result of decreased income or increased expense, or both, the renal failure patient and his family almost invariably experience some financial hardship. Not everyone has access to a source of alternate income, so that when the patient has been the breadwinner, income can abruptly cease. Disability benefits or retirement income, when these are available, seldom equal the earned income they replace. There is almost always an extended period, usually of months, between establishing eligibility for such benefits and actual receipt of funds. In the meantime, while medical expenses mount alarmingly, savings are depleted, obligations may go unmet, and creditors press for payment.

Some families are forced to seek welfare payments to tide them over, and others end up drawing welfare on a permanent basis. Many persons, who have taken pride in being independent and meeting their responsibilities, experience the need to accept public assistance as a crushing humiliation.

Loss of income is only one side of the coin; the enormous cost of maintenance dialysis and kidney transplantation is the other. The cost of in-center dialysis for one patient for a year, approximately $25,000, exceeds total predialysis income for the vast majority of patients.

A cataloging of resources available to renal failure patients and their hard-pressed families must necessarily remain very general in content. The availability of resources varies extensively from state to state and frequently from one locality to another within the same state. Even resources provided by the federal government such as Medicare and Veterans Administration hospitals, which are generally presumed to be uniform throughout the country, are subject to strict or liberal interpretation of the regulations governing them, and hence will show some variation. In short, it matters a great deal where the renal failure patient happens to live. It is the responsibility of the social worker as social broker in each location to become thoroughly familiar with all the resources available to patients in his local area, and to know at least how to go about exploring the possibilities in other localities for transient patients who come within his purview.

If the direct and indirect costs of being on a program of maintenance dialysis are to be met, it is usually necessary to look to a variety of resources for assistance.

1. Medicare

Beginning in 1972 with the passage of Public Law 92-603, the Medicare End-Stage Renal Disease (ESRD) Program was established as the main funding source for the provision of maintenance dialysis. Eligibility for help through Medicare depends on being permanently or currently insured by virtue of one's contributions to the Social Security system, or on being the spouse or dependent child of someone so insured. This is a more liberal policy than is applied to other disabled persons, who must qualify on the basis of their own contributions and are subject to a 2 year waiting period for benefits to begin. Not everyone is eligible for ESRD Medicare benefits, even under these liberal provisions. A self-employed person may never have made Social Security contributions. A child who has once gained independence from his parents, even for so brief a period that he cannot qualify on his own, can never again be presumed to be dependent on his parents, regardless of how disabled he becomes. (This was true, for example, in the case of Miss N., cited previously, who became blind after having been self-supporting for only a few months.)

In general, Medicare pays the first 80% of out-patient treatment costs for eligible recipients, as well as all covered in-patient costs after a deductible amount is met in each benefit period. At present, there is a waiting period of 3 months from the date of the first dialysis for benefits to begin, although this waiting period is waived for those patients who begin training for home dialysis or who receive a kidney transplant within that period. Medicare offers no help with the cost of necessary medicines other than those administered to hospitalized patients.

For those patients receiving in-center dialysis who do not qualify for waiver of the waiting period, treatment costs *not* covered by Medicare can easily exceed $11,000 in the first year, with an additional $5000–$6000 annually thereafter.

With the growth in the number of ESRD Medicare beneficiaries from 11,000 in 1973 to 50,000 at present, and with 90,000 projected by 1995, shrinking governmental resources for health care have demanded reappraisal of the cost burden of this program. As this is being written, both houses of Congress are considering separate proposals for budgetary reductions in the ESRD provisions of Medicare. While the final form of the new Senate and House Budget proposals remains to be seen, it is certain that the effects will be far-reaching.

2. Private Insurance

Provisions of health care insurance plans differ from company to company and from policy to policy. Most plans place a total dollar limit on coverage which, even when they appear to be quite liberal, can be exhausted. Some group coverage provided by employers terminates when the patient's employment ends; other policies can be continued in force if the patient assumes the payment of premiums. With income severely reduced, patients can be faced with a choice between paying premiums and providing for the necessities of daily living. In such cases, insurance coverage usually goes by the board.

3. Medicaid

Medicaid programs are, at present, administered by the individual states, and funded jointly by state and federal appropriations. These programs vary widely in their eligibility requirements, as well as in the amount and kinds of assistance provided to dialysis patients. For certain eligible recipients, Medicaid offers limited help with the cost of some of the necessary medicines, i.e., those listed in the various state Medicaid formularies. In general, Medicaid assistance as it now stands is based on low income and is linked with the receipt of welfare or Supplementary Security Income (SSI).

It has been proposed that, beginning in October 1982, responsibility for Medicaid be assumed by the federal government. All that can be said of that proposal with any certainty is that such a change would be a major move toward uniformity of eligibility requirements and benefits countrywide. Whether such uniformity, once achieved, would improve or worsen the resource picture for renal failure patients is open to conjecture.

4. State Renal Programs

Thirty-five of the 50 states maintain additional programs offering financial assistance with the cost of dialysis. Generally speaking, these are last resort resources for patients with inadequate funding from other providers. Eligibility requirements vary considerably, as do the services covered. Total annual funding for these programs in 1979–1980 ranged from a low of $20,000 in one state to a high of $12.7 million in another (3).

5. Veterans Administration

The Veterans Administration provides maintenance dialysis and transplantation services at no cost to eligible veterans, i.e., those whose kidney failure arises from a condition originating in or made worse by service in the armed forces, or others with a service-connected disability that has been rated as 50% or more disabling. Non-service-connected veterans may also be served on a space available basis. The Veterans Administration does not coinsure with any other provider.

6. Other Needs, Other Resources

The life situation of maintenance dialysis patients generates a profusion of collateral needs. The cost of special diets, medicines, and transportation are significant treatment-related items. Reduced income produces crises involving housing, utilities, and other day-to-day costs that run the gamut of human experience.

There is little uniformity of resources across the country to offer help with these persistent problems. Medicare and private insurance do not address the issue of the cost of transportation to and from dialysis clinics, although Medicaid does offer help in some states. Medicaid, private insurance, and state renal programs usually provide partial assistance with the expense of medicines for eligible beneficiaries, but vary widely in the specific items covered. Some necessary preparations, however, are considered to be "over-the-counter" drug items (vitamins, laxatives, acetaminophen, and, in some localities, phosphate binders, for example) and are thus excluded from reimbursement under any plan. Some few state programs offer help with transportation, but most do not. None of these agencies provides for assistance with renal-failure-related emergencies of daily living.

The American Kidney Fund has been able to provide limited transportation grants where hardship can be demonstrated, and to assist with other emergency needs of kidney patients. However, the ability of this organization to help depends on funds available at a given time in relation to the number of applicants requesting aid, i.e., very heavy demands may result in reduction of grants.

In general, the National Kidney Foundation channels its funds toward promoting research, the education of medical professionals, and the early detection and prevention of kidney disease through public education. Some local chapters have established modest emergency funds for direct aid to kidney patients; in a very few localities, chapters have addressed the problem of transportation by lobbying successfully for state funds to aid dialysis patients with these costs.

By and large, the needs of this growing population of patients far exceed the capacities of existing resources to deal with them. Budgetary curtailments at all governmental levels offer little prospect of improvement in the future.

III. CONCLUDING STATEMENT

We live in a time of immense social change. Traditional values are undergoing searching scrutiny; accepted social roles, notably ascribed roles arising from sex, age, race, and physical condition, are in the process of reappraisal; new roles are emerging. What the result will be cannot be predicted. It is cold comfort to those who find themselves adrift between two worlds, never fully able to identify with or take their bearings from either, that they may be the pioneers of some possibly better future social order. At present, they are primarily aware of the pain and isolation of their marginal state. It is clear that chronic renal failure patients struggling to adapt to the confusion and conflict of being cast in the "sick/not sick" role belong to this category. Unfortunately, recognition of the life paradox of such persons is only a small and frustrating step. Neither health care professionals nor patients themselves can, by individual effort, hasten the tedious process of assimilating a new role, produced by technology, into the social order. Like explorers on a strange social continent, we are still mapping behavioral topography, emotional currents, and role boundaries. In an address at the Southern Illinois University School of Medicine in 1974, Joe C. Eades, Ph.D., pointed out that what is required is resocialization, "a very difficult task which involves profound changes in the individual's perception of self and in his activities and values." In addition, it must be emphasized that the process is not confined to patients alone: the social framework must become restructured to accommodate the new role and its reciprocals. The task for patients of becoming acquainted with a changed self and reorienting that self in an altered world is a complex one that must be shared by health care professionals, family, and the community as a whole.

GENERAL REFERENCES

Bracht, N. F. "Social Work in Health Care: A Guide to Professional Practice." Haworth Press, New York, 1978.
Strauss, A. L. "Chronic Illness and the Quality of Life." Mosby, St. Louis, Missouri, 1975.
"Perspectives: The Journal of the Council of Nephrology Social Workers," Vol. 1, No. 1. National Kidney Foundation, New York, 1977ff.

REFERENCES

1. Doremus, B. L. The four r's: Social diagnosis in health care. *Health Soc. Work* **1**, 120–139 (1976).
2. Nisbet, R. A. "The Social Bond." Alfred A. Knopf, New York, 1970.
3. "State Renal Programs." National Association of Patients on Hemodialysis and Transplantation, Great Neck, New York, 1980.

The Problem of Vascular Access
in the Management
of End-Stage Renal Disease:
The Various Possibilities
of Producing a Shunt

ROBERT E. RICHIE

I. ACCESS FOR HEMODIALYSIS

A. Historical Perspective

In 1944 Kolff reported the use of hemodialysis to treat renal failure (*1*). From the beginning it became apparent that maintaining access to the vascular system was difficult and would be the limiting factor for hemodialysis.

165

END-STAGE RENAL DISEASE

In some of these early reports, the inferior vena cava was utilized and the blood was returned via a peripheral vein (2). Others preferred to cannulate an artery directly, and with this technique the blood vessel could be used several times because each time the vessel was used it could be cannulated at a higher level (3). Teschan et al. (4) reported the use of plastic cannulae in 1960. At that time, blood vessels were preserved for repeated use by filling the cannulae with heparinized saline between dialyses. With this method, the length of time each vessel could be used was less than 2 weeks. Long-term hemodialysis became a reality in 1960 when Scribner reported the creation of an external arteriovenous shunt using Teflon cannulae and Silastic tubing to connect the arterial and venous circulation (5). In the original Scribner shunt, the tubing was curved so that the shunt could be placed as close to the wrist as possible. This permitted preservation of the length of the vessels so that should revision become necessary, it could be accomplished easily. On the other hand, this curve made it more difficult to remove a clot using the Fogarty embolectomy catheter. Subsequently, several modifications of the external shunt have been reported. In 1966, Ramirez et al. (6) introduced a shunt comprised of straight tubing with wings to permit fixation. This modification allowed removal of thrombi with an embolectomy catheter. Brescia and Cimino introduced the forearm arteriovenous fistula in 1966 (7). They performed a side-to-side anastomosis between the distal radial artery and the cephalic vein at the wrist. This led to an increased blood flow in the cephalic vein, which, because of its superficial location, could be easily cannulated with large bore needles and connected to the dialyzer. Some have advocated a modification of the fistula with creation of an end-to-side anastomosis whereby there would be a maximal blood flow proximally and less to the hand (8). Others have advocated an end-to-end anastomosis, the advantage being that all the blood from the radial artery is diverted directly into the vein (9, 10). No single method has been exclusively adopted. Thus, successful hemodialysis is dependent on the establishment of adequate access to the patient's circulation by means of an external arteriovenous shunt or an internal arteriovenous fistula. Each method has its advantages and disadvantages and it is incumbent on those individuals responsible for long-term management of the uremic patient to be familiar with the alternatives.

B.   External Arteriovenous Shunts

An external arteriovenous shunt is the use of a prosthetic device tubing connected to both arterial and venous systems, which permits shunting of the blood directly from the artery to the vein in order to maintain patency of the cannulae in these vessels (Fig. 1).

This method of access to the circulation is applicable to all patients who require hemodialysis for treatment of acute renal failure. It may also be preferred in certain instances for the management of the patient with chronic renal failure. The most noteworthy advantage of this type of shunt is that it enables performance of dialysis immediately following its placement. This type of access allows a patient to dialyze while waiting for a fistula to mature. The external shunt can be utilized chronically in those patients who do not have adequate vessels for creation of a fistula. Furthermore, patients in the older age group frequently have very thin skin, which cannot sustain the repeated trauma of multiple venipunctures with the large gauge needles required for the use of a fistula. Also, if the superficial veins are thin walled and do not become thickened with increased flow from the fistula, puncture with a needle will result in leakage of blood around the needle with subsequent hematoma formation. The external shunt tubing makes connection to the dialyzer easy and is often preferred by home dialysis patients, especially those individuals who do not become proficient at venipuncture. If the shunt clots it can frequently be declotted with the use of the Fogarty embolectomy catheter (11). Unfortunately, there are disadvantages to the external shunt. While some external shunts may function satisfactorily for years, the average duration is 6–9 months; therefore, the necessity for revision is omnipresent. The shunt is a foreign body that increases the likelihood of an infection, not only at the skin exit site, but also at the point where the vessels are cannulated. This may lead to a septicemia or the formation of a mycotic aneurysm, which can bleed and cause exsanguination. If an infection occurs at the shunt site, then the shunt must be removed, the patient placed on appropriate antibiotics, and vascular access established elsewhere. Because of the ease with which the shunt can deliberately or accidentally be disconnected with subsequent exsanguination, this type of shunt should be avoided if at all possible.

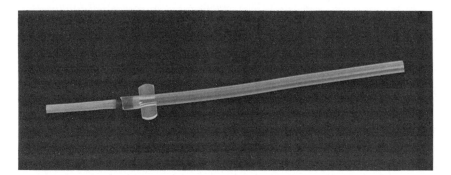

Fig. 1. External shunt silicone rubber cannula with Ramirez wing and Teflon tip.

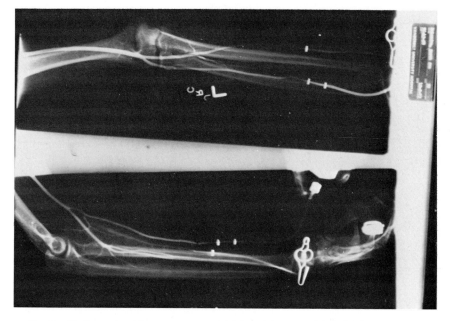

Fig. 2. Radiograph with contrast material injected into arterial limb of external shunt showing narrowing of the radial artery at the tip of the cannula.

Thrombosis is probably the most common complication. Radiographic studies usually will show a narrowing of the vessel at the site where the shunt has been inserted (Fig. 2). This may be seen at either the arterial or the venous end although it is more common at the venous end. Subintimal fibrosis of the vessel may develop, probably due to the "jet effect" of the blood from the artery being shunted directly to the low flow venous circulation (Fig. 3). Recannulation at a higher level will establish an effective shunt in this situation. If there is no narrowing of the vessel at the cannula tip, removal of the clot with a Fogarty embolectomy catheter can be accomplished. Thereafter, the shunt should be irrigated with heparinized saline and subsequently warfarin can be used to prevent recurrence of thrombosis.

Choice of Site

Once it has been determined that the patient is a candidate for placement of an external shunt, a thorough assessment of the peripheral arteries and veins of all the extremities should be made. The concept of adequate collateral circulation to the extremities distal to the shunt is of paramount importance because the technique of cannulation involves ligating both the artery and the vein distally. The site most frequently selected is the distal radial artery

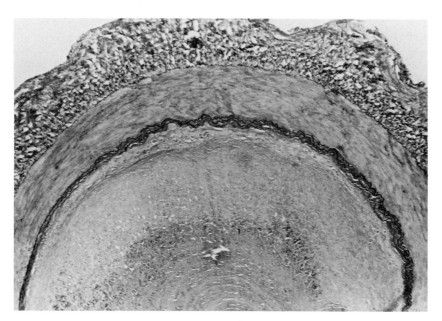

Fig. 3. Photomicrograph of arterial vessel in Fig. 2 showing subintimal fibrosis of the artery.

and distal cephalic vein in the forearm (Fig. 4). In the lower leg, the posterior tibial artery and the long saphenous vein are utilized (Fig. 5). Therefore, the patency of the ulnar artery should be determined if the forearm is to be used, and the patency of the dorsalis pedis artery, if the leg is to be used. If the clinical examination is not conclusive, arteriography can be performed to ascertain the integrity of the circulation. The status of the

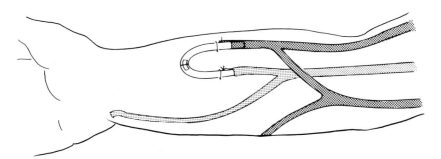

Fig. 4. Diagram of forearm showing cannulation of radial artery and cephalic vein to create external A-V shunt.

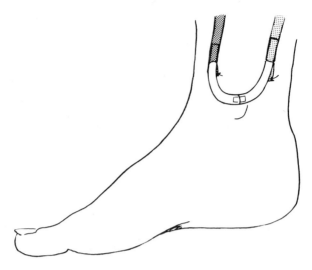

Fig. 5. Diagram of lower leg showing cannulation of posterior tibial artery and long saphenous vein to create external A-V shunt.

venous circulation is also important. This can be established first by application of a tourniquet proximally to see if the vein will distend with blood, and second, with release of the tourniquet to ascertain the rapidity of venous blood flow. All too often, the superficial veins have been previously used for an indwelling intravenous catheter with subsequent thrombophlebitis and obliteration of the lumen by thrombosis and fibrosis. This will render the superficial vein unusable and it may be necessary to use the deep vein usually found adjacent to the artery for shunt placement.

C. Internal Arteriovenous Fistulae

An internal arteriovenous fistula is the creation of a vascular communication by suturing a vein directly to an artery so that adequate blood flow to a dialyzer can be obtained by venipuncture.

The preferred method of vascular access in a patient who needs long-term hemodialysis is the arteriovenous fistula of the Brescia–Cimino type. Most of the problems seen with external shunts, i.e., infection, thrombosis, bleeding, and the need for frequent revision, are less commonly seen with an arteriovenous fistula. In addition, the patient is spared the constant worry about dislodgement during daily activities. Probably the biggest advantage of the fistula is the length of time it can be used successfully. There are reports describing successful dialysis for several years with this method of access (*12–15*). At our institution, we have had some patients who have used

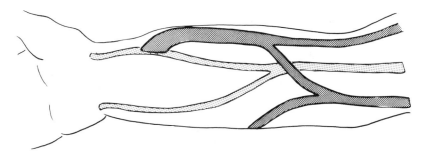

Fig. 6. Diagram of forearm showing end to side anastomosis of cephalic vein to radial artery in order to create an arteriovenous fistula.

the same fistula for more than 10 years. The average life expectancy of a fistula approaches 5 years.

Sites of Arteriovenous fistulae

The usual site chosen for creation of the arteriovenous fistula is the lower forearm utilizing the distal radial artery and cephalic vein (Fig. 6). Examination should be done to assure patency of both the radial artery and ulnar artery. This is not as imperative as in the case of an external shunt because the artery is not interrupted when the fistula is created and occlusion is only temporary. The vein should be patent and large enough to carry the increased flow. The nondominant arm is chosen because this will permit the patient to perform self-cannulation, particularly if home dialysis is considered. If there is not a suitable vein in the forearm, a fistula can be created above the elbow between the cephalic vein and the brachial artery (Fig. 7).

Complications can occur. Bleeding is seen infrequently. In the first 24 hr following the operative procedure, bleeding may be related to inadequate hemostasis at the anastomotic suture line. Reoperation may be required

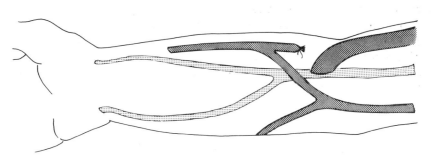

Fig. 7. Diagram of forearm showing end to side anastomosis of cephalic vein and brachial artery in order to create an arteriovenous fistula.

with evacuation of the hematoma and suture of the bleeding site. Occasionally, there is prolonged bleeding at the venipuncture site. If this is felt to be due to the heparin given during dialysis, then prolonged external pressure will result in hemostasis. Protamine has also been helpful in this situation. Sometimes the needle puncture site is in an area of scarring from repeated usage. Then it may be necessary to insert a fine suture of nonabsorbable material to stop the bleeding. Occasionally, a perivascular hematoma develops. This may be the result of insertion of the needle into the side of the vein or of not applying enough pressure on the insertion site following removal of the needle. The hematoma usually resolves following conservative management consisting of localized application of heat and elevation of the limb.

Thrombosis may complicate the immediate postoperative period. This will necessitate revision of the fistula. Should it occur later, it may be necessary to create a new anastomosis at a more proximal level. In our experience, it is quite common to see a fistula that has been functioning well for years, suddenly clot following any major surgery such as a kidney transplant, nephrectomy, or parathyroidectomy. The reason for this is unclear. Attempts to remove the thrombus by means of a Fogarty embolectomy catheter through venotomy have not been successful. Again, a more proximal fistula site will be required if the same extremity is selected.

Aneurysmal dilatation of the vein may develop. This usually occurs just distal to the arterial anastomosis. If the site is not infected, successful treatment can be accomplished by excision of the dilated portion of the vein with a venovenous anastomosis. On the other hand, when there is a mycotic aneurysm, the arterial inflow must be ligated and the aneurysm and surrounding vein excised. Access will need to be established at another site. If the fistula is of the side-to-side type, distention of the veins on the dorsum of the hand and thumb area will occasionally lead to the "sore thumb" syndrome (16). This can be managed by ligating the distal vein going to the hand, shunting all the blood proximally to the cephalic vein. A small percentage of patients will have cephalic veins which will not develop to the point where the blood flow is adequate for dialysis. In this situation an alternative method of creating a fistula using a synthetic material may be necessary. Polytetrafluoroethylene (PTFE), Dacron, and bovine carotid artery xenografts have been used (17–22).

D.   Creation of Vascular Access in the Problem Patient

We are beginning to see a group of patients in whom it is not possible to utilize the standard means of access as previously described. Many of these patients have been on dialysis for over 10 years and have required numerous and varied access procedures. Some have had a transplant that failed after a period of time and have returned to dialysis without a suitable functioning access site. In these individuals it is often necessary to utilize a secondary or even a tertiary procedure in order to create a usable vascular access.

1. Alternative External Shunts

In 1969, Thomas (23) introduced a variation of the external shunt which consists of a Silastic cannula with an attached piece of Dacron which can be sutured end-to-side to a vessel, and thus not interrupt the flow of blood distally. The cannula can then be brought out through the skin to function as an external shunt. The Allen–Brown shunt is similar (Fig. 8). It consists of a small piece of knitted Dacron attached to a Silastic tube. A Dacron velour sleeve is attached proximally to the knitted Dacron and this acts as a bacterial barrier. This also preserves the artery distally and can function as an external shunt. Both of these shunts can be sutured to large vessels such as the femoral artery, superficial femoral artery, or brachial artery. Complications seen with these are the same as with the Scribner external shunt but are often more severe. If an infection develops around the tubing and it involves the anastomosis with the artery, the shunt must be removed. The artery should be ligated above and below the anastomotic area in order to prevent hemorrhage. With prolonged use of the Allen–Brown shunt a pseudo-intima may develop in the Dacron sleeve which will occlude the lumen and cause thrombosis (Fig. 9).

2. Alternative Methods of Creating an Arteriovenous Fistula

a. BRACHIOBASILIC FISTULA. Dagher, in 1976, established an arteriovenous, fistula by mobilizing the basilic vein in the upper arm, placing it in a

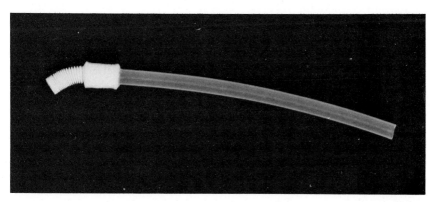

Fig. 8.   Allen–Brown external shunt cannula with 4 mm diameter Dacron graft and Dacron velour sleeve.

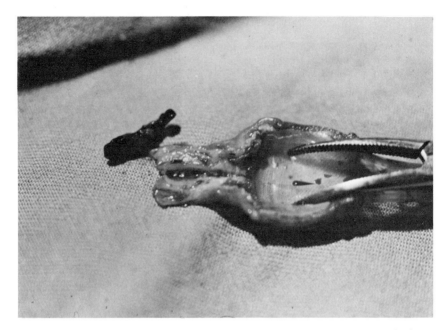

Fig. 9. Allen–Brown shunt showing pseudointima in Dacron sleeve with thrombosis as a result.

subcutaneous tunnel, and then suturing it to the brachial artery (*24*). Our experience indicates that a very short segment is created which often is difficult to puncture. We have rarely used this type of access.

    b. FEMORAL ARTERY TO SAPHENOUS VEIN FISTULA WITH A SAPHENOUS VEIN LOOP. In 1972 Perez-Alvarez developed a fistula between the saphenous vein and femoral artery by mobilizing the saphenous vein, dividing it below the knee, looping it back through a subcutaneous tunnel, and anastomosing it to the superficial femoral artery (*25*). Satisfactory long-term use from this may be obtained. However, frequently the vein becomes fibrosed and will subsequently clot.

    c. CREATION OF AN ARTERIOVENOUS SHUNT WITH AN INTERPOSITION GRAFT. Chinitz, in 1972, described a technique of creating an arteriovenous fistula in the upper arm by using a bovine xenograft interposed between the brachial artery and the cephalic vein (*17*). It was tunneled beneath the skin and could be punctured with needles. Subsequently, this technique has been modified and similar fistulae have been created in the forearm and in the thigh (Figs. 10 and 11). In our experience with this type of graft, 53% were patent at 6

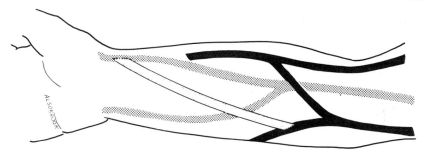

Fig. 10. Diagram showing a Bovine xenograft interposed between radial artery and basilic vein in order to create an A-V fistula. (Reprinted from ref. *26*, by permission from the *Southern Medical Journal*, **71**, 386–388, 1978.

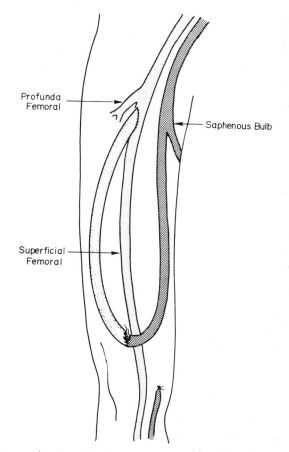

Fig. 11. Diagram showing a Bovine xenograft interposed between superficial femoral artery and saphenous vein in order to create an A-V fistula. (Reprinted from ref. *26*, by permission from the *Southern Medical Journal*, **71**, 386–388, 1978.

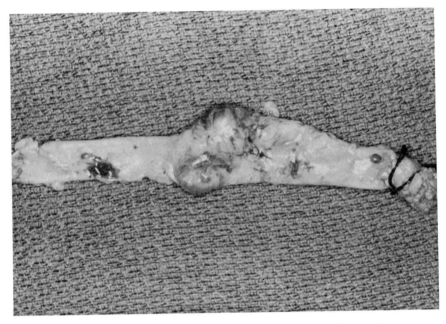

Fig. 12.   Excised Bovine xenograft showing two aneurysms of the graft.

months, 36% patent at 12 months, and only 15% patent at 24 months (26). The most common cause of graft failure was thrombosis. Other complications included false aneurysms, infection, ischemia of the distal extremity, and bleeding (Fig. 12). Infection is particularly serious because it can cause arterial rupture and potential exsanguination. Modified umbilical veins have been used instead of the bovine xenograft, but experience with this technique is limited. Because of the problem with aneurysmal dilatation of the bovine xenografts, synthetic materials have been used to establish an interposition graft. At present, the material that has most widespread use is polytetrafluoroethylene (PTFE). PTFE has the advantage over the bovine xenograft in that there is less tendency to form aneurysms. If an abscess develops at a puncture site, the graft, being a foreign body, will usually have to be excised. In a few instances, however, it may be possible to bypass the infection and only remove the infected portion. Unlike bovine grafts, PTFE does not tend to erode in the presence of infection. Thrombosis is a common complication and is usually related to stenosis of the vein at the site of the venous anastomosis. Frequently, this can be managed by using a patch of PTFE to widen the outflow tract and then declotting the graft.

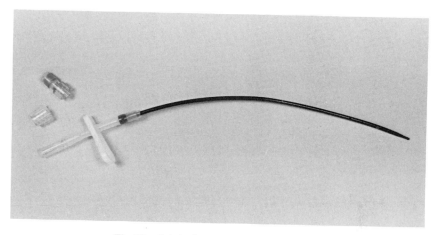

Fig. 13. Subclavian vein hemodialysis catheter.

3. Direct Cannulation of Vessels

Direct cannulation of the femoral vein or the subclavian vein may be used if a patient is in need of immediate dialysis and there are no sites for an external arteriovenous shunt or if a fistula or interposition graft fistula needs time to mature (27, 28). This technique can be successful on a temporary basis until a more permanent method of access can be established (Fig. 13). If the catheter is left in place, as is the case with the subclavian method, it may be necessary to flush the catheter frequently with small doses of heparin to prevent clot formation. When a femoral vein catheter is used, a separate puncture is necessary for insertion before each dialysis. With either site, thrombosis and infection are major complications. Should either occur, the catheter must be removed and replaced or reinserted in the contralateral side (29). Air embolism is also more dangerous when venous cannulae are used for hemodialysis.

II. ACCESS FOR PERITONEAL DIALYSIS

For a variety of reasons, peritoneal dialysis may be chosen for long-term management. Inability to secure adequate vascular access is one indication for peritoneal dialysis. Recently, continuous ambulatory peritoneal dialysis (CAPD) has been introduced and has gained in popularity. Using CAPD the patients are more mobile and are less restricted in their activity. Also, CAPD can be carried out at home by the patient without the constant threat of bleeding from dislodgement of an external shunt or bleeding while on hemodialysis with a fistula. Tenckhoff, in 1968, described the use of a Silastic catheter for this purpose (*30*) (Fig. 14).

Under local anesthesia the catheter can usually be placed into the peritoneal cavity without any difficulty, especially if the patient has not had a previous laparotomy. In individuals who have adhesions from previous laparotomies, the procedure may be more involved and requires freeing up of adhesions in order to place the catheter properly. Initially, a lower midline site approximately 4–6 cm below the umbilicus was utilized. However, more recently we have chosen to place the catheter either in the right or left lower

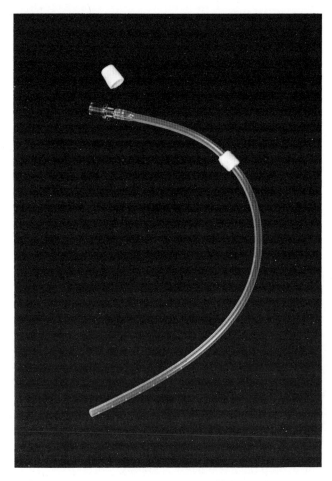

Fig. 14.   Adult Tenckhoff peritoneal dialysis catheter.

quadrant at the lateral border of the rectus muscle. At the time of placement, it is necessary to be certain that there is a free flow of fluid in and out of the catheter. If this is not present, then the catheter must be replaced. The most frequent cause of malfunction is secondary to omentum wrapping around the catheter. In this event, when the catheter is removed, the omentum can occasionally be pulled out through the peritoneum and amputated, in part. Infection is another frequent complication of the Tenckhoff catheter, and usual management consists of instilling antibiotics in the peritoneal dialysate (*31*). However, if this fails to control the infection, then the catheter must be removed and the patient treated with antibiotics for several days before reinserting another catheter. Temporary hemodialysis may be necessary during this period of time.

III. CONCLUSION

We have discussed the options available for obtaining and maintaining access to the circulation necessary for acute and chronic hemodialysis. Internal arteriovenous fistulae and external shunts are described. The associated advantages and complications are given. Alternative methods are detailed for patients in whom access to the circulation has been compromised. The methodology and complications associated with access routes for chronic peritoneal dialysis are described.

GENERAL REFERENCES

Bell, P. R. F., and Coleman, K. C., "Surgical Aspects of Haemodialysis." Churchill-Livingston, Edinburgh and London, 1974.
Legrain, M., ed. "Continuous Ambulatory Peritoneal Dialysis," Proc. Int. Symp., Paris, Nov. 2, 3, 1979. Excerpta Medica, Amsterdam, 1980.

REFERENCES

1. Kolff, W. J., and Beck, H. T. J. The artificial kidney: A dialyzer with a great area. *Acta Med. Scand.* **117,** 121–134 (1944).
2. Anderson, A., and Kolff, W. J. Artificial kidney in the treatment of uremia associated with acute glomerulonephritis (with a note on regional heparinization). *Ann. Intern. Med.* **51,** 476–487 (1959).
3. Alwall, N. On the artificial kidney. I. Apparatus for dialysis of the blood in vivo. *Acta Med. Scand.* **128,** 317–325 (1947).
4. Teschan, P. E., Baxter, C. R., O'Brien, T. F., Freyhof, J. N., and Hall, W. H. Prophylactic hemodialysis in the treatment of acute renal failure. *Ann. Intern. Med.* **53,** 992–1016 (1960).

5. Quinton, W. E., Dillard, D., and Scribner, B. H. Cannulation of blood vessels for pro-
    longed hemodialysis. *Trans. Am. Soc. Artif. Intern. Organs* **6,** 104–113 (1960).
6. Ramirez, O., Swartz, C., Onesti, G., Mailloux, L., and Brest, A. N. The winged inline
    shunt. *Trans. Am. Soc. Artif. Intern. Organs* **12,** 220–228 (1966).
7. Brescia, M. J., Cimino, J. E., Appel, K., and Hurwich, B. J. Chronic hemodialysis using
    venipuncture and a surgically created arteriovenous fistula. *N. Engl. J. Med.* **275,** 1089–
    1092 (1966).
8. Bussell, J. A., Abbott, J. A., and Lim, R. C. A radial steal syndrome with arteriovenous
    fistula for hemodialysis. *Ann. Intern. Med.* **75,** 387–394 (1971).
9. Salomon, J., Vidne, B. Robson, M., Rosenfeld, J., and Levy, M. J. Our experience with
    the use of arteriovenous fistula in chronic dialysis: Modified surgical technique. *Surgery*
    (*St. Louis*) **63,** 899–902 (1968).
10. Lawton, R. L., and Gulesserian, H. P. New technique for creating buried arteriovenous
    fistulae. *Proc. Eur. Dial. Transolant Assoc.* **6,** 53–58 (1969).
11. Fogarty, T. J., Cranley, J. J., Krouse, R. J., Strasser, E. S., and Hofner, C. D. A method
    for extraction of arterial embolis and thrombi. *Surg., Gynecol. Obstet.* **116,** 241–244 (1963).
12. Hodson, J. M., Menno, A. D., and McMahon, J. Radial arteriovenous fistula as a sub-
    stitute for the conventional external prosthesis in maintenance hemodialysis. *J. Urol.*
    103, 5–8 (1970).
13. Lytton, B., Goffinet, J. A., May, C. J., and Weiss, R. M. Experience with arteriovenous
    fistula in chronic hemodialysis. *J. Urol.* **104,** 512–517 (1970).
14. Kuruvila, K. C., and Beven, E. G. Arteriovenous shunts and fistulas for hemodialysis.
    Surg. Clin. North Am. **51,** 1219–1234 (1971).
15. Haimov, M., Singer, A., and Schupak, E. Access to blood vessels for hemodialysis:
    Experience with 87 patients on chronic hemodialysis. *Surgery* (*St. Louis*) **69,** 884–889
    (1971).
16. Butt, K. M. H., Friedman, E. A., and Kountz, S. C. Angio-access. *Curr. Probl. Surg.*
    13, 9–11 (1976).
17. Chinitz, J. L., Yokoyama, T., Bower, R., and Swartz, C. Self sealing prosthesis for arterio-
    venous fistula in man. *Trans. Am. Soc. Artif. Intern. Organs* **18,** 452–456 (1972).
18. Richie, R. E., Johnson, H. K., Walker, P., and Ginn, H. E. Creation of an arteriovenous
    fistula utilizing a modified bovine artery graft: Clinical experience in fourteen patients.
    Proc.—Clin. Dial. Transplant Forum **2,** 86–87 (1972).
19. Merickel, J. H., Anderson, R. C., Knutson, R., Lipschultz, M. L., and Hitchcock, C. R.
    (1974). Bovine carotid artery shunts in vascular access surgery. *Arch. Surg.* (*Chicago*)
    109, 245–250.
20. Anderson, C. V., Etheredge, E. E., and Sicard, G. A. One hundred polytetrafluoroethylene
    vascular access grafts. *Dial. Transplant.* **9,** 237–238 (1980).
21. Shack, R. B., Neblett, W. W., Richie, R. E. *et al.* Expanded polytetrafluoroethylene as
    dialysis access grafts: Serial study of histology and fibrinolytic activity. *Am. Surg.* **43,**
    817–825 (1977).
22. Flores, L., Dunn, I., Frunkin, E. *et al.* Dacron arteriovenous shunts for vascular access in
    hemodialysis. *Trans. Am. Soc. Artif. Intern. Organs* **19,** 33–37 (1973).
23. Thomas, G. I. A large vessell applique arteriovenous shunt for hemodialysis. *Trans.
    Am. Soc. Artif. Intern. Organs* **15,** 288–292 (1969).
24. Dagher, F., Gelver, R., Ramos, E. *et al.* The use of basilic vein and Brachial artery as an
    A–V fistula for long term hemodialysis. *J. Surg. Res.* **20,** 373–376 (1976).
25. Perez-Alvarez, J. J., Vargas-Rosendo, R., Gutierrez-Bosque, R. *et al.* A new type sub-
    cutaneous arteriovenous fistula for chronic hemodialysis in children. *Surgery* **67,** 355–359
    (1970).

26. Richie, R. E., Withers, E. H., Petracek, M. R., and Conkle, D. M. Vascular access for chronic hemodialysis: Use of bovine xenografts to create arteriovenous fistulas. *South. Med. J.* **71**, 386–388 (1978).

27. Shaldon, S., Chiandussi, L., and Higgs, B. Hemodialysis by percutaneous catheterization of the femoral artery and vein with regional heparinization. *Lancet* **2**, 857–859 (1961).

28. Uldall, P. R., Woods, F., Merchant, N. *et al.* Two years experience with the subclavian cannula for temporary vascular access for hemodialysis and plasmapheresis. *Proc.—Clin. Dial. Transplant Forum* **9**, 32–35 (1979).

29. Uldall, P. R., Merchant, W., and Woods, F. Changing subclavian hemodialysis cannulas to reduce infection. *Lancet* **1**, 1373 (1981).

30. Tenckhoff, H., and Schechter, H. A bacteriologically safe peritoneal access device. *Trans. Am. Soc. Artif. Intern. Organs* **14**, 181–187 (1968).

31. Tenckhoff, H. Home peritoneal dialysis. *in* "Clinical Aspects of Uremia" S. G. Massy, and A. L. Sellers, eds.), Thomas, p. 583. Springfield, Illinois, 1976.

Dialysis

RICHARD L. GIBSON

I. INTRODUCTION

Dialysis was first proposed as a treatment for renal failure by Abel, Rowntree, and Turner in 1913 (*1*). Technical problems such as lack of a safe anticoagulant hampered the development of hemodialysis and it was not until 1943 that the first patient was successfully dialyzed (*2*). Hemodialysis is

Copyright © 1983 by Academic Press, Inc.
All rights of reproduction in any form reserved.
ISBN 0-12-672280-3

END-STAGE RENAL DISEASE

now widely available and is nearly synonymous with treatment of kidney failure. However, other dialytic methods are available and peritoneal dialysis now rivals hemodialysis in importance, primarily because of the development of continuous ambulatory peritoneal dialysis (CAPD) (3).

Chronic hemodialysis became possible in 1960 when Quinton and Scribner introduced the external arteriovenous shunt (4). Earlier, each dialysis had required surgical insertion of an arterial cannula, which was removed at the end of dialysis. Only a few dialyses could be performed before arteriotomy sites were exhausted.

Application of chronic peritoneal dialysis, like hemodialysis, was initially constrained by lack of an access device that could be used repeatedly. Peritoneal dialysis required insertion of a catheter into the peritoneal space through a trocar each time the dialysis was done. In 1971 Tenckhoff introduced a catheter that could remain permanently in the peritoneal cavity (5). The nearly simultaneous introduction of automated peritoneal dialysis equipment eliminated the need for constant attention during the procedure and decreased the incidence of peritonitis. However, peritoneal dialysis was still considered a "second rate" form of dialysis, useful mainly in patients unable to undergo hemodialysis.

With the introduction of CAPD, peritoneal dialysis has begun to assume a position of importance equal to hemodialysis. Since CAPD was first described by Popovich, Moncrief, and Nolph in 1976, it has become the most rapidly growing form of dialysis. Worldwide, as many as 250 new patients per month are being placed on CAPD (6).

Between 1960 and 1972 entry of patients into a chronic end-stage renal disease (ESRD) program was limited by financial considerations. Few patients had private resources sufficient to pay for dialysis, and public resources were almost nonexistent. In 1972 Public Law 92-603 was passed which provides that the federal government will underwrite the cost of dialysis and transplantation. At the time the law was passed there were approximately 1000 patients receiving treatment for ESRD. Over 50,000 patients are currently being treated in ESRD programs (7).

A.   Indications for Dialysis

It is necessary to consider indications for dialysis from the standpoint of (a) acute dialysis for relief of problems occurring in acute renal failure, and (b) chronic dialysis to maintain patients for the long term. Specific guidelines are given in Tables I and II.

TABLE I

Indications for Dialysis in Acute Renal Failure

Absolute	
Clinical uremia[a]	
Guidelines	
BUN	> 100 mg/dl
Serum creatinine	> 10 mg/dl
Serum potassium	> 6.5, not controllable by simpler measures
pH	< 7.2, not controllable by simpler measures
pH	> 7.5, not controllable by simpler measures
Serum sodium	< 120 mEq/liter, dilutional
Serum sodium	> 160 mEq/liter
Fluid overload	Persistently elevated central venous pressure, pulmonary artery wedge pressure, S_3, S_4, rales, effusion

[a] See Chapter 2.

TABLE II

Indications for Dialysis in Chronic Renal Failure

Absolute	
Clinical uremia[a]	
Guidelines	
BUN	> 100–150 mg/dl
Serum creatinine	> 10–15 mg/dl
Clinical criteria	
"Soft"	Irritability
	↓ Memory
	Sensory neuropathy, "restless legs"
Other	Soft tissue calcification
	Motor neuropathy
	Anemia
	Anorexia
	Malaise

[a] See Chapter 2.

B. Methods of Dialysis

Once the decision to dialyze is made, a method is chosen. Most patients can be treated equally well by either hemodialysis or peritoneal dialysis, although the majority of patients receiving ESRD therapy are on hemodialysis (6). As previously mentioned, the number of patients on peritoneal dialysis is rapidly increasing, mainly due to the popularity of CAPD.

TABLE III

Indications for Hemodialysis or Peritoneal Dialysis

Hemodialysis
Hypercatabolic state
Drug intoxication (hemoperfusion may be better)
Marked abdominal distension, multiple previous abdominal operations
Hyperkalemia, severe
Colostomy
Peritoneal dialysis
Cardiovascular instability
Hemorrhagic diathesis
Infants
Lack of vascular access
Diabetes mellitus (?)

Relative indications for choosing one form of dialysis over another are listed in Table III.

The choice of method is made on the basis of availability, physician preference, or patient preference. Selection of a method of dialysis is generally the first major decision facing the patient with ESRD. Unfortunately, too often discussion of dialysis methods is left until the patient has become uremic and in need of emergency dialysis. At that point the patient may be unable to participate meaningfully in choosing a method of dialysis, and the decision is left to family and physician. Ideally, the patient should participate.

C. Location of Dialysis

1. Hemodialysis

There has long been a debate about whether center or home hemodialysis is preferable. Proponents of home hemodialysis point to its lower cost and improved life-style. Advocates of center hemodialysis describe higher mortality rates and greater family stresses in home hemodialysis patients. The debate often becomes emotionally charged, with accusations of profiteering leveled against those favoring center dialysis, and charges that those favoring home dialysis are insensitive to the needs of their patients (8). There is probably some truth on both sides. To date, there is no clear evidence to indicate that the location of dialysis has an adverse effect on patient survival. Home hemodialysis does cost less than center dialysis, and the preponderance of the evidence indicates that home dialysis patients fare at least as well as center patients. If patient safety is not a factor, then home dialysis should be encouraged for economic reasons. However, there has been a progressive decline in patients on home dialysis from 43% in 1973 to only 11% in 1978 (8). This decrease may represent both lack of physician interest in home training and inadequate support of home dialysis training programs by the government. Although center hemodialysis costs at least twice as much as home hemodialysis, until 1979 there were considerable financial *disincentives* for patients to dialyze at home, and there is now little *incentive* for patients to choose home hemodialysis.

2. Peritoneal Dialysis

Peritoneal dialysis offers the same choices as hemodialysis, but center peritoneal dialysis has disadvantages. Patients on intermittent peritoneal dialysis dialyze 36–40 hr per week, much longer than the 9–12 hr required for hemodialysis. To make center peritoneal dialysis a cost effective procedure, dialysis must be performed on a 24 hr basis; patients who go to the center must remain 18–20 hr. Staffing such a unit is practically impossible except in a hospital setting. Since patients spend 18–20 hr twice a week dialyzing, it may not be possible for them to continue to work or carry on a normal family relationship. Center peritoneal dialysis is therefore not widespread and is unlikely to grow. Home peritoneal dialysis, however, has several advantages and is growing rapidly. The time requirement is less of a disadvantage at home because, with automated equipment, dialysis can be done safely at night while a patient is asleep. Unlike hemodialysis, the patient can perform peritoneal dialysis without assistance.

Continuous ambulatory peritoneal dialysis (CAPD), almost by definition, is performed at home.

D. Cost of Dialysis

Cost of the ESRD treatment program is not insignificant; the cost in 1980 was estimated to be one billion dollars (8) and with the dialysis population still increasing the cost also will increase in the years to come. Cost must therefore be considered when planning the future direction of ESRD treatment. Home hemodialysis costs $10,000 to $15,000 per year; center hemodialysis $25,000 to $30,000 per year; home peritoneal dialysis using a reverse osmosis machine costs only $10,000 to $12,000 per year. Home peritoneal dialysis using a cycler machine may cost as much as center hemodialysis, i.e., $25,000 to $30,000 per year. The cost of CAPD is uncertain. Estimates range from $8000 to $30,000 per year. One reason for the great range is that some people feel that the expense of hospitalization for peritonitis should be included in calculating the cost of CAPD (9, 10).

II. HEMODIALYSIS

The basic hemodialysis system is illustrated in Fig. 1 and consists of three parts: (1) a hemodialyzer, which is the membrane separating blood from dialysate, and across which diffusion of solutes and transfer of water will occur; (2) the dialysate delivery system which produces and delivers dialysate of appropriate composition to the dialyzer; and (3) the blood circuit from the patient through the dialyzer and back to the patient.

Delivery systems are available from several different manufacturers. Basically, a delivery system presents dialysate to the dialysis membrane. Two systems are available: a batch system in which a measured amount of concentrate is mixed in a tank with water, and a proportioning system that utilizes a pump to mix water and concentrate to yield dialysate. The delivery system also monitors the system for the presence of blood leaks and air leaks. Delivery systems are constantly being changed and will not be reviewed in detail here.

A.   Principles of Hemodialysis

In simplest terms, dialysis is the removal of solute, waste products, and excess fluid from a patient. Hemodialysis is accomplished by circulating the

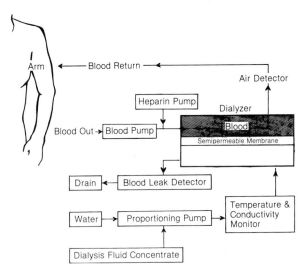

Fig. 1.   Components of a typical hemodialysis system. Reprinted by permission from C. K. Colton and E. G. Lowrie. Hemodialysis: Physical principles and technical considerations. In "The Kidney" (B. M. Brenner and F. C. Rector, eds.), 2nd ed., p. 2427. Saunders, Philadelphia, Pennsylvania, Copyright 1981.

patient's blood through a dialyzer, the dialyzer being a device containing a semipermeable membrane that separates blood from a balanced electrolyte solution (dialysate). Transfer of solute across a membrane involves two basic mechanisms: diffusion and ultrafiltration (convective transfer). Diffusive transfer is quantitatively the more important and depends on several factors including net membrane permeability, membrane surface area, and the solute concentration gradient. These factors in turn depend on other variables such as solute size and charge, blood flow rate, and dialysate flow rate. Figure 2 shows dialyzer clearance plotted against blood flow. Note that the clearance of small molecules is quite flow dependent, whereas the clearance of larger molecules is far less flow dependent. Blood flow rates of 200 ml/min are commonly used. Figure 3 shows the relationship of dialyzer clearance to dialysate flow. Note once more that small molecules are flow dependent, larger molecules are not. Standard dialysate flow rate is 500 ml/min.

Ultrafiltration refers to the transfer of solvent across a membrane. The solvent will contain some of the dissolved solutes; therefore, an increase in ultrafiltration will increase solute transfer. This convective effect is quantitatively less important than diffusion for solute transfer.

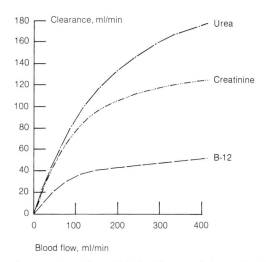

Fig. 2. Solute clearance during hemodialysis. Clearance is inversely related to molecular size. The clearance of large molecules is not so flow dependent as the clearance of small molecules. Reprinted by permission from Extracorporeal Medical Specialties, Inc., King of Prussia, Pennsylvania; S. T. Boen, Kinetics of peritoneal dialysis: A comparison with the artificial kidney. *Medicine* (*Baltimore*) **40**, 240 (1961). Williams & Wilkins Co., Baltimore, Maryland, Copyright, 1961.

Ultrafiltration rate depends on the effective surface area of the membrane, the hydraulic permeability of the membrane, and the total transmembrane pressure (TMP). TMP is the sum of the mean positive pressure in the blood circuit (venous pressure, or pressure of blood actually in the dialyzer as it returns to the patient) minus the mean pressure in the dialysate circuit. Some dialysis systems generate a vacuum in the dialysate circuit and are called negative pressure systems. The effect of the negative pressure is to pull fluid from the blood across the dialysis membrane. This "pull" force is additive to the ultrafiltration pressure generated by a positive pressure on the blood side of the membrane (a "push" force).

Clearance refers to the volume of blood cleared of a particular substance per unit time. Dialyzer clearance is a useful measure of dialyzer performance which can be employed to compare the performance of various dialyzers. The quantity of solute removed is equal to the product of the blood flow (Q_B) and the difference between the concentrations in the blood flowing into (C_{B_i}) and out of (C_{B_o}) the dialyzer.

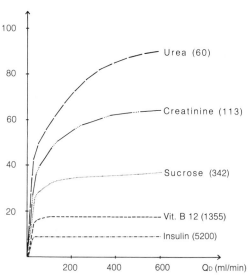

Fig. 3. Relationship between dialysate flow and dialyzer clearance according to solute molecular weight. Reprinted by permission from P. Jungers, J. Zingraff, N. K. Man, T. Drueke, and B. Tardieu, "The Essentials in Hemodialysis: Basic Principles of Hemodialysis," p. 25. The Tardieu Series. Distributed by Martinus Nijhoff Medical Division, Boston, Massachusetts, Copyright 1978.

Clearance is equal to solute removed divided by blood concentration of the solute. Therefore, clearance can be defined as in Eq. (1).

$$\text{Dialyzer clearance} = \frac{Q_B(C_{B_i} - C_{B_o})}{C_{B_i}} \tag{1}$$

Dialyzer performance may also be defined in terms of dialysance, which is similar to clearance but slightly more complex.

B. Types of Dialyzers

Selection of a particular dialyzer for an individual patient is currently as much an art as a science and, in practice, may be based on availability of dialyzers within a given unit. Factors to consider in selecting a dialyzer are the patient's need for fluid removal (some dialyzers have a much more permeable membrane than others) and the clearance required. If a patient has a significant residual renal clearance, less dialyzer clearance is necessary and a smaller surface area dialyzer can be used. The amount of fluid a patient gains between dialyses, and thus the amount of fluid to be removed during each dialysis, varies tremendously from patient to patient. Most nephrologists recommend that patients regulate their fluid intake so that they gain less than $1-1\frac{1}{2}$ kg between dialyses. It is not uncommon for less compliant patients to gain 5–7 kg between dialyses, necessitating massive ultrafiltration. Ultrafiltration rates in ml/mm Hg transmembrane pressure are given in the package insert accompanying a dialyzer. Typical ultrafiltration rates are 2–4 ml/mm Hg transmembrane pressure.

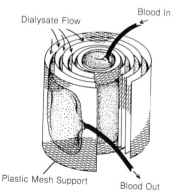

Fig. 4. Coil dialyzer. Redrawn by permission from C. L. Hampers, E. Schupak, E. G. Lowrie, and J. M. Lazarus, "Long-Term Hemodialysis: The Management of the Patient with Chronic Renal Failure," 2nd ed., p. 21. Grune & Stratton, Inc., New York, Copyright 1973.

Coil dialyzers (Fig. 4) are constructed by wrapping one or two tubular cellulose membranes around a central mesh support. Blood is pumped through the tubes and dialysate circulates around the tubes. The coil sits in a tank of dialysate so as dialysis proceeds, the concentration of solutes in the dialysate increases, thereby decreasing the gradient for continued solute removal. This effect is minimized by changing the dialysate midway through the procedure or by using a recirculating single pass system where dialysate is pumped from a large reservoir into a smaller tank holding the coil. The dialysate that has already circulated through the coil is discarded as the fresh dialysate is added.

The major problem with the coil dialyzer is its high internal resistance to

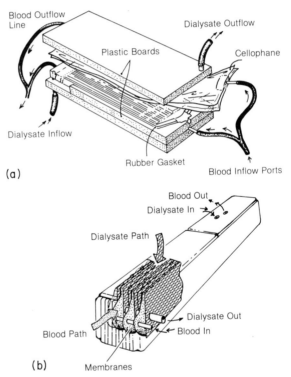

Fig. 5. (a) Parallel plate dialyzer (nondisposable). Redrawn by permission from C. L. Hampers, E. G. Schupak, E. G. Lowrie, and J. M. Lazarus, "Long-Term Hemodialysis: The Management of the Patient with Chronic Renal Failure," 2nd ed, p. 23. Grune & Stratton, Inc., New York, Copyright 1973. (b) Parallel plate dialyzer (disposable). Redrawn by permission from C. L. Hampers, E. Schupak, E. G. Lowrie, and J. M. Lazarus, "Long-Term Hemodialysis: The Management of the Patient with Chronic Renal Failure," 2nd ed., p. 23. Grune & Stratton, Inc., New York, Copyright 1973.

blood flow which creates an intrinsic ultrafiltration rate of 3–5 ml/min; that is, there is an obligatory loss from the patient of 3–5 ml/min during dialysis. Hypotension may thus be a serious problem, especially in patients with an unstable cardiovascular system. A second problem is that the membranes are extremely compliant and coil volume (blood volume inside the coil and outside the patient) may vary from 150 to 350 ml. Some patients are unable to tolerate such large volumes of blood outside the body.

Advantages of the coil are its price (cheapest of the disposable dialyzers), good washout characteristics, and the high ultrafiltration rate, which may be an advantage in an overhydrated patient with a stable blood pressure.

Coil dialyzers do not generate a negative pressure in the dialysate compartments. Ultrafiltration is entirely dependent on the positive pressure on the blood side of the membrane.

Parallel plate dialyzers (Fig. 5) consist of a series of membranes stretched over a supporting structure. Blood flows inside the membranes and dialysate between the membranes and supporting structure. The system tends to be less compliant than the coil system. The rate of ultrafiltration is controlled by applying a negative pressure to the dialysate side of the compartment if ultrafiltration is desired. The internal resistance of a parallel plate dialyzer is very low so in the absence of applied negative pressure the ultrafiltration rate depends on the pressure generated by resistance of blood returning to the body (the venous pressure).

Hollow fiber dialyzers (Fig. 6) are the most recently developed type of dialyzer and are gaining in popularity. A hollow fiber dialyzer consists of

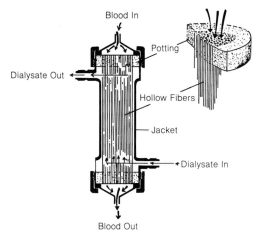

Fig. 6. Hollow fiber dialyzer. Redrawn by permission from C. L. Hampers, E. Schupak, E. G. Lowrie, and J. M. Lazarus, "Long-Term Hemodialysis: The Management of the Patient with Chronic Renal Failure," 2nd ed., p. 24. Grune & Stratton, Inc., New York. Copyright 1973.

10,000–15,000 cellulosic capillary tubes, each 200–300 μm in diameter. The ends of the fibers are encased in a potting material that prevents blood from going between the fibers. Blood flows through the fibers and dialysate circulates between the fibers. These dialyzers have a high ratio of membrane surface area to blood volume, and solute clearances may be higher than with other types of dialyzers. These dialyzers are also used with negative pressure systems.

It is an advantage to be able to control the rate of ultrafiltration. Negative pressure systems are thus more versatile than positive pressure systems (coils) where there is an intrinsic high rate of ultrafiltration.

C. Dialysate Composition

Dialysate is now relatively standard and the usual composition is shown in Table IV. Potassium concentration can be varied from 0 to 4 mEq/liter as needed, calcium concentration from 0 to 6.5 mg%, and glucose is either absent from the dialysate or present at 200 mg%.

1. Sodium

A sodium concentration lower than plasma sodium was used originally in the belief that negative sodium balance was desirable to prevent hypertension and congestive heart failure. While it is true that hypertension and its complications are major causes of death in dialysis patients (11), it has not been shown that low dialysate sodium concentrations prevent hypertension or its complications. It has lately been postulated that higher sodium concentrations may be beneficial in preventing certain troublesome dialysis-related problems such as weakness, nausea, vomiting, hypotension, and

TABLE IV

Composition of Dialysate Used
in Hemodialysis

Na	130–146 mEq/liter
K	0–4 mEq/liter
Cl	96–115 mEq/liter
Acetate	35–39 mEq/liter
Mg	1.0–1.5 mEq/liter
Ca	2.5–3.25 mEq/liter
	(5.0–6.5 mg(dl)
Glucose	0–200 mg/dl

cramps (*12*). The most suitable dialysate sodium concentration has yet to be determined but may be between 135 and 145 mEq/liter. A sodium concentration higher than 140 mEq/liter may be particularly beneficial when rapid ultrafiltration is desired (*13*).

2. Potassium

Control of potassium is critical because of its effects on the cardiovascular system. Generally, the problem in renal failure is hyperkalemia and potassium concentrations of 0–3 mEq/liter are used to lower serum potassium. Concentration of dialysate potassium for routine outpatient dialysis is usually 1–2 mEq/liter, the low $[K^+]$ allowing the patient a more liberal diet. For hospitalized patients who are less stable, a concentration of 3 mEq/liter is preferable. For extremely ill patients with cardiovascular instability a K^+ of 4 mEq/liter may be used. Any patient with renal failure, acute or chronic, may develop hyperkalemia requiring dialysis against a zero K^+ bath. It is important to keep in mind that if the concentration of K^+ is extremely high, a rapid drop may produce cardiac irritability (*14*). Therefore, in cases of profound hyperkalemia, especially in patients on digitalis preparations, it may be preferable to begin dialysis with a dialysate containing K^+ (3–4 mEq/liter) and decrease dialysate concentration as the K^+ falls. The effect of dialysis on the serum K^+ is complex and depends not only on removal of K^+ from the blood but on movement of K^+ into the cells produced by the base (and sometimes glucose) contained in the dialysate (*15*). The rate of K^+ movement out of the cell will also influence the final serum K^+. Thus, although K^+ is removed from the body at the rate of 25–50 mEq/hr, there is no good rule of thumb to be used in estimating how quickly the serum K^+ will be lowered. It is necessary to monitor the EKG closely and check serum K^+ values frequently.

3. Calcium

Bone disease in renal failure is multifactorial (*16*). Disordered calcium metabolism is common, and calcium balance is usually negative. If no calcium is present in dialysate, additional calcium will be lost by dialysis. Calcium is therefore raised in the dialysate to the point where it will be transferred into the patient, thereby helping to correct the negative calcium balance (*17*). Usual levels are 5.0–6.5 mg/dl, as shown in Table IV. Although this concentration is less than total blood calcium, it is all in the ionic form and higher than the ionized calcium concentration of the blood. Therefore, calcium balance is positive during most hemodialyses. Maintaining fairly high calcium levels may decrease secretion of parathyroid hormone, another factor of importance in the genesis of renal osteodystrophy (*18*).

4. Magnesium

Dialysate usually contains 0.5–1.5 mEq/liter magnesium. There is little reason to add magnesium since the dialysance of magnesium is low (*19*) and sufficient magnesium is contained in a standard dialysis patient's diet to prevent deficiencies. There is some evidence that lowering the magnesium in dialysate may ameliorate itching, which is a major problem for many patients. It is necessary to remove the magnesium from the dialysate if patients must be treated with magnesium-containing antacids.

5. Acetate

Except in acid solutions, bicarbonate precipitates with calcium to form insoluble calcium carbonate. In the early years of chronic dialysis this problem was solved by bubbling CO_2 into the dialysate to lower the pH. In 1964, acetate, which *in vivo* is metabolized to bicarbonate, was substituted for bicarbonate in dialysate, making possible the preparation of a concentrated solution. This, in turn, made it feasible to ship dialysate so that patients and small hospitals did not have to work with chemicals to prepare dialysate. The use of acetate was considered a major advance in the history of dialysis. Lately, investigations concerning the metabolism and side effects of acetate have raised the possibility that acetate could be contributing to cardiovascular morbidity and mortality in dialysis patients (*20, 21*). Additionally, some investigators feel that use of bicarbonate dialysate in critically ill patients may help prevent dialysis-associated hypotension (*22*). Therefore, there has been a revival of interest in use of bicarbonate as the base in hemodialysis. Several newer delivery systems make it possible to substitute bicarbonate for acetate.

6. Chloride

Chloride in dialysate is determined by the equation:

Total cations (mEq/liter) = acetate (or bicarbonate) + chloride (both in MEq/liter)

7. Glucose

Originally glucose was added to dialysate to facilitate ultrafiltration (*23*). Today, glucose is added to dialysate either to prevent hypoglycemia in diabetic patients (glucose is dialyzable, insulin is not) or to add calories and thereby help prevent negative nitrogen balance. There is no consensus among nephrologists as to whether glucose should be added to the dialysate except in the case of the insulin-dependent diabetic patient where it is clearly desirable.

8. Water

Dialysate is prepared from commercial concentrate, which is diluted 1:34 with water. Purified water must be used or various contaminants can pass from water to patient with undesirable consequences (see Chapter 9 for technical aspects).

Mixing of water and the concentrated electrolyte solution is done by the machine itself (proportioning system), in a large tank connected to an individual machine (batch system), or in a large reservoir from which dialysate is pumped to individual stations (central system).

D. Complications

Complications of hemodialysis may be related to the dialysis procedure or to the underlying renal disease. Medical complications of renal disease are considered in another section and only procedural complications of dialysis are considered here.

1. Cardiovascular

The most common cardiovascular complication is hypotension, which may occur in up to 25% of dialyses (24). There may be no single cause. Sometimes, it is clearly related to rapid fluid removal. At other times, it occurs with minimal ultrafiltration and may be due to a fall in osmolality, accumulation of acetate, or autonomic neuropathy (25–27). Treatment includes normal saline, hypertonic saline, albumin, slowing the blood flow rate, or changing dialyzers. Any or all may be effective. Hypertonic dialysate and hemofiltration have been proposed as preventive measures and show promise (14, 28, 29). Closely related to hypotension, and often accompanying it, are muscle cramps, which are extremely distressing to patients but of unknown etiology. Again, hypertonic dialysate shows promise of being an effective treatment (30, 31).

2. Neurological

Neurological complications include disequilibrium syndrome, dialysis dementia, and subdural hematoma. Disequilibrium syndrome is felt to be secondary to rapid solute removal (32, 33). It may be prevented by slowing the rate of solute removal; in practice this means initiating dialysis with brief periods (2–3 hr of dialysis) at low blood flow rates (100–125 ml/min). Once patients reach a steady state, i.e., where solute removal equals solute generation in the interdialytic interval, clinical disequilibrium syndrome is seldom seen. Dialysis dementia is reviewed in Chapter 2 of this volume.

Subdural hematoma may occur in 3% of hemodialysis patients and may be extremely difficult to diagnose (34). The presence of focal neurologic deficits should alert one to its presence but these are not always present. Computed tomographic scan may confirm the diagnosis but often arteriography is necessary (35). Treatment is by surgical drainage.

3. Infections

Vascular access infections are frequently the cause of fever in dialysis patients. A benign-appearing fistula may be the source of sepsis (36). Infections are most often due to staphylococci but gram negative infections are also observed (37). Fever during the course of dialysis due to contaminated equipment or endotoxemia is no longer common but is still possible (38, 39).

Viral hepatitis is a particular problem among dialysis patients (40–41a). The infection may be anicteric; dialysis unit personnel may be affected with serious consequences (42, 43). Regular screening of patients and personnel for HB_sAg should be done in all chronic dialysis centers. Once patients are identified as HB_sAg positive, they should be isolated from other patients. Hepatitis B immune globulin may be useful in reducing the incidence of this type of hepatitis (43). A vaccine has been developed and will soon be released; indications for the vaccine are still uncertain.

4. Hemorrhagic

There is an increased incidence of spontaneous bleeding in chronic dialysis patients. Underlying responsible factors include heparinization during dialysis, oral anticoagulation to maintain shunt patency, and the bleeding tendency due to uremia (44). Sites of bleeding include the GI tract (44), the CNS (subdural hematoma), the pericardium, the pleura (45), and the retroperitoneum (46). If bleeding occurs, heparin use during dialysis should be minimized by regional heparinization or by calculating the lowest dose of heparin necessary to keep the dialyzer from clotting.

5. Air Embolism

Air embolism is always a potential hazard because of the combination of an extracorporeal blood circuit and blood pump. The incidence of air embolism is uncertain because many cases of air embolism are not reported. Clinically, patients may have shortness of breath, cough, tightness in the chest, or loss of consciousness. If air embolism occurs, the first step is to stop the infusion of air by clamping the venous return line and turning off the pump. The patient should then be turned onto the left side with the head and chest down. Oxygen should be given. The use of a compression chamber to drive the air into solution should be considered in serious cases of air embolism (47). Prevention, by attention to detail and by use of air detection alarms, is of primary importance.

Other uncommon problems include electrolyte imbalance due to improperly mixed dialysate [which may result in death (48)] and hemolysis due to copper, overheated dialysate (49), hypotonic dialysate, nitrates, or chloramines (50–52).

E. Modifications of Standard Hemodialysis

Standard hemodialysis treatment consists of three treatments per week, for 3–6 hrs per session, employing a dialyzer with 1–2 m² of surface area. Several modifications of the standard regimen have been proposed, either to prevent problems or in a search for better methods of dialysis:

1. Sequential Ultrafiltration Dialysis

Ultrafiltration across semipermeable membranes without simultaneous dialysis was used by Alwall in 1947 (53) and by Skeggs in 1952 (54), both in animal studies. In 1975, Ing performed isolated ultrafiltration in humans and observed that blood pressure did not fall during ultrafiltration nor in the following diffusion dialysis treatment (55). Sequential ultrafiltration dialysis involves separating fluid removal (ultrafiltration) from diffusive dialysis. Observations from many centers indicate that if dialysis is separated from ultrafiltration, blood pressure during the procedure is better preserved. The reasons are not completely understood. It is possible that hypotension during standard dialysis results from a fall in the plasma osmolality (25) or from an increase in blood acetate (20). Whatever the reason, sequential ultrafiltration dialysis is a useful modification to aid in fluid removal from a volume-overloaded patient with an unstable blood pressure. Ultrafiltration must be followed by a period of dialysis in order to effect adequate solute removal. During ultrafiltration solute removal is entirely by convection and is limited to the ultrafiltration rate (UFR), i.e., if UFR is 25 ml/min, clearance of urea is 25 ml/min, versus urea clearances of 150–200 ml/min during standard dialysis. Ultrafiltration alone may occasionally be useful in nonuremic patients with fluid overload.

2. Hemodiafiltration

Hemodiafiltration is a currently experimental technique developed because it was thought to more nearly mimic the performance of the human kidney than conventional hemodialysis (56). The technique involves use of an extremely permeable (noncellulosic) membrane, which allows removal of large amounts of water (UFR 100 ml/min) and larger molecular weight solutes (up to 50,000 daltons). The ultrafiltrate is replaced by a physiological electrolyte solution to prevent dehydration. Dialysate is not necessary. Advantages claimed are better control of fluid balance, better control of hypertension, and better removal of middle molecules; expense of equipment and solutions is a major disadvantage (57). The role of hemodiafiltration has not yet been established.

3. Hemoperfusion

Hemoperfusion involves perfusing the blood through a column of activated charcoal or resin absorbents rather than through a standard dialyzer. Using this procedure, solutes are removed by adherence to the column. The procedure has been used in uremia but appears to be unpromising as a method of treatment (58). Its current role is in the treatment of selected patients with drug intoxications. Hemodialysis in drug intoxication is useful only in the case of drugs that are water soluble, of small molecular weight, not highly protein bound, and present in significant concentrations in extracellular fluid. Hemoperfusion, on the other hand, may effectively remove drugs of higher molecular weight which are lipid soluble and/or bound to protein. It has been used successfully in intoxication due to digoxin (59), theophylline (60), and tricyclic antidepressants (61). The role of any form of dialytic therapy in drug intoxication may be limited (62).

TABLE V

Guidelines for Dialysis or Hemoperfusion in Intoxicated Patients[a]

Severe clinical intoxication (hypotension, hypothermia, apnea)
Ingestion or absorption of potentially lethal dose (after gastric lavage)
A drug level in blood within the lethal range
Impaired drug excretion by the normal routes, e.g., the patient is anuric or has liver disease
Circulating toxin which is metabolized to a worse substance, e.g., methanol, ethylene glycol
Progressive clinical deterioration despite less invasive treatment
Prolonged coma
Presence of an underlying disease increasing the hazards of coma: aspiration, pneumonia, chronic lung disease, etc.
Ingestion of specific agents associated with very high morbidity/mortality: methanol, ethylene glycol, paraquat, mushrooms, acetaminophen

---

[a] Adapted from "Criteria for dialysis or perfusion of intoxicated patients" with permission from J. F. Winchester, M. C. Gelfand, J. H. Knepshield, and G. E. Schreiner, Dialysis and hemoperfusion of poisons and drugs. *Trans. Am. Soc. Artif. Intern. Organs* **23,** 762–842 (1977).

Survival following drug intoxication appears to depend on supportive care to pulmonary and other complications rather than on dialytic removal (63). Table V contains guidelines which may aid in deciding whether or not to begin hemoperfusion or dialysis.

4. Immunoabsorption

Selective removal of plasma components may be the next step in the development of dialytic techniques, and, indeed, promising results have been obtained in early experiments.

A DNA collodion charcoal system was developed by Terman and associates and used for removal of immune complexes from the circulation of a patient with severe lupus glomerulonephritis (64). Serum complement normalized; serum creatinine and proteinuria improved. Postperfusion renal biopsy demonstrated a reduction in subendothelial glomerular deposits compared to a preperfusion biopsy.

Staphylococcal protein A has a strong affinity for immunoglobulin G (65). If protein A is placed in a column or in a membrane filter, IgG can be safely and effectively removed from blood perfusing the column or filter.

Such techniques may find application in the therapy of malignancies such as carcinoma, myeloma, and leukemia, as well as autoimmune diseases such as lupus.

III. PERITONEAL DIALYSIS

Peritoneal dialysis is an alternative form of renal replacement therapy which is becoming more widely used because of recent technical advances. Peritoneal dialysis was a standard method of treatment for acute renal failure in the 1940s and 1950s (66) but could not be used on a regular basis to maintain patients with chronic renal failure because of the difficulties of repeatedly inserting the dialysis catheter. Maintenance peritoneal dialysis became possible in 1972 with the development of the Tenckhoff catheter (Fig. 7), a soft, flexible, nonirritating Silastic catheter, which provided chronic access to the peritoneum and was therefore equivalent to the external shunt in hemodialysis (5, 67). At about the same time as the Tenckhoff catheter was developed, automated methods for performing peritoneal dialysis also became available and contributed to the growing popularity of the procedure by decreasing the incidence of infection and by eliminating the need for constant attention during the procedure.

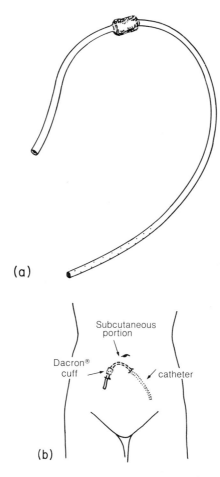

(a)

(b)

Fig. 7. (a) Tenckhoff catheter. (b) Tenckhoff catheter *in situ*. Note that the catheter exits at a point different than the insertion site via a subcutaneous tunnel.

A. Principles of Peritoneal Dialysis

The surface area of the peritoneum is probably $1-2$ m², about the same surface area as standard hemodialyzers. Solute removal occurs by diffusion from blood in peritoneal capillaries to dialyzing solution. To enter the dialyzing solution, solutes must cross the capillary wall, the capillary basement membrane, and the mesothelium. It is known that solutes up to molecular weights of 30,000 may cross the peritoneum although the mechanisms of transport have not been determined (*68, 69*). Several factors influence solute removal, including dialysate flow rate, temperature of the solution, its pH, and osmolality. Increasing dialysate flow rate increases removal of small molecules rather than large molecules. Increasing the temperature of the dialysate from room temperature (20°C) to body temperature (37°C) increases clearance by about 35% (70). Adjustments of pH have limited usefulness in increasing clearances but acid solution may cause pain on inflow which can be relieved by neutralizing it (71). Increasing the dialysate osmolality has been shown to increase solute clearances, presumably by a solvent drag effect (72).

Fluid removal in peritoneal dialysis occurs by osmosis. Dialysate has a dextrose content of 1.5 or 4.25%. The osmolality of the 1.5% solution is 345 mOsm/kg and of the 4.25% solution 490 mOsm/kg. The dextrose is poorly absorbed across the peritoneal membrane and therefore creates an osmotic gradient for fluid removal. Uremic plasma is hypertonic to normal plasma because of the presence of urea, and diabetics undergoing peritoneal dialysis may have markedly hypertonic plasma because of increases in serum glucose, making fluid removal very difficult in either case.

B. Types of Peritoneal Dialysis

Peritoneal dialysis may be considered as acute or chronic. Acute peritoneal dialysis is performed in a hospital setting and, as the name implies, is a temporary measure. Insertion of a catheter for acute peritoneal dialysis and conduct of the dialysis is covered in Section III,C.

Chronic peritoneal dialysis may be separated into chronic intermittent peritoneal dialysis (CIPD) and continuous ambulatory peritoneal dialysis. CIPD is accomplished using a machine of some type to deliver dialysate to the peritoneal cavity. The two types of machines available are the cycler and the reverse osmosis (RO) machine. The major advantage of the cycler is simplicity. A patient can be taught to perform dialysis using the cycler in 1 or 2 weeks. Basically, it operates by gravity. A number of bottles (or bags) of peritoneal dialysate, usually eight 2-liter bottles, are hung on an octopus head stand (see Fig. 8). The bottles empty simultaneously into a heater bag. The volume can be set at 1000, 1500, or 2000 ml. The solution runs from the heater bag into the patient's peritoneal cavity, remains for a preset dwell time, and then is automatically drained.

The RO machine is slightly more complex, resembling a hemodialysis machine in operation. Fluid is pumped into the peritoneal space; inflow time is set by a timer. There is a second timer that allows dwell time to be set, and a third timer that controls drain time. Dialysate is produced by the machine from a concentrate in much the same manner that dialysate is generated for hemodialysis using a proportioning pump. Learning the operation of the RO machine takes 3–4 weeks for most patients. The major

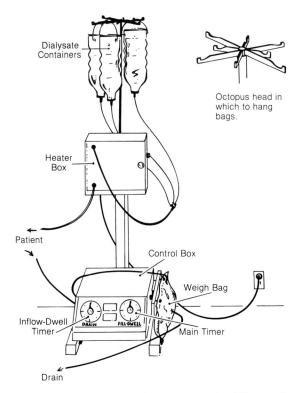

Fig. 8. Cycler dialysis machine. "Octopus" head illustrated.

advantage of the RO machine is the fact that dialysate is made from concentrate, thereby eliminating the expense of shipping or storing finished dialysate, as is necessary if the cycler is used.

Continuous peritoneal dialysis may be performed using a cycler machine, continuous cyclic peritoneal dialysis (CCPD), or without a machine using the technique of continuous ambulatory dialysis (CAPD).

CAPD is a new concept of dialysis in which patients continually dialyze themselves by infusing 2 liters of dialysate from a flexible plastic container into the peritoneum; the container is then folded and carried in a pocket or pouch for the dwell time of 4–6 hr, or overnight. During the dwell time the patient can walk about and carry on usual daily activities. At the end of the dwell time the dialysate is drained and replaced with fresh dialysate. The drainage and reinfusion usually takes 20–30 min.

The advantages of CAPD are simplicity, mobility, freedom from machinery, and an increased sense of well-being. The disadvantages are

TABLE VI

Clearance (liters/week) for Different Solutes by Various Dialysis Techniques[a]

	CCPD (4 exchanges)			CAPD (5 exchanges)	CIPD (40 hr/week)	Hemodialysis (15 hr/week)	Normal kidney
	Nocturnal	Diurnal	Total				
Urea	54.0 ± 8.2	12.7 ± 2.7	66.7	76	60	135	604
Creatinine	46.2 ± 6.8	12.5 ± 2.1	58.7	58	28	90	1008
B$_{12}$	34.8 ± 10.7	10.1 ± 1.8	44.9	50	15	30	1008

[a] Adapted from ref. 74, by permission.

susceptibility to peritonitis, lack of nondialysis days, and the fact that long-term effects of CAPD are not yet known.

CCPD is a modification of CAPD which allows patients to use a machine (cycler) to dialyze at night. When disconnecting the morning-after dialysis, 2 liters of dialysate are infused into the peritoneal space; the dialysate remains until connection is made at night for the next dialysis.

Table VI shows clearance data for the various methods of dialysis.

C. Acute Peritoneal Dialysis Procedure

Peritoneal dialysis is a relatively simple procedure which can be life saving if hemodialysis is not available. As it is a skill which most physicians caring for hospitalized patients should possess, the technique of catheter insertion and conduct of an acute peritoneal dialysis will be reviewed in detail.

Technique (*Acute Peritoneal Dialysis*)

1. Preparation
   a. Weigh patient before beginning procedure.
   b. Shave and scrub abdomen from side to side, xiphoid to pubic hair.
   c. Patient and circulating nurse wear masks. Operator and first assistant wear mask, cap, gown, and gloves (sterile procedure).
   d. Have patient void. Catheterize if necessary. Bladder must be empty.
   e. Prepare abdomen with Betadine.
   f. Thoroughly drape to create a large sterile field.

2. Insertion of the catheter
   a. Choose a spot in the midline 1–3 cm below the umbilicus. Move a few centimeters to the side of an old scar or recent wound. Unless necessary, do not traverse the rectus muscles or any other site outside the midline. Avoid reusing a recent puncture site.
   b. Infiltrate the skin, subcutaneous tissues, and the peritoneum with a local anesthetic. The peritoneum may often be found by slowly advancing the needle until the patient feels pain, and then infiltrating as the needle is withdrawn.
   c. Insert a 16 gauge needle (of the type with a plastic sheath over the needle) into the peritoneal cavity. Run in 500–1000 ml of dialysate.
   d. Make a small stab wound through the skin with a #11 blade.
   e. Heparinize the catheter-stylet to minimize clotting in the small holes in the sides of the catheter.
   f. Using firm pressure, *slowly* advance the catheter-stylet combination, using a rotating motion, at an almost perpendicular angle.
   g. *Immediately* stop forward motion when the stylet pops through the peritoneum. At this point it may be helpful to pull back the stylet a few millimeters so that the blunt catheter is now leading.
   h. Lower the catheter to a 45° angle or less, and advance it under the anterior peritoneal surface and to one side of the midline (usually the left) to avoid the bladder. Some authorities recommend advancing the catheter at nearly a perpendicular angle. Advance the catheter until all holes are within the peritoneal cavity.
   i. Quickly attach tubing (after flushing air) and infuse heparin-containing dialysate while securing cannula.
   j. A purse-string suture about the cannula may be used, but is not necessary, and is *not* sufficient to anchor the cannula.
   k. Apply local antibiotic ointment about the cannula if the patient is not allergic.
   l. Apply a bulky dressing, tape securely, and then anchor cannula with heavy tape secured to the dressing to prevent upward or downward movement.
3. Conduct of dialysis (acute)
   a. Sterile technique.
   b. Keep fluid in incubator at body temperature until ready for use. Use masks and gloves when adding medications to bottles or spiking bottles.
   c. Each 2-liter exchange should take about 50–60 min: 10 min inflow, 20–30 min dwell, 20 min outflow.
   d. Remove as much fluid as possible with each exchange and use oral and IV fluids to make up for losses if indicated.

e. Do not waste time attempting to increase fluid return volume by manipulating the patient. Fluid left in the abdomen can usually be removed on future exchanges. Occasional exchanges of 4.25% dialysate will facilitate fluid removal.

f. Detailed flow sheets of fluid balance for each exchange and a running total for the entire dialysis must be kept. Weigh patient at least every 24 hr. Weights are a better measure of fluid balance than flow sheets; the volume of a "2-liter" container of dialysate varies from 1800 to 2200 ml.

g. Culture the effluent daily.

h. Check SMA-6 and creatinine every 12 hr.

i. Stop dialysis after 48 hr because of increasing risk of peritonitis.

j. Manipulation of the catheter may occasionally be necessary for poor outflow but is best avoided.

k. Do not give prophylactic antibiotics.

l. Add 100 units of heparin to each 2-liter bottle.

m. Specify concentration of K^+ desired.

D. Complications of Peritoneal Dialysis

Complications of peritoneal dialysis may be divided into six major areas as shown in Table VII.

1. Mechanical

Pain is the most common mechanical complication. Pain in the rectal or bladder area is due to the catheter and can be corrected by repositioning it. Pain in the shoulder is referred from the diaphragm and occurs from abdominal distention due to air or excessive dialysate. Air will be absorbed over a period of days. Free air under the diaphragms is seen during every peritoneal dialysis and thus is not useful as a sign of bowel perforation. If the pain is due to excessive volume of dialysate, the volume should be reduced. Pain may occur on inflow or after drainage. Inflow pain is of uncertain etiology but often responds to 10 ml of 1% xylocaine. Pain occurring after the dialysate has drained out usually resolves spontaneously.

Bleeding is usually insignificant but may be alarming since only a small amount of blood will cause the dialysate to appear grossly bloody. If the hematocrit of the bloody effluent is greater than 1%, there is reason for concern and the patient should be watched closely (75). Transfusions or even surgical intervention may be required.

Leakage of dialysate may sometimes be so extensive as to make keeping an accurate balance impossible. Sometimes leakage can be stopped with a

TABLE VII

Complications of Peritoneal Dialysis

Mechanical
  Pain
  Bleeding, including perforation of major vessels
  Inadequate drainage
  Leakage of dialysate
  Bowel or bladder perforation
  Dissection of dialysate leading to edema or pleural effusion
  Pneumoperitoneum
Infectious
  Peritonitis
  Wound and catheter abscesses
Metabolic
  Hyperglycemia
  Hypoglycemia
  Hypertriglyceridemia
  Protein loss
  Hypokalemia
  Metabolic acidosis or alkalosis
Cardiovascular
  Overhydration or dehydration
  Arrhythmias
Pulmonary
  Atelectasis
  Pleural effusion
  Pneumonia
Neurological
  Seizures

---

purse-string suture around the catheter. In the case of a Tenckhoff catheter, leakage will often stop if dialysis is discontinued for 24 hr.

Bowel perforation is the most serious mechanical complication and occurs in about 0.1% of percutaneous peritoneal catheter insertions (76). The incidence of perforation can be minimized by a few simple precautions such as instilling 500–1000 ml of dialysate into the peritoneal cavity prior to attempting insertion of the catheter, not attempting catheter placement in an area of previous surgery, and not attempting catheter placement in anyone with a distended abdomen.

If perforation does occur, it may be recognized by failure of dialysate return, feculent peritoneal drainage, or watery diarrhea. Optimal management is not settled. Surgical exploration may be necessary. Alternatively, patients may be managed by inserting a catheter at another site and performing continuous peritoneal dialysis with intraperitoneal and systemic antibiotics. Failure to respond to medical management is certainly an indication for surgical exploration.

Subcutaneous dissection of dialysate may occur if the catheter holes are not entirely within the peritoneal cavity or may result from movement of dialysate through the hole in the peritoneum into the subcutaneous tissue. Scrotal or labial edema is the usual result. The edema usually resolves with temporary discontinuation of dialysis.

2. Infections

Peritonitis is the most important infectious complication and is also the major factor limiting widespread acceptance of peritoneal dialysis as a method of treating chronic renal failure.

The incidence of peritonitis varies from 6% in acute dialysis to 1% in CIPD, with two to six episodes per patient per year for continuous ambulatory dialysis (10, 77, 78). Bacteria appear to gain entry to the peritoneum *through* the catheter, not outside the catheter along the catheter tract; thus, using sterile technique during dialysis is the most important step to take in preventing peritonitis. Masks and gloves should be worn when spiking bottles or adding medication to bottles.

Peritonitis should be suspected in any patient with fever, abdominal pain, tenderness, discomfort, or cloudy peritoneal fluid. A specimen of fluid should be immediately sent for gram stain, cell count, and culture. Cell counts of greater than $300/mm^3$ in the initial outflow are usually found with peritonitis. If the dialysis has been running for some time, fewer than 300 cells may indicate infection. The proportion of polymorphonuclear cells and mononuclear cells is also important; mononuclear cells appear to be a peritoneal defense mechanism so an increase in cell count due to an increase in mononuclear cells may indicate resolution of the infection.

Treatment of peritonitis should be started once appropriate cultures have been obtained. In mild episodes of peritonitis there may be only a small number of bacteria in the peritoneal fluid. The larger the volume of fluid cultured, the greater the chance of a positive culture. Specimens may be concentrated by centrifugation or Millipore filter, making it possible to culture 50–100 ml of fluid (79). If gram-positive cocci are present, the organism is almost certain to be a staphylococcus and treatment is begun with a penicillinase-resistant penicillin, cephalosporin, or vancomycin. If gram-negative organisms are seen, treatment is with an aminoglycoside. If no organisms are seen on gram stain, both an aminoglycoside and an anti-staphylococcal drug should be used. The antibiotics are added to the dialysate in a concentration that equals the desired serum concentration (see Table VIII). For instance, 5 mg/liter of gentamicin produces a serum level of 5 μg/ml, the therapeutic level. Likewise, 50 mg/liter of cephalothin produces

TABLE VIII

Antibiotic Concentrations in Peritoneal Fluid
for Treatment of Peritonitis

	Recommended dose	
Antibiotic	IPD (mg/liter)	CAPD (mg/liter)
Cephalothin	50	200–250
Ampicillin	50	50
Kanamycin	10	100
Gentamicin	5–8	5–8
Tobramycin	5–8	5–8
Carbenicillin	200	[a]
Penicillin	8–50,000 U	50,000
	(1 U = 1.6 mg)	
Cloxacillin	100	100
Methicillin	100	100
Vancomycin	15	30
5-Fluorocytosine	50	50
Amphotericin	2–4	[a]
Chloramphenicol	[b]	
Clindamycin	[a]	

[a] No data.
[b] Ineffective.

a serum level of 50 μg/ml. Where possible, it is a good idea to check serum levels frequently. Parenteral loading doses should probably be used although some investigators feel they are unnecessary.

Infections may also occur along the catheter tract including the exit site. Such infections are difficult to eradicate but may respond to meticulous local care and systemic antibiotics. Catheter replacement should be undertaken only after failure of medical therapy.

Infection with hepatitis B virus is a serious problem since the virus is contained in high concentrations in the peritoneal fluid and can be transmitted (80). Patients on chronic peritoneal dialysis should be regularly tested for the virus and the test should be performed on patients undergoing acute peritoneal dialysis as well.

3. Pulmonary

Pneumonia and atelectasis are thought to occur because of abdominal distention limiting respiratory excursion (81). Patients should be encouraged to cough and breathe deeply. It may be necessary to decrease the exchange volume to one liter if abdominal distention occurs. Pleural effusion is most frequent on the right side and is thought to occur because of movement of dialysate through diaphragmatic defects (82).

4. Cardiovascular

Cardiovascular complications can generally be prevented by close attention to detail. The patient's volume status should be assessed frequently for signs of overhydration or volume depletion. Bradyarrhythmias may occur because of increased vagal tone due to abdominal distention and can be prevented by using a smaller exchange volume (83).

5. Neurological

Neurological complications are infrequent with peritoneal dialysis. The disequilibrium syndrome, common in hemodialysis, is uncommon in peritoneal dialysis. The slow rate of solute removal probably prevents dialysis-associated neurological syndromes. When neurological disturbances are seen in peritoneal dialysis, an infection or metabolic disturbance should be suspected.

6. Metabolic

Hyperglycemia is a common complication of peritoneal dialysis. During a 1 hr exchange, about 10 g of glucose are absorbed from 2 liters of 1.5% solution, and up to 50 g from 2 liters of 4.25% solution (84, 85). To prevent hyperglycemia it is necessary to monitor the serum glucose closely (every 12–24 hr, initially and use insulin if necessary.

Hypoglycemia may result if insulin is added to the dialysate due to delayed absorption of insulin compared to glucose (86). This is not necessarily a contraindication to the use of intraperitoneal insulin, and many patients on chronic peritoneal dialysis use intraperitoneal insulin safely and effectively. Reactive hypoglycemia due to *endogenous* insulin has been reported (87).

Protein loss during peritoneal dialysis may be severe enough to cause nephrotic syndrome, but usually protein losses become minimal with repeated dialysis. Patients who are stable on chronic intermittent peritoneal dialysis lose only 0.1 g protein per liter of effluent, an amount that can be replaced by diet without great difficulty. Patients on CAPD may lose about 9 g of protein per 24 hr. Most patients eating 1.0 g/kg/day of protein are in positive nitrogen balance, so to err on the side of safety, patients on chronic peritoneal dialysis are encouraged to ingest 1.2–1.5 g/kg/day of protein (88).

IV. RESULTS OF DIALYSIS

There is no doubt that survival of patients on hemodialysis has improved dramatically over the past few years. It is a national disgrace that since 1977, when the Health Care Financing Administration took over the ESRD program, medical information about dialysis patients in the United States has been practically nonexistent. Current morbidity and mortality data are therefore only available from scattered reports of individual centers and from the European Dialysis and Transplant Association statistics. In Europe, mortality of hemodialysis patients during the first year of dialysis has decreased from 36.2% in 1965 to 15% in 1978 (*89*). In the United States, the mortality rate among chronic dialysis patients appears to be about 10% per year. Certain groups of dialysis patients fare less well than others; thus, older patients have a poorer survival rate than younger patients (*90*); patients with diabetes mellitus have a much poorer survival rate on hemodialysis. There are not many data regarding survival of diabetics on peritoneal dialysis but some investigators feel CAPD offers some hope of improved survival and improved quality of life for the diabetic patient (*91*). There is surprisingly little information about rehabilitation of patients with ESRD. Gutman and colleagues (*92*) gathered data on some 2482 patients at 18 dialysis centers scattered across the United States and analyzed it in terms of physical activity and employment. They found only 60% of the nondiabetic patients and 23% of the diabetic patients to be capable of physical activity beyond caring for themselves at home. Twenty percent of the nondiabetics and 51% of the diabetics were unable to care for themselves. Twenty-five percent of patients worked outside the home. They concluded that debilitation among dialysis patients was much more severe than previously suspected. A previous report (*93*), for instance, suggested that as many as 60–80% of patients on hemodialysis were able to achieve a "nearly normal life style." Since Gutman's study is broad based, it is likely that the figures more nearly reflect the true situation than the earlier study dealing with a selected population.

It appears, then, that rehabilitation lags far behind improved survival and is deserving of increased attention from all health professionals working in renal-related fields. In addition, the severe debilitation has profound implications regarding the psychological health of the patient on chronic dialysis.

REFERENCES

1. Abel, J. J., Rowntree, L. G., and Turner, B. B. On the removal of diffusible substances from the circulating blood by means of dialysis. *Trans. Assoc. Am. Physicians* **28**, 51–62 (1913).
2. Kolff, W. J. First clinical experience with the artificial kidney. *Ann. Intern. Med.* **62**, 608–619 (1965).
3. Popovich, R. P., Moncrief, J. W., Decherd, J. F., Bomar, J. B., and Pyle, W. K. The definition of a novel portable/wearable equilibrium peritoneal dialysis technique. *Trans. Am. Soc. Artif. Intern. Organs* **5**, 64 (abstr.) (1976).

4. Quinton, W., Dillard, D., and Scribner, B. H. Cannulation of blood vessels for prolonged hemodialysis. *Trans. Am. Soc. Artif. Intern. Organs* **6**, 104–107 (1960).

5. Tenckhoff, H., and Schechter, H. A bacteriologically safe peritoneal access device. *Trans. Am. Soc. Artif. Intern. Organs* **14**, 181–187 (1968).

6. Moncrief, J. Guest interview. *Contemp. Dial.* **5**, 22–31 (1981).

7. Rettig, R. A. "Implementing the End-Stage Renal Disease Program of Medicare," R-2505-HCFA/HEW, pp. 1–255. Rand Corp., 1980.

8. Rettig R. A. The politics of health cost containment: End-stage renal disease. *Bull. N. Y. Acad. Med.* [2] **56**, 115–138 (1980).

9. Nolph, K. D. Continuous ambulatory peritoneal dialysis. *Am. J. Nephrol.* **1**, 1–10 (1981).

10. Rubin, J., Rogers, W. A., Taylor, H. M., Everett, D., Prowant, B. F., Fruto, L. V., and Nolph, K. D. Peritonitis during chronic ambulatory peritoneal dialysis. *Ann. Intern. Med.* **92**, 7–13 (1980).

11. Rostand, S. G., Gretes, J. C., Kirk, K. A., Rutsky, R. A., and Andreoli, T. E. Ischemic heart disease in patients with uremia undergoing maintenance hemodialysis. *Kidney Int.* **16**, 600–611 (1979).

12. Van Stone, J. C., Bauer, J., and Carey, J. The effect of dialysate sodium concentration on body fluid distribution during hemodialysis. *Trans. Am. Soc. Artif. Intern. Organs* **26**, 383–386 (1980).

13. Ogden, D. A. A double blind crossover comparison of high and low sodium dialysis. *Proc.—Clin. Dial. Transplant Forum* **8**, 157–164 (1978).

14. Kohn, R. M., Kiley, J. E. Electrocardiographic changes during hemodialysis, with observations on contribution of electrolyte disturbances to digitalis toxicity. *Ann. Intern. Med.* **39**, 38–50 (1953).

15. Johny, K. V., Lawrence, J. R., O'Halloran, M. W., and Wellby, M. L., Effect of haemodialysis on erythrocyte and plasma potassium, magnesium, sodium, and calcium. *Nephron* **8**, 81–90 (1971).

16. Eastwood, J. B., Bordier, P. J., and DeWardener, H. Some biochemical, histological, radiological, and clinical features of renal osteodystrophy. *Kidney Int.* **4**, 128–140 (1973).

17. Johnson, W. J. Optimum dialysate calcium concentration during maintenance hemodialysis. *Nephron* **17**, 241–258 (1976).

18. David, D. S. Calcium metabolism in renal failure. *Am. J. Med.* **58**, 48–56 (1975).

19. Catto, G. R. D., Reid, I. W., and MacLeod, M. The effect of low magnesium dialysate on plasma, ultrafilterable erythrocyte and bone magnesium concentrations from patients on maintenance haemodialysis. *Nephron* **13**, 372–381 (1974).

20. Aizawa, Y., Ohmari, T., Imai, K., Nara, Y., Matsuoka, M., and Hirasawa, Y. Depressant action of acetate upon the human cardiovascular system. *Clin. Nephrol.* **8**, 477–480 (1977).

21. Kirkendol, P. L., Devia, C. J., Bower, J. D., and Holbert, R. D. A comparison of the cardiovascular effects of sodium acetate, sodium bicarbonate, and other potential sources of fixed base in hemodialysate solutions. *Trans. Am. Soc. Artif. Intern. Organs* **23**, 399–405 (1977).

22. Graefe, U. J., Milutinovich, W. C., Follette, J. E., Nizzo, J. E., Babb, A. L., and Scribner, B. H. Less dialysis-induced morbidity and vascular instability with bicarbonate in dialysate. *Ann. Intern. Med.* **88**, 332–336 (1978).

23. Kolff, W. J. "New Ways of Treating Uremia." Churchill, London, 1947.

24. Henderson, L. W. Symptomatic hypotension during hemodialysis. *Kidney Int.* **17**, 571–576 (1980).

25. Kjellstrand, C. M. Current problems in long-term hemodialysis. *Dial. Transplant.* **9**, 295–299 (1980).

26. Kersh, E. S., Kronfield, S. J., Unger, A. Popper, R. W., Cantor, S., and Cohn, K. Autonomic insufficiency in uremia as a cause of hemodialysis-induced hypotension. *N. Engl. J. Med.* **290**, 650–653 (1974).

27. Lilley, J. J., Golden, J., and Stone, R. A. Adrenergic regulation of blood pressure in chronic renal failure. *J. Clin. Invest.* **57**, 1190–1200 (1976).

28. Bergstrom, J., Asaba, H., Furst, P., and Oules, R. Dialysis, ultrafiltration, and blood pressure. *Proc. Eur. Dial. Transplant Assoc.* **13**, 243–305 (1976).

29. Shaldon, S., Deschodt, G., Bean, M. C., Claret, G., Mion, H., and Mion, C. Vascular stability during high-flux haemofiltration. *Proc. Eur. Dial. Transplant Assoc.* **16**, 695–697 (1979).

30. Stewart, W. K., and Fleming, Mannel, M. A. Muscle cramps during haemodialysis. *Lancet* **1**, 1049–1051 (1972).

31. Van Stone, J., and Cook, J. Decreased postdialysis fatigue with increased dialysate sodium concentration. *Proc.—Clin. Dial. Transplant Forum* **8**, 152–155 (1978).

32. Arieff, A. I., Massry, S. G., Barrientos, A., and Kleeman, C. R. Brain water and electrolyte metabolism in uremia: Effects of slow and rapid hemodialysis. *Kidney Int.* **4**, 177–187 (1973).

33. Kennedy, A. C., Linton, A. L., Luke, R. G., Renfrew, S., and Dinwoodie, A. The pathogenesis and prevention of cerebral dysfunction during dialysis. *Lancet* **1**, 790–793 (1964).

34. Leonard, A., and Shapiro, F. L. Subdural hematoma in regularly hemodialyzed patients. *Ann. Intern. Med.* **82**, 650–658 (1975).

35. Bechar, M., Lakke, J. P., Van der Hem, G. K., Beks, J. W. F., and Penning, L. Subdural hematoma during long-term hemodialysis. *Arch. Neurol.* (*Chicago*) **26**, 513–516 (1972).

36. Latos, D. L., Stone, W. J., and Alford, R. H. Staphylococcus aureus bacteremia in hemodialysis patients. *J. Dial.* **1**, 399–418 (1977).

37. Dobkin, J. F., Miller, M. H., and Steigbigel, N. H. Septicemia in patients on chronic hemodialysis. *Ann. Intern. Med.* **88**, 28–33 (1978).

38. Hindman, S. H., Carson, L. A., Favero, M. S., Petersen, N. J., Schonberger, L. B., and Solano, J. J. Pyrogenic reactions during haemodialysis caused by extramural endotoxin. *Lancet* **2**, 732–734 (1975).

39. Raij, L., Shapiro, F. L., and Michael, A. F. Endotoxemia in febrile reactions during hemodialysis. *Kidney Int.* **4**, 57–60 (1973).

40. Hourani, M. R., Mayor, G. H., Greenbaum, D. S., Hugget, D. O., and Patterson, M. J. Hepatitis B surface antigen in urine of hemodialysis patients. *Kidney Int.* **13**, 324–328 (1978).

41. Szmuness, W., Prince, A. M., Grady, G. F., Mann, M. K., Levine, R. W., Friedman, E. A., Jacobs, M. J., Josephson, A., Ribot, S., Shapiro, F. Stenzel, K., Suki, W. N., and Vyas, G. Hepatitis B infection: A point-prevalence study in 15 U.S. hemodialysis centers. *JAMA* **227**, 901–906 (1974).

41a. Garibaldi, R. A., Forrest, J. N., and Bryan, J. A. Hemodialysis-associated hepatitis. *JAMA* **225**, 384–389 (1973).

42. London, W. T., DiFiglia, M., Sutnick, A. I., and Blumberg, B. S. An epidemic of hepatitis in a chronic hemodialysis unit: Australian antigen and differences in host response. *N. Engl. J. Med.* **281**, 571–578 (1969).

43. Prince, A. M., Szmuness, W., Mann, M. K., Vyas, G., Grady, G. F., Shapiro, F. L., Suki, W. N., Friedman, A., and Stenzel, K. H. Hepatitis B "immune" globulin: Effectiveness in prevention of dialysis-associated hepatitis. *N. Engl. J. Med.* **293**, 1063–1067 (1975).

44. Stewart, J. H., Tuckwell, L. A., and Sinnett, P. F. Peritoneal and haemodialysis: A comparison of their morbidity and of the mortality suffered by dialyzed patients. *Q. J. Med.* **35**, 407–420 (1965).

45. Galen, M. A., Steinberg, S. M., Lowrie, E. G., Lazarus, J. M., Hampers, C. L., Merrill, J. P. Hemorrhagic pleural effusion in patients undergoing chronic hemodialysis. *Ann. Intern. Med.* **82,** 359–361 (1975).

46. Milutinovich, J., Follette, W. C., and Scribner, B. H. Spontaneous retroperitoneal bleeding in patients on chronic hemodialysis. *Ann. Intern. Med.* **86,** 189–192 (1977).

47. Ward, M. K., Shadfurth, M., Hill, A. V., and Kerr, D. N. S. Air embolism during haemodialysis. *Br. Med. J.* **3,** 74–78 (1971).

48. Weiner, M., and Epstein, F. H. Signs and symptoms of electrolyte disorders. *Yale J. Biol. Med.* **43,** 76–109 (1970).

49. Berkes, S. L., Kash, S. I., Chazan, J. A., and Garella, S. Prolonged hemolysis from overheated dialysate. *Ann. Intern. Med.* **83,** 363–364 (1975).

50. Carlson, D. J., and Shapiro, G. L. Methemoglobinemia from well water nitrates: A complication of home dialysis. *Ann. Intern. Med.* **73,** 757–759 (1970).

51. Eaton, J. W., Kolpin, C. F., Swofford, H. S., Kjellstrand, G. M., and Jacobs, H. S. Chlorinated water: A cause of dialysis-induced hemolytic anemia. *Science* **181,** 463–464 (1973).

52. Orringer, E. P., and Mattern, W. D. Formaldehyde-induced hemolysis during chronic hemodialysis. *N. Engl. J. Med.* **294,** 1416–1420 (1976).

53. Alwall, N. On the artificial kidney. I. Apparatus for dialysis of the blood in vivo. *Acta Med. Scand.* **128,** 317–325 (1947).

54. Skeggs, L. T., Leonards, J. R., and Kahn, J. R. Removal of fluid from normal and edematous dogs by continuous ultrafiltration of fluid. *Lab. Invest.* **1,** 488–494 (1952).

55. Ing, T. S., Ashbach, D. L., Kanter, A., Oyama, J. H., Armbruster, K. F. W., and Merkel, F. K. Fluid removal with negative-pressure hydrostatic ultrafiltration using a partial vacuum. *Nephron* 1975; **14,** 451–455 (1975).

56. Henderson, L., Besarab, A., Michaels, A., and Bluemle, L. W. Blood purification by ultrafiltration and fluid replacement (diafiltration). *Trans. Am. Soc. Artif. Intern. Organs* **12,** 216–226 (1967).

57. Kopp, K. F. Hemofiltration. *Nephron* **20,** 65–74 (1978).

58. Chang, T. M. S. Microencapsulated absorbent hemoperfusion for uremia, intoxication, and hepatic failure. *Kidney Int.* **7,** S387–S392 (1975).

59. Smiley, J. W., March, N. M., and Del Anercio, E. T. Hemoperfusion in the management of digoxin toxicity. *JAMA* **20,** 2736–2737 (1978).

60. Russo, M. E. Management of theophylline intoxication with charcoal column hemoperfusion. *N. Engl. J. Med.* **30,** 24–26 (1979).

61. Diaz-Buxo, J. A., Farmer, C. D., and Chandler, J. T. Hemoperfusion in the treatment of amitriptyline intoxication. *Trans. Am. Soc. Artif. Intern. Organs* **24,** 699–703 (1978).

62. Farrell, P. C. Acute drug intoxication and extracorporeal intervention. *ASAIO J.* **3,** 39–42 (1980).

63. Lorch, J. A., and Garella, S. Hemoperfusion to treat intoxications. *Ann. Intern. Med.* **91,** 301–303 (1979).

64. Terman, D. S., Buffaloe, G., Maltioli, C., Cook, G., Tilquist, R., Sullivan, M., and Ayus, J. C. Extracorporeal immunoabsorption: Initial experience in human systemic lupus erythematosus. *Lancet* **2,** 824–826 (1979).

65. Bansal, S. C., Bansal, B. R., Thomas, H. L., Siegel, P. D., Rhoads, J. E., Cooper, D. R., and Terman, D. S. Ex vivo removal of serum IgG in a patient with colon carcinoma: Some biochemical, immunological, and histological observations. *Cancer* **42,** 1–18 (1978).

66. Maxwell, M. H., Rockney, R. E., Kleeman, C. R., and Twiss, M. R. Peritoneal dialysis. I. Technique and applications. *JAMA* **170,** 917–924 (1959).

67. Striker, G. E., and Tenckhoff, H. A. A transcutaneous prosthesis for prolonged access to the peritoneal cavity. *Surgery* **67,** 70–74 (1971).

68. Putnam, T. J. The living peritoneum as a dialyzing membrane. *Am. J. Physiol.* **63**, 54–65 (1922).

69. Karnovsky, M. J. The ultrastructural basis of capillary permeability studied with peroxides as a tracer. *J. Cell Biol.* **35**, 213–236 (1967).

70. Miller, R. B., and Tassistro, C. R. Peritoneal dialysis. *N. Engl. J. Med.* **281**, 945–949 (1969).

71. Tenckhoff, H. "Chronic Peritoneal Dialysis Manual." Division of Kidney Diseases, Department of Medicine, University of Washington School of Medicine, Seattle, Copyright 1974.

72. Brown, E. A., Kliger, A. S., Goffinet, J., and Finkelstein, F. O. Effect of hypertonic dialysate and vasodilators on peritoneal dialysis clearances in the rat. *Kidney Int.* **13**, 271–277 (1978).

73. Price, C. G., and Suki, W. N. Newer modifications of peritoneal dialysis: Options in the treatment of patients with renal failure. *Am. J. Nephrol.* **1**, 97–104 (1981).

74. Diaz-Buxo, J. A., Farmer, C. D., Walker, P. J., Chandler, J. T., and Holt, K. L. Continuous peritoneal dialysis: A preliminary report. *Int. Soc. Artif. Organs* **5**(2) (1981).

75. Henderson, L. W. Hemodialysis. *In* "Strauss and Welt's Diseases of the Kidney" (L. E. Earley and C. W. Gottschalk, eds.), 3rd ed.,pp. 421–462. Little, Brown, Boston, Massachusetts, 1979.

76. Rubin, J., Oreopoulos, D. G., Lio, T. T., Mathews, R., and DeVeber, G. A. Management of peritonitis and bowel perforation during chronic peritoneal dialysis. *Nephron* **16**, 220–225 (1976).

77. Vaamonde, C. A., and Perez, G. O. Peritoneal dialysis today. *Kidney* **10**, 31–35 (1977).

78. Robson, M. D., and Oreopoulos, D. G. Continuous ambulatory peritoneal dialysis, a revolution in the treatment of chronic renal failure. *Dial. Transplant.* **7**, 999–1003 (1978).

79. Nolph, K. D., and Serbin, M. I. Diagnosis and treatment of peritonitis. *In* "CAPD Update" (J. W. Moncrief and R. P. Popovich, eds.), pp. 265–272. Masson, New York, 1981.

80. Oreopoulos, D. G. Hepatitis and treatment of chronic renal failure by peritoneal dialysis. *Lancet* **2**, 1256 (1972).

81. Berlyne, G. M., Lee, H. A., Ralston, A. J., and Woolcock, J. A. Pulmonary complications of peritoneal dialysis. *Lancet* **2**, 75–78 (1966).

82. Edwards, S. R., and Unger, A. M. Acute hydrothorax—A new complication of peritoneal dialysis. *JAMA* **199**, 853–855 (1967).

83. Rutsky, E. A. Bradycardic rhythms during peritoneal dialysis. *Arch. Intern. Med.* **128**, 445–447 (1971).

84. Boyer, J., Gill, G. M., and Epstein, F. H. Hyperglycemia and hyperosmolality complicating peritoneal dialysis. *Ann. Intern. Med.* **67**, 568–573 (1967).

85. Rubin, J. Comments on dialysis solution composition, antibiotic transport, poisoning, and novel uses of peritoneal dialysis. *In* "Peritoneal Dialysis" (K. Nolph, ed.), pp. 240–274. Martinus Nijhoff, The Hague, 1981.

86. Shapiro, D. J., Blumenkranz, M. J., Levin, S. R., and Coburn, J. Absorption and action of insulin added to peritoneal dialysate in dogs. *Nephron* **23**, 174–180 (1979).

87. Greenblatt, D. J. Fatal hypoglycemia occurring after peritoneal dialysis. *Br. Med. J.* **2**, 270–271 (1972).

88. Blumenkranz, M. J., and Gakl, G. M. Protein loss during peritoneal dialysis. *Kidney Int.* **19**, 593–602 (1981).

89. Wing, A. J., Brunner, F. P., Brynger, H., Chantler, C., Donckerwolcke, R. A., Gurland, H. S. Hathway, R. A., Jacobs, C., and Selwood, N. H. Combined report in regular dialysis and transplantation in Europe. *Proc. Eur. Dial. Transplant Assoc.* **15**, 3–77 (1978).

90. Walker, P. J., Ginn, H. E., Johnson, H. K., Stone, W. J., Teschan, P. E., Latos, D., Stouder, D., Lamberth, E. L., and O'Brien, K. Long-term hemodialysis for patients over 50. *Geriatrics* **31,** 55–61 (1976).
91. Amair, P., Khanna, R., Leibel, B., Pierratos, A., Vas, S., Meema, E., Blair, O. Chisholm, L., Vas, M., Zingg, W., Digenis, O., and Dimitrios, O. Continuous ambulatory peritoneal dialysis in diabetes with end stage renal disease. *N. Engl. J. Med.* **306,** 625–630 (1982).
92. Gutman, R. A., Stead, W. W., and Robinson, R. R. Physical activity and employment status of patients on maintenance dialysis. *N. Engl. J. Med.* **304,** 309–313 (1981).
93. Jenkins, P. G., Gutmann, F. D., and Rieselbach, R. E. Self-hemodialysis: The optimal mode of dialytic therapy. *Arch. Intern. Med.* **136,** 357–361 (1976).

9

Technical Aspects of Dialysis

PATRICK E. HOPKINS

I. INTRODUCTION

Dialysis is a treatment in which technical knowledge and skills are of the utmost importance. This chapter will describe ways and means in which technical expertise is invaluable in understanding and operating dialysis systems. These skills and knowledge also may be taught to the patient and his assistant in home or limited-care dialysis. Reuse of dialyzers and effective methods of water treatment are two examples of the technological contributions to safer and less costly dialysis. Well-trained dialysis technologists and

219

END-STAGE RENAL DISEASE

ISBN 0-12-672280-3

technicians are an essential component of any end-stage renal disease (ESRD) treatment program.

II. WATER TREATMENT

The preparation of large volumes of water suitable for hemodialysis has become a problem for many hemodialysis centers. This is due to the varying minerals and other contaminants in tap water. Hemodialysis patients are exposed to 100 times the normal daily intake of water during an average hemodialysis treatment. Therefore, it is necessary to carefully plan a water purification system capable of removing the minerals and other contaminants.

A. Filters

Filters can provide adequate removal of particulate matter from water used to prepare dialysate and are of three types: (a) Sand filters consist of a layer of sand of varying size to remove suspended particles that range from 25 to 100 μm. (b) Cartridge filters are usually the honeycomb or cellulose type that are capable of removing particles that vary from 1 to 100 μm in size. (c) Submicron or membrane filters which are capable of removing particles down to 0.25 μm. It is generally accepted that 5 μm filters are necessary to provide protection for water treatment and proportioning equipment.

B. Activated Carbon Filters

Carbon filters will absorb chlorine, chloramines, odor-producing materials, and pyrogens from water. These carbon filters will not remove salts since there are no charged groups to bond with the salt ions. Since carbon filters are highly porous and have a high affinity for organic material, they can become contaminated with bacteria if they are not serviced properly or exchanged frequently.

C. Water Softeners

Water softening is a method used to remove calcium, magnesium, and certain other polyvalent cations from the water supply. Water softeners are usually sodium forms of cation exchange resins. The resins are charged with sodium ions which exchange with calcium and magnesium. The latter are removed from the water and the sodium goes into the water in equivalent amounts. In instances in which the water is extremely hard (high calcium and magnesium content), the amount of sodium released may become a serious problem. The amount of sodium added to the water supply will need to be checked in order to determine if additional water treatment is necessary. The amount of sodium that is released can be calculated by the following formula.

Na (mEq/liter) = Total hardness as $CaCO_3$ (mg/liter)/50

When all the available sodium ions have been exchanged, the resin is exhausted. Regeneration is accomplished by using a brine solution produced from sodium chloride, usually in the form of rock salt.

D. Deionizers

Deionizers also work on the ion exchange principle; however, the deionizer removes all types of cations and anions. Deionization is accomplished by using both a cation exchange and an anion exchange resin (mix-bed system). The cation exchange resin is in the hydrogen ion (H^+) form instead of the sodium ion (Na^+) form used in water softeners. The anion exchange resin is in the hydroxyl ion (OH^-) form. As the water enters the mix-bed system, the cations (e.g., Na^+, K^+, Mg^{2+}) are exchanged for the H^+ on the cation resin and the anions (e.g., HCO_3^-, Cl^-, SO_4^{2-}, F^-) are exchanged with the OH^- ion on the anion resin. The hydrogen and hydroxyl ions released combine to form water.

The dual-bed system consists of two tanks. One tank contains the cation resin and the other tank contains the anion resin. This type of treatment does not result in as good a quality of water as the mix-bed system; however, since more water is treated before the tank exhausts, it is less expensive. In the mix-bed tank, as the name implies, the cation and anion resins are mixed together in the same tank. This system will produce a water quality considerably in excess of one million ohms specific resistance, whereas the dual-bed results in water with a specific resistance of 200,000–500,000 ohms. Deionization is effective and generally safe; however, significant problems can occur in these systems. Deionization tanks that are near exhaustion will allow ions to pass through that were previously absorbed on the resin. As more ions become available the incoming chloride ions will displace fluoride ions on the resin. The result is a higher concentration of fluoride in the treated than in the untreated water, subjecting the patient to a great exposure to this ion. In a similar manner other cations can displace aluminum from the resin, resulting in exposure to toxic levels of aluminum. The cation and the anion resins generally will not become exhausted at the same time. For example, if the cation resin continues to exchange the H^+ ion for the Na^+ ion and the

H^+ ion is passed into an exhausted anion (OH^-) resin, the increasing H^+ concentration will markedly decrease the pH of the water.

E. Reverse Osmosis

The use of reverse osmosis in dialysis units has increased substantially during recent years. Reverse osmosis utilizes a semipermeable membrane, which will remove bacterial and pyrogens as well as a great percentage of dissolved salts. The dissolved salt ions are rejected by the reverse osmosis membrane in direct relation to their valences. Therefore, 90–95% of the univalent ions (e.g., Na^+ and K^+) and 95–98% of the divalent ions (e.g., Ca^{2+} and Mg^{2+}) are rejected by the membrane. Accordingly, 2–10% of the dissolved ions will pass through the membrane into the product water to be made into dialysate. Reverse osmosis generally produces water that is safe for dialysis, but in some instances the quantity of the dissolved salts allowed to pass may exceed the maximum safety concentrations.

The reverse osmosis membranes are sensitive to several factors: (a) The temperature of the incoming water supply. Cold feed water to the system will result in a decrease in the volume of product water. The feed water may need to be warmed in order to achieve adequate water production. (b) Cellulose acetate (spiral wound) and the polyamide aromatic (hollow fiber) are the two types of membranes most commonly used in reverse osmosis systems. Both of these membranes are affected by excessive amounts of hardness and chlorine in the feed water. The cellulose acetate membrane is more sensitive to pH changes than the hollow fiber. A pH in excess of 8 deacetylates this membrane. The hollow fiber membrane is insensitive to bacterial attack; however, plugging of the membrane fibers may occur. A relatively new type of reverse osmosis membrane (thin-film composite membrane), which shares some of the properties of both the cellulose acetate and polyamide membranes, has recently become available. This membrane will tolerate a wider pH range (3–11) than the cellulose acetate membrane and is more resistant to chlorine than the polyamide membrane. In view of the above limitations, reverse osmosis should not be used as the only system for treating water unless the feed water is of exceptionally high quality. If adequate pretreatment is employed, such as filtration and softening, reverse osmosis will often produce water of adequate purity without the necessity of subsequent deionization.

To determine what type of water treatment equipment will be needed, an analysis must be obtained to determine which minerals and chemicals exist in the water supply. Figure 1 shows a water treatment that will be suitable for hemodialysis.

The American Society for Artificial Internal Organs and Association for the Advancement of Medical Instrumentation Kidney Standards subcom-

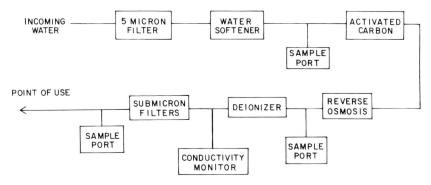

Fig. 1. Water purification system for hemodialysis.

mittee has suggested that water used to prepare dialysate should meet the following requirements:

1. Total viable microbial count shall not exceed 200 per ml.
2. If a deionizer system is used to prepare water for dialysate, the product water should be monitored continuously to produce water of 1 megohm or greater specific resistivity at 25°C.
3. If a reverse osmosis system is used to prepare water for dialysate, the system should be monitored continuously. The salt passage rate (i.e., 100%

TABLE I

Maximum Allowable Concentrations of Solutes in Water Used to Prepare Dialysate

Contaminant	Maximum allowable level (mg/liter)
Calcium	2 (0.1 mEq/liter)
Magnesium	4 (0.3 mEq/liter)
Sodium	70 (3 mEq/liter)
Potassium	8 (0.2 mEq/liter)
Fluoride	0.2
Chlorine	0.5
Chloramines	0.1
Nitrates (N)	2
Sulfate	100
Copper, barium, zinc	Each 0.1
Aluminum	0.01
Arsenic, lead, silver	Each 0.005
Cadmium	0.001
Chromium	0.014
Selenium	0.09
Mercury	.0002

minus the rejection rate) should not exceed two times the salt passage rate of the equipment at the time of the initial testing.

4. The chemical contaminants in the water used to prepare dialysate shall not exceed those in Table I, except where the physician in charge of dialysis has directed.

III. HEMODIALYSIS SYSTEMS

Current dialysate delivery systems are of two basic types: the recirculating single pass and the single pass. Both systems can be designed to deliver dialysate to one or more hemodialyzers at the proper temperature, conductivity, pressure, and flow. Monitors are also incorporated into each system to control fluid removal across the dialyzer membrane surface and to detect blood leaks in the membrane and pressure changes in the blood circuit.

A. Recirculating Single Pass

This system mixes used dialysate in a circuit with fresh dialysate which is being pumped continuously from a supply tank. This constant infusion of fresh dialysate causes the dialysate in the circuit to overflow to a drain (Fig. 2).

Recirculating single pass systems generally use the coil dialyzers and are referred to as a positive pressure system. The dialysate pressure in the coil dialyzer is zero or slightly positive. The blood compartment pressure is positive, but is inadequate for much fluid removal. Venous line clamps

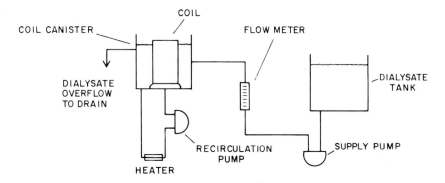

Fig. 2.   Flow diagram of a recirculating single pass system.

and/or addition of dextrose to the dialysate will result in ultrafiltration at acceptable levels.

B. Single Pass

In the single pass system purified water and concentrated electrolyte solution are mixed together in correct proportions by a pumping mechanism to form dialysate or proper concentration. The concentration of salt in the dialysate is continuously monitored by a conductivity meter, which indicates the ionic content (Fig. 3).

The single pass systems are used in conjunction with hollow fiber or flat plate dialyzers, and are referred to as negative pressure systems since the pressure in the dialysate compartment is negative. The negative pressure pump creates a vacuum or negative hydrostatic pressure, which pulls water through the membrane. The pressure in the blood compartment is positive, and forces water across the membrane from the blood into the dialysate. When necessary the positive pressure in the blood compartment can be increased by placing a clamp on the venous line. The average pressure in the blood compartment minus the average pressure in the dialysate compartment is the transmembrane hydrostatic pressure (TMP).

The single patient negative pressure system is located at the patient's bedside. The dialysate preparation can be adjusted according to the patient's needs. In addition to monitoring the conductivity and temperature, the blood circuit is also monitored with accessories which have been integrated into the system. Typical devices are heparin pumps, blood pumps, air detectors, blood leak detectors, drip chamber holders, and dialyzer holders.

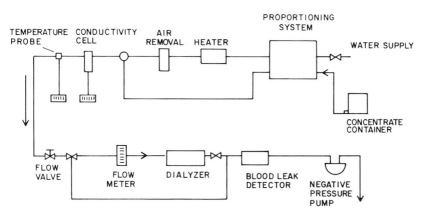

Fig. 3. Flow diagram of a single pass system.

C. Central Systems

These multipatient systems prepare dialysate at the central system located away from the patient's bedside. They have the capacity to deliver dialysate to several patient bedside stations and generally control and monitor the conductivity and temperature.

The dialysate is delivered to the patient's bedside station through insulated pipe to prevent heat loss. The bedside station controls flow rate and pressure and incorporates the accessories to monitor the blood circuit. Multipatient systems are usually more cost efficient than individual patient systems; however, a major disadvantage of the multipatient system is that dialysate preparation for individual patients cannot be varied. If the central system malfunctions, dialysis will have to be discontinued for all patients, unless a backup central system is provided for use when repairs to the main system are required (Fig. 4).

The following are necessary components of any system which is employed in hemodialysis:

1. Temperature Monitors

The temperature of the dialysate solution must be continuously monitored and maintained between 36° and 40°C as it enters the dialyzer. Audio and visual alarms are required in the event that the temperature exceeds these limits. If it should, the system must prevent dialysate from reaching the dialyzer by diverting it into a bypass circuit.

2. Concentration Monitor

The proportioning system continuously monitors the dialysate solution being produced. If dialysate concentration varies more than 5% of its normal value, the system must go into bypass. Recirculating single pass

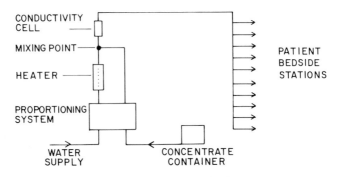

Fig. 4. Flow diagram of a multipatient system.

systems need not have the dialysate monitored continuously because it is prepared in batches. However, each batch should be tested with a conductivity meter before it is used.

3. Dialysate Pressure Monitors

Pressure monitors in the dialysate circuit are necessary to prevent negative-pressure-related excess ultrafiltration, which may result in hypotension. The reverse may also occur if the pressure in the dialysate compartment becomes more positive than in the blood compartment, causing dialysate to be infused into the blood. To prevent these occurrences a direct pressure monitor should be provided as a backup to the negative pressure controller.

4. Blood Pressure Monitors

Monitors are used to measure pressures at various points in the blood circuit. The three locations where pressures can be measured are (a) between the patient's arterial access and the blood pump, usually a negative pressure; (b) between the blood pump and dialyzer; (c) between the dialyzer and the patient's venous access. The postpump and postdialyzer pressures are usually positive.

The postdialyzer pressure is the one most generally used and provides a means of calculating the amount of TMP necessary for fluid removal. TMP is calculated by averaging the pressures in the positive blood compartment and in the negative dialysate compartment. However, since the pressure drop in the blood compartment is only 25–30 mm Hg, the postdialyzer pressure is used for the blood compartment pressure in most dialysis units. Monitors should have high and low limits to prevent the pressure from exceeding the desired range. They must be guarded against blood backup by a transducer protector. Predialysis blood pressure monitors are useful in detecting clotted dialyzers but have the disadvantage of being a source of air entry.

5. Blood Leak and Air Detectors

All hemodialysis systems must have a blood leak detector to prevent blood loss in the event of a membrane rupture. This detector should alarm when the blood loss is 0.35 ml/min and clamp off the venous line. If a blood pump is used, the blood detector must also be able to shut the pump off to minimize the amount of blood loss.

Air detectors prevent the patient from receiving an air embolus. Air can enter the blood circuit through disconnected arterial needles, saline administration sites, dialyzers, and from the pre- and postdialyzer traps. In an alarm condition the air detector shuts off the blood pump and clamps the venous line after the point of monitoring.

IV. DIALYZER REUSE

Dialyzer reuse is becoming increasingly popular as a means of reducing the cost of hemodialysis. Processing the dialyzer for reuse involves removing blood products from the dialyzer membrane followed by a sterilization procedure. However, in order to implement a successful reuse program, criteria for reuse should be established to protect the patients and staff.

Numerous methods of cleaning and sterilizing dialyzers are now available. Some of the problems that arise when dialyzers are reused are the following: (a) Inadequate removal of the blood products that remain in the dialyzer. Blood products that accumulate on the membrane will reduce the surface area, thereby causing a decrease in blood clearance and ultrafiltration rate. (b) If the dialyzer is not properly sterilized the patient may suffer pyrogen reactions or become septic. (c) If the sterilizing agent (usually formaldehyde) is not adequately removed the patient may suffer a toxic reaction. (d) Use of the solutions involved can cause membrane rupture resulting in patient blood loss. (e) Hepatitis can be transmitted to unit personnel.

The reuse procedures we employ are effective and simple. Both the plate and hollow fiber dialyzer are reused in our dialysis unit. Our goal is to employ each plate or hollow fiber dialyzer six times. While it is possible to reuse dialyzers more than six times, cost effectiveness begins to diminish at this point due to the amount of personnel time required to process the dialyzers and to the decreased solute clearance rates.

A. Reuse Procedure for Hollow Fiber Dialyzers

1. The reverse osmosis water source is connected to the arterial blood compartment of the dialyzer and flushed at a flow rate of 1000–1500 ml/min for a few minutes to remove the residual blood. After the initial flushing of the blood compartment has been completed, the water supply is turned off and disconnected from the blood port (Fig. 5).

2. Next, reverse osmosis water is connected to the dialysate port and the dialysate compartment is filled. The other dialysate port is capped and the compartment is pressurized to 20 psi. This pressure forces the residual blood and fibrin out both ends of the blood compartment and is maintained in the dialysate compartment for 15–20 min. After this reverse filtration procedure has been completed, the water supply is turned off and disconnected from the dialysate port (Fig. 6).

3. The water source is connected to the blood compartment and flushed at a flow rate of 1000–1500 ml/min to remove blood components that might have been loosened but not pushed out of the capillaries in the first rinse.

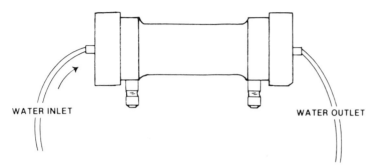

Fig. 5.   Reuse procedure for hollow fiber dialyzer, initial rinse. (Used with permission from *Nephrology Nurse*, January/February 1982.)

4.   After the final rinse has been completed, the water supply is turned off and a finger placed over the outlet blood port. Water is forced out of the dialyzer with a pressure bulb into a graduated cylinder. The volume is recorded. If the volume falls below 85% of its original value, the dialyzer is discarded as this indicates loss of surface area via clotted capillaries (Fig. 7).

5.   The dialyzer is then filled with 1.5% formaldehyde that has been colored with an indicator dye (brilliant blue F.C.F.) for easy detection of residual formaldehyde. The formaldehyde lines are connected to the dialyzer blood ports and dialysate ports. The vacuum is increased in the chamber to 12–15 psi. The formaldehyde lines are opened to the blood compartment to allow the formaldehyde to flow through until all of the small bubbles are removed. The formaldehyde lines to the blood compartment are closed

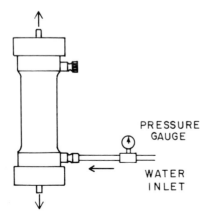

Fig. 6.   Reuse procedure for hollow fiber dialyzer, reverse filtration. (Used with permission from *Nephrology Nurse*, January/February 1982.)

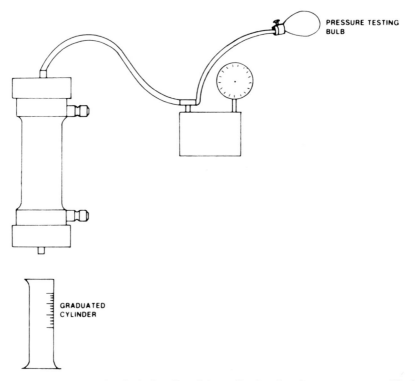

Fig. 7. Reuse procedure for hollow fiber dialyzer, fiber bundle volume measurement. (Used with permission from *Nephrology Nurse*, January/February 1982.)

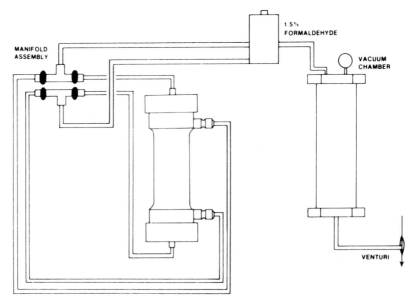

Fig. 8. Reuse procedure for hollow fiber dialyzer, sterilization with formaldehyde. (Used with permission from *Nephrology Nurse*, January/February 1982.)

and the lines to the dialysate compartment are opened to allow that compartment to fill. The formaldehyde lines to the dialysate compartment are closed and sterilizing lines removed. The ports are capped and the dialyzer labelled with the patient's name, date, volume and number of reuses. The dialyzer will remain in this state until its next use (Fig. 8).

B. Reuse Procedure for Plate Dialyzers

1. A reverse osmosis water source is connected to the arterial end of the blood compartment and flushed at a flow rate of 1000 ml/min for 10 min to remove residual blood. After the initial rinsing procedure the water source is disconnected from the arterial blood port (Fig. 9).

2. A 1% sodium hypochlorite (Clorox) feed line is connected to the arterial blood port and pumped into the blood compartment at a flow rate of 200 ml/min for 3 min. While this solution is being pumped into the dialyzer, the venous line is manually crimped two or three times. (This helps to expand the blood sac and remove any air or residual blood trapped in the dialyzer.) After the Clorox solution has beer. pumped through the dialyzer the pump is turned off and the line disconnected from the arterial blood port. Exposure of the Clorox to the membranes for greater than 3 min can result in etching and thus contribute to weakening and membrane rupture (Fig. 10).

3. The reverse osmosis water source is connected to the arterial end of the blood compartment. The venous end of the blood compartment is attached to a Hansen connector on the lower dialysate port. A Hansen

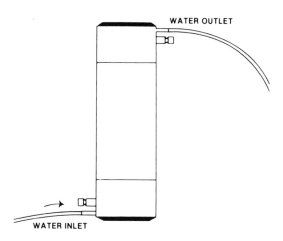

Fig. 9. Reuse procedure for parallel plate dialyzer, initial rinse. (Used with permission from *Nephrology Nurse*, January/February 1982.)

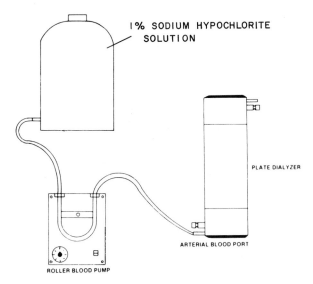

Fig. 10. Reuse procedure for parallel plate dialyzer, cleaning with sodium hypochlorite. (Used with permission from *Nephrology Nurse*, January/February 1982.)

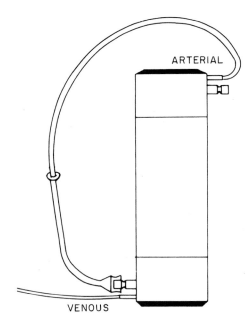

Fig. 11. Reuse procedure for parallel plate dialyzer, final rinse. (Used with permission from *Nephrology Nurse*, January/February 1982.)

connector joined to a small piece of latex tubing at the upper dialysate port provides egress from the system. The blood and dialysate compartments are flushed with reverse osmosis water at a flow rate of 1000 ml/min for 15 min. We have found that this rinse procedure removes any Clorox solution that may have passed through the membrane into the dialysate compartment. During the final rinse, the venous line is again manually crimped two or three times to remove any air or Clorox trapped in the dialyzer. After the final rinse has been completed, the water source is disconnected from the blood and dialysate ports (Fig. 11).

4.   Next, the formaldehyde sterilization line is connected to the arterial end of the blood compartment. A 1.5% formaldehyde solution colored with brilliant blue dye is pumped into the blood compartment. The arterial and venous ends of the blood compartment are capped. The dialysate compartment is also filled with a 1.5% formaldehyde solution (Fig. 12).

The formaldehyde solution must remain in the dialyzer for 8 hr to insure proper sterilization. The dialyzer will remain filled with formaldehyde until its next use.

Before the reused dialyzer can be connected to the patient the formaldehyde must be removed. This is accomplished in the following manner:

1.   Connect the dialysate lines to the dialyzer and set the negative pressure gauge at − 150 mm Hg.

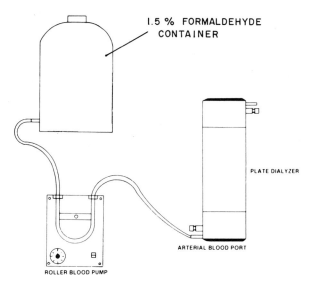

Fig. 12.   Reuse procedure for parallel plate dialyzer, sterilization with formaldehyde. (Used with permission from *Nephrology Nurse*, January/February 1982.)

2.   Allow 500 ml of isotonic saline to flow through the blood compartment of the dialyzer forcing the formaldehyde out the venous end.

3.   Clamp the venous line and allow the saline to drip into the dialyzer
for 10 minutes. During this period maintain a negative pressure of -150
mm Hg in the dialysate compartment.

4.   After 10 min, pump the remaining saline through the dialyzer. Connect
the second liter of heparinized saline and pump 500 ml through the dialyzer.

5.   Connect the venous and arterial lines together and recirculate for
10 min ($Q_B = 200$ ml/min). Pump the remaining saline through the dialyzer.

6.   Connect the third liter of saline and remove the pump segment from
the blood pump. Clamp the arterial and venous lines and allow the saline to
continue to drip into the dialyzer through the saline administration site.

7.   Collect a sample for the formaldehyde test from the top of the drip
chamber.

Residual formaldehyde levels are measured in each dialyzer. The Clinitest
is unsatisfactory for this purpose because of its inability to measure formaldehyde levels less than 50 μg/ml. Therefore, we use the Hantzsch test to
measure residual formaldehyde. This test detects formaldehyde concentration as low as 0.5 μg/ml. A safe level is less than 10 μg/ml.

Bacteriological cultures of the reverse osmosis water, formaldehyde, and
Clorox solutions are performed once a week. We also culture 15% of the
reused dialyzers chosen at random.

Dialyzers are not reused on patients with acute renal failure, hepatitis,
febrile illnesses, or when patients are new to our unit.

V.   PERITONEAL DIALYSIS

The two types of peritoneal dialysis currently in use are intermittent
peritoneal dialysis (CIPD) and continuous peritoneal dialysis (CAPD,
CCPD). CIPD utilizes a machine that prepares dialysate as it is used, or a
cycler that infuses peritoneal dialysate from bags or bottles on a timed basis.

The machines developed for on-line preparation of dialysate generate
water that is essentially sterile and nonpyrogenic by reverse osmosis. This
purified water is then mixed with sterile dialysate concentrate in a ratio of
19 parts of water to 1 part of concentrate by the machine, and pumped at
0.5 liter/min into the patient's peritoneal cavity through an indwelling
catheter that has been surgically placed in the abdomen. Usually, 1–2 liter
volumes are employed per exchange. The machine is equipped with three
timers, so that the inflow, dialysis, and outflow cycles can be separately
regulated. After the fluid has spent a sufficient period of time within the

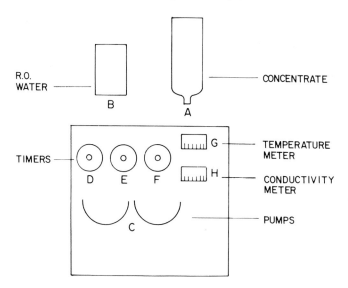

Fig. 13.   Automatic peritoneal dialysis machine.

peritoneal cavity, it drains back through the machine, where the outflow volume can be monitored (Fig. 13).

These machines are equipped with a variety of monitors for both the reverse osmosis water and the dialysate. The product water of the reverse osmosis modules is continuously monitored by means of its electrical conductance. When the produce water falls below 85% rejection of solutes within the feed water, the reverse osmosis modules are not functioning correctly and require replacement.

As is the case with hemodialysis, the composition of the dialysate is measured by means of a conductivity meter. The usual components and concentrations are listed in Table II. The water is heated after going through the reverse osmosis module, and can at times cool to below body temperature if there is a delay in infusion of fluid. This problem is not serious but may provide some discomfort for the patient. The machine is also equipped with an inflow pressure monitor to avoid forcing fluid through the inflow circuit if the line is clamped or if the peritoneal catheter is blocked.

The available machines for on-line proportioning of peritoneal dialysate require extensive maintenance. They must be regularly sterilized with formaldehyde and also must be frequently cleaned with sodium hypochlorite. Failure to sterilize the reverse osmosis modules as well as the remainder of the dialysate circuit can result in bacterial growth within the machine, causing peritonitis in the patient. The machines generate a significant amount of

TABLE II

Constituents of Peritoneal Dialysate

Constituent	Concentrations
Automated peritoneal dialysate (CIPD)	
Sodium	119–130 mEq/liter[a]
Potassium	0
Calcium	3.5 mEq/liter
Magnesium	1.0 mEq/liter
Chloride	90.5–102 mEq/liter[a]
Acetate	34 mEq/liter
Dextrose	1.5–2.5 g/dl
Continuous ambulatory peritoneal dialysate (CAPD, CCPD)	
Sodium	132–141 mEq/liter
Potassium	0
Calcium	3.5 mEq/liter
Magnesium	1.5 mEq/liter
Chloride	101–106 mEq/liter
Lactate	35–45 mEq/liter
Dextrose	1.5–4.25 g/dl

[a] Lower concentrations are used in the 2.5% dextrose dialysate to prevent hypernatremia.

noise, which can be bothersome to the patient, since many programs attempt to have the patient sleep during the peritoneal dialysis procedure. Most patients adjust to the noise.

In recent years intermittent peritoneal dialysis has been almost completely replaced by two forms of continuous peritoneal dialysis. These are known as continuous ambulatory peritoneal dialysis (CAPD) and continuous cyclic peritoneal dialysis (CCPD). Both types infuse dialysate from bottles or plastic bags, and rely on lengthy dwell times of each exchange to provide continuous dialysis.

In the case of CAPD, the dialysate is infused from a bag into the peritoneal cavity. The bag remains attached to the tubing and is carried with the patient until the exchange is completed, usually 3–6 hr later. The fluid is then drained into the bag. Then the bag is disconnected and discarded, and another bag is hung for the next infusion. The longest dwell time occurs at bedtime when the exchange remains in throughout sleep, to be drained upon awakening.

In the case of CCPD, a cycler (the same machine employed in some CIPD patients) is used to infuse three or four exchanges while the patient is asleep. The dwell time for each exchange is $2\frac{1}{2}$–3 hr, and a final exchange is infused in the morning when the patient awakens. The cycler is then disconnected

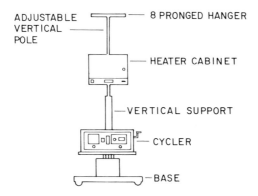

Fig. 14. Continuous ambulatory peritoneal dialysis machine.

and the patient spends the day with a full exchange of fluid within the peritoneal cavity. That exchange is then drained in the evening when the patient attaches to the cycler again (Fig. 14).

In both cases, the dialysate fluid that is used contains 1.5–4.25% dextrose in addition to the usual electrolytes. Because continuous peritoneal dialysis provides greater total clearance than does intermittent peritoneal dialysis, these two forms of continuous peritoneal dialysis are replacing intermittent peritoneal dialysis in current therapy.

The major complication of any type of peritoneal dialysis is peritonitis, or bacterial infection of the peritoneal cavity. Meticulous sterile technique can eliminate most cases of peritonitis. In the case of the cycler, the machine can malfunction. But because the cycler is an extremely simple machine, malfunctions are very uncommon. The cycler offers the advantage of the fluid being warmed when it enters the patient's body. In addition, it offers the convenience of performing the exchanges automatically while the patient sleeps, rather than occupying time during the day. Perhaps the most significant advantage of CCPD is a lower incidence of peritonitis with this technique, because there are fewer connect and disconnect procedures during each 24 hr interval. Probably both CAPD and CCPD will be the preferred forms of peritoneal dialysis in the future, with CIPD being infrequently used.

VI. PATIENT EDUCATION

The majority of dialysis centers have found that home dialysis is most effective when the patient assumes the primary responsibility for his care.

Therefore, he is taught both the technical and medical aspects of home dialysis.

Since the technical procedures cause the patient the most anxiety, these are taught first. He learns about the maintenance of equipment as well as the proper procedures for setting up each dialysis and appropriate cleanup after the treatment. In most cases a dialysis assistant, usually a spouse, is also an active participant in the instruction.

Instruction is accomplished by starting step-by-step procedures, along with reasons for each action. The patient should be able to perform each step of the procedure and understand the purpose of each step. A home training manual is used to provide written instructions that he may refer to during the training at the center and at home. Pictures and diagrams supplied by equipment manufacturers also aid in helping him understand the concept of the technical aspects of his therapy. Any training program must be designed to provide the "student" with the ability to conduct a safe dialysis, and the "instructor" must feel confident of the patient's ability and understanding. Adequate competence must be demonstrated by the patient and documented by the nurse and technician before the patient ever leaves the center.

A reasonable training period is 6 weeks. Our program is geared to the individual needs of the patient depending upon his educational and cultural background. All procedures are demonstrated by the instructor in a simple and methodical manner. When the instructor judges that ample explanation and demonstration of a given procedure have been done, he then requires that the patient and assistant demonstrate these procedures. Continuous support by the instructor and practice on the part of the patient contributes to his eventual understanding and confidence.

Each patient is taught on an individual basis the proper procedure for preparing his equipment for each dialysis and how to clean it after each use. Each procedure is taught step-by-step with reasons given for each one until the patient can perform the procedure and understand the reasons for it.

Besides learning dialysis procedures and equipment maintenance, the patient and assistant are taught how to order supplies in order to keep a sufficient amount at home at all times. Instructions are also given explaining how to contact the necessary personnel in the event of equipment malfunction or any other emergency.

When the patient and assistant are reasonably comfortable with the technical procedures, the medical aspects of home dialysis are emphasized. They are given a basic understanding of the most important functions of the kidney, and are taught the causes of high blood pressure, anemia, and other complications of kidney failure. Considerable emphasis is placed on the correct diet for each patient, and the reasons for each part of the diet are explained. They also receive instruction in the types of medicine being administered, and are made aware of why they are important. The major side effects of each medicine are explained.

Only after the patient and his assistant have become thoroughly familiar with both the technical and medical aspects of dialysis is the decision made that they are ready to dialyze at home. In many programs, a member of the training term visits the patient's home to install the equipment and/or to assist with the first dialysis, to be certain that the patient performs well in the new setting. However, if instruction has been adequate, a home visit for the first dialysis is not essential.

The patients and assistants are seen back at the center about two weeks after they go home, and then at monthly intervals. In addition, thorough instruction is given in how to reach a member of the training team should technical problems arise, and also in how to reach a physician should medical problems arise. Continued monitoring is an extremely important part of performing dialysis at home.

REFERENCES

1. Levin, N. Dialyzer re-use in a hospital. *Dial. Transplant.* **9**, 40–46 (1980).
2. Lanning, J. T. Multiple use of hollow fiber dialyzers in a free-standing center. *Dial. Transplant.* **9**, 36–38 (1980).
3. Clark, M., and Diener, M. Professional platform: A second look at dialyzer reuse. *Contemp. Dial.* December, p. 10 (1980).
4. "Dialysis Manual." VA Medical Center, Nashville, Tennessee, 1979.
5. Kant, K. S., Pollak, V. E., Cathey, M. *et al.* Multiple use of dialyzers: Safety and efficacy. *Kidney Int.* **19**, 728–738 (1981).
6. Deane, N. Renal physicians association survey on re-use. *Dial. Transplant.* **9**, 21–22 (1980).
7. Crystal, R. C. The Health Care Financing Administration's position on re-use. *Dial. Transplant.* **9**, 23–26 (1980).
8. Cotter, D. The Food and Drug Administration's position on kidney re-use. *Dial. Transplant.* **9**, 31–32 (1980).
9. Clark, M. Dialyzer re-use: Home dialysis. *Dial. Transplant.* **9**, 39–46 (1980).
10. Roushey, G. W. Water treatment: Easier said than done. *Dial. Transplant.* **8**, 668–671 (1979).
11. Comty, C. M., Luehmann, D., Wathan, R., and Shapiro, F. Water treatment for hemodialysis. *Dial. Transplant.* **3**, 26–37 (1974).
12. Klein, G., Autian, J., Bower, J. D. *et al.* Evaluation of hemodialyzers and dialysis membranes. *Artif. Organs* **2**, 35–44 (1978).
13. Nash, T. The colorimetric estimation of formaldehyde by means of the Hantzsch reaction. *Biochem. J.* **55**, 416–421 (1953).

14. "Issues in Hemodialysis. Systems Performance, Water Purity and Treatment, Cost Reimbursement and Regulation," pp. 17–19, 30–32, 47–48. Association for the Advancement of Medical Instrumentation, Arlington, Virginia, 1981.
15. "Investigation of the Risks and Hazards Associated with Hemodialysis Devices," pp. 12–38, 89–128, 338–344. U.S. Department of Health, Education, and Welfare, Bureau of Medical Devices, Silver Springs, Maryland, 1980.
16. Walker, P. J., Johnson, H. K., Ginn, H. E., and Hopkins, P. Water treatment for hemodialysis. *Proc.—Clin. Dial. Transplant Forum* **3**, 135–140 (1973).

10

The Case
for Renal Transplantation

H. KEITH JOHNSON, ROBERT E. RICHIE,
and GARY D. NIBLACK

241

Copyright © 1983 by Academic Press, Inc.
END-STAGE RENAL DISEASE
ISBN 0-12-672280-3

I. THE CONCEPT OF TRANSPLANTATION

A. History

The concept of transplantation has attracted man's interest for as long as there is recorded history. The story of modern transplantation, however, may be thought to have been initiated by Alexis Carrel in the early twentieth century. In 1905 he described a method for anastomosing blood vessels for which he received the Nobel Prize for Medicine in 1912 (*1*). It was this discovery that made possible subsequent organ transplants by providing the surgical technique that would allow revascularization of the graft. Between 1906 and 1914 several surgeons utilized this technique in attempts to transplant kidneys from other species into humans with kidney failure. Predictably none of these grafts worked and for a period of time interest in this kind of surgery waned. The first allograft, that is, the first transplant of a human kidney into another human, was performed in 1936 by Veronay. This Russian surgeon treated a patient with acute renal failure secondary to mercury poisoning with the attempted transplant of a cadaveric kidney to the vessels in the patient's groin. The kidney never functioned and the patient subsequently died of his acute renal failure (*2*). In 1945, Hume attempted the grafting of a cadaveric kidney to the arm vessels of a patient who also had acute renal failure. This kidney likewise did not function, although the patient recuperated spontaneously from his acute renal failure and was discharged from the hospital with life-sustaining renal function from his own kidneys (2). In the late 1940s, Küss in Paris transplanted several cadaveric kidneys into patients with end-stage renal disease (ESRD). None of these kidneys survived; however, Küss utilized the surgical technique currently in practice, that is, placing the kidney in the right or left iliac fossa and anastomosing the renal artery to the hypogastric artery, the renal vein to iliac vein, and implanting the ureter into the bladder (3). In the early 1950s Hume and his associates utilized the technique established by Küss to perform 17 cadaveric transplants in Boston. Nine of these transplants were reported in 1955 and, although none of the transplants attained permanent or long-term function, one of the kidneys functioned for 6 months with only the help of what must be considered homeopathic doses of immunosuppression by today's standards (4).

By this time it had become apparent that even when the transplant functioned, a serious reaction took place between the host and the foreign tissue which inevitably caused the destruction of that tissue. In 1953, Hamburger and his group in Paris performed the first transplant from a living-related donor. The kidney functioned immediately and continued to function well for about 2 weeks, then rejection occurred, the kidney abruptly ceased functioning, and the patient died of renal failure (3). In 1954, Murray, Merrill, and their colleagues performed the first transplant between identical twins. As expected, because the tissues of the donor and recipient were genetically identical, the kidney functioned well without any evidence of rejection and the patient was discharged home with normal kidney function 3 weeks after the transplant (3). Increasingly transplanters appreciated that technical considerations were not so much the hindrance to a clinically successful transplant as was the rejection process itself. The search was on for improved methods of immunosuppression. Corticosteroids alone were discovered not to be satisfactory for the long-term survival of the grafted tissue. In 1959, Murray, in Boston, and Hamburger, in Paris, utilized whole body irradiation as an additional approach to immunosuppression in an attempt to suppress the rejection process. In the two patients that were transplanted, initial renal function was good and rejection did not occur. However, as more patients were treated with this methodology, it became apparent that this amount of irradiation was quite hazardous to the patient because of the high risk of bone marrow suppression, leukopenia, infection, and death.

In 1958, 6-mercaptopurine (6-MP) was demonstrated by Schwartz and Dameshek to be an effective immunosuppressant in laboratory animals (5). An analogue of 6-mercaptopurine, azathioprine (Imuran), was subsequently developed and utilized for transplant purposes. This drug was first utilized in clinical transplantation by Murray and his associates in 1961 (6). The combination of corticosteroid and azathioprine proved to be a great improvement on any prior immunosuppressive regimen.

During 1966, Starzl and co-workers first utilized an antilymphocyte globulin (ALG) preparation as an adjunct immunosuppressant in addition to azathioprine and prednisone (7). Since that time the effectiveness of ALG has been debated in transplant circles. The most current information, however, would suggest that ALG is a most effective immunosuppressant and its discovery must take its place as one of the milestones of organ transplantation.

Since 1966 the evolution of clinical transplantation has largely concerned itself with refining the surgical techniques and the immunosuppressive medications that have already been defined. During this period tissue matching has refined so that it is now possible to match the tissues of donor and recipient and thereby decrease rejection and improve graft survival. During this interval methods of kidney retrieval and preservation have also been improved so that currently kidneys can be maintained *ex vivo* for periods up to 72 hr prior to transplantation. All these disciplines have combined to make renal transplantation a clinical reality, an option for the patient with ESRD. In the rest of this chapter we shall look at each of the important aspects of renal transplantation in turn and relate these to the context of the ESRD patient.

B.   Histocompatibility

Today's generally accepted concept that genetic factors play an important part in the likelihood that a transplant will not be rejected evolves from work that far antedates clinical transplantation. Years before the first clinical transplant, workers in the field of tumor immunology demonstrated that tumor cells from one mouse could be successfully transferred to another mouse with the same genetic makeup (8). The chance that such a tumor could be transferred, however, was shown to decrease as the recipient of the tumor became more genetically dissimilar from the tumor's original host. This concept of compatibility was again demonstrated in the infancy of clinical transplantation when it was observed that transplants from identical twins were successful whereas transplants from nonidentical family members or from individuals unrelated to the recipient were rejected. It was readily apparent that the ability to measure these differences prior to transplantation might well affect the result after transplantation and, indeed, determine which donor–recipient pairs were appropriate for renal transplantation.

The first human histocompatibility antigen was reported by Jean Dausset in 1954 (9). A variety of workers have subsequently collaborated to identify multiple histocompatibility antigens and to characterize the major histocompatibility complex (MHC) in humans. It is this genetic complex that is currently thought to determine the characteristics of an individual (the donor) that may be recognized as foreign by another individual (the recipient), thus initiating the rejection process. This segment of genetic material is located on the small arm of the sixth chromosome in man and consists of several different loci (Fig. 1). The antigens defined within this complex are called the HLA (human leukocyte antigen) system. The HLA system contains two categories of antigens: those antigens that can be determined by serological techniques, the so-called serologically defined (SD) antigens, and those antigens that may be defined only by reactions in mixed lymphocyte culture (MLC), the so-called lymphocyte defined (LD) antigens. The antigenic products of the A, B, and C loci are serologically determined while

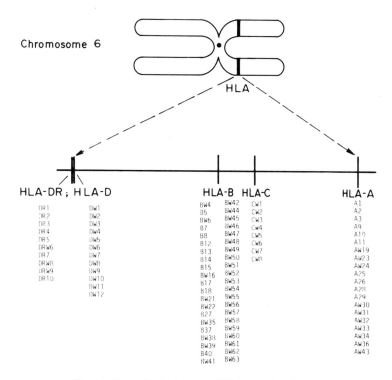

Fig. 1. The major histocompatibility complex of man.

the antigen products of the *D* locus are lymphocyte defined. The antigen products of a fifth locus, the *DR* (*D*-related) locus, are also serologically determined. The *DR* locus is unique in that it is located very close to the *D* locus, and in that its antigenic products are found only on a few cell types including B lymphocytes, endothelial cells and sperm. By comparison, the *A*, *B*, and *C* locus antigens are expressed on all nucleated cells.

The role of HLA antigens in the rejection process continues to be under investigation. It appears, however, that incompatibility at the *D* locus is responsible for T-cell stimulation resulting in proliferation of T cells and the production of various helper factors while SD antigens appear to be the target structures for cytotoxic cells which evolve during the process. There is no doubt that matching the donor with the recipient at these loci by the appropriate serological and lymphocyte proliferative techniques leads to improvement in allograft survival (*10–14*).

As mentioned, the antigens of the *A*, *B*, and *C* region are expressed on all nucleated cells of the body. The concentration of the HLA antigens on the cell surface, however, depends on the cell type. The concentration of antigens on the lymphocyte is rather high and, because these cells are easily isolated from peripheral blood, it is the lymphocyte that has been found most suitable for determining the serologically defined HLA specificities in humans. The process of determining these specificities is called histocompatibility testing or *tissue typing*. Antigens of the *A*, *B*, and *C* loci are determined serologically by exposing purified lymphocytes to antibodies specific for the HLA antigens in the presence of complement. If the antibody to which the cells are exposed is directed against an antigenic specificity on the lymphocyte, in the presence of complement, cell death occurs. This may be determined microscopically following the addition of eosin dye which stains the dead cells. DR typing is also determined serologically according to the same serological cytotoxicity techniques. DR antigens, however, are present on B lymphocytes; therefore, the laboratory procedure for determining the DR antigen must first involve isolation of the B lymphocyte population from the sample obtained from the individual to be typed.

D locus antigen identification depends on the phenomenon that two populations of lymphocytes, when mixed together in tissue culture, will undergo blast formation and proliferate if the two populations of lymphocytes differ at the *D* locus. The amount of proliferation is measured by the addition of tritiated thymidine, which is incorporated into the DNA of the dividing cells. The degree of incorporation of tritiated thymidine is proportional to the amount of proliferation in the culture. In general individuals differing for two *D* locus antigens will proliferate twice as much as those differing for only one.

Since identification of *D* locus antigens involves testing against a number of cells, the usual procedure is to only assess compatibility between donor and recipient. Even this procedure is quite lengthy and the total time lapse between the isolation of the lymphocytes and the final result is 6–7 days. Thus, assessing *D* locus compatibility may be of considerable assistance in assessing live donor–recipient pairs but, because of the time limitations of preservation, is not presently applicable to cadaveric renal transplantation.

Because the *DR* locus is physically located so close to the *D* locus, in many cases it is possible to match donor and recipient for the *DR* locus and in the process match for *D* locus antigens. This is useful since *DR* typing can be accomplished within the time constraints of preservation. Unfortunately, DR antigen identification is not as well established as A, B, or C antigen identification and not all transplant programs have the capability to test for *DR* locus antigens.

The HLA system is remarkably polymorphic. Currently 42 antigenic specificities have been identified at the *B* locus, 20 at the *A* locus, 8 at the *C* locus, 12 at the *D* locus, and 10 at the *DR* locus. Because the genetic determinants are expressed in a co-dominant fashion, the genotype of the individual with respect to the HLA complex is the same as the individual's phenotype. Thus, each individual possesses two identifiable antigens at the *A* locus, two at the *B* locus, two at the *C* locus, and two at the *D* locus. Individuals in whom fewer than two antigens are definable at each locus can be found. These "missing antigens" are referred to as "blanks" and may occur because the individual is homozygous for that antigen, has a rare antigen that has not been defined, or theoretically, has genetic material that does not produce an antigenic product.

At present only antigens at the *A, B, D,* and *DR* loci are considered significant in improving renal transplant results. The tissue match between donor and recipient pairs may be expressed in haplotypes, particularly in the living donor situation. A haplotype is a group of genes present on a single chromosome. Thus, a perfect donor–recipient match would be a two-haplotype match, which would mean that all antigens at the *A, B, D* and *DR* loci are identical. A one-haplotype match indicates that the chromosomal information on one of the chromosomes of the donor is identical to that of the recipient, while the second chromosome is dissimilar. This translates to a one antigen match at the *A* locus, a one antigen match at the *B* locus, a one antigen match at the *D* locus, and a one antigen match at the *DR* locus. These techniques of histocompatibility testing or tissue typing have gained increasing importance as collective transplant results have indicated that improving the match at the various loci improves the results after transplant. Attempting to match the donor with the recipient then makes good sense and plays a significant part in the selection of the appropriate kidney for the appropriate recipient.

II. RECIPIENT SELECTION

The identification of suitable candidates for transplantation is a process of mutual selection involving three participants. Key to the selection is the patient who, after being suitably informed, must decide that transplantation is the desired form of therapy. The nephrologist who has cared for the patient on dialysis is the second key individual involved with the selection process. The nephrologist can help the patient make a realistic comparison between transplant and long-term dialysis treatment. The third participant in the selection process is the representative from the transplant service. This individual is most knowledgeable about transplantation itself and, therefore, must accept the responsibility for educating and informing the patient and the patient's nephrologist regarding the everchanging techniques of transplantation and how they affect the specific patient being considered for that form of therapy. To be effective and appropriate, the counseling phase of recipient acceptance must be preceded by careful evaluation of the patient's prior medical history in order to assess the potential benefit that patient may accrue from transplantation, and that patient's specific risk of the procedure.

A. Patient Risk Factors

There are few absolute contraindications to renal transplantation. Many medical problems can be modified by pretransplant therapy to make the patient acceptable for transplant.

1. Peptic Ulcer Disease

The presence of active peptic ulcer disease is an absolute contraindication to transplantation until it is effectively treated either medically or surgically. Because the immunosuppressants used after transplantation can worsen any preexisting ulcer disease, it is imperative that an ulcer be healed before transplant surgery is entertained. Even then the development of an ulcer after transplantation is more likely in a patient who has previously been so affected than in a patient who has been ulcer free. The risks and hazards of perforation and bleeding after transplant are significant and the patient must weigh these factors in the decision to seek renal transplantation.

2. Diverticulitis–Diverticulosis

The presence of diverticulitis is also an absolute contraindication to transplant surgery until the condition is successfully treated. In the patient with inflammatory bowel disease of this kind, it is wise to consider removal of the area of inflamed bowel prior to transplantation so that infection will not recur in that area during immunosuppressive therapy. For patients without active inflammatory disease but with asymptomatic diverticulosis, the risk to the patient is related to the number of diverticula present. Such patients have an increased risk of perforation of these diverticula with resultant peritonitis because of the immunosuppressive drugs given to prevent rejection after transplantation. They need to be counseled about this hazard and, if multiple diverticula are present, pretransplant resection of the involved areas of bowel may well be the most prudent course.

3. Pancreatitis

Active pancreatitis contraindicates transplantation, and a past history of pancreatitis is a very significant risk factor for the patient desiring transplant. A pancreatitis-free period of at least 1 year should elapse before such a patient is seriously considered for transplant and even then the patient should be aware of the possibility that the pancreatitis might recur following transplant with devastating results. The concern about recurring pancreatitis may be somewhat lessened, however, if the patient who has contracted this problem in the past can identify a specific inciting event which has been removed. Such an inciting event might include certain medications, the presence of a penetrating duodenal ulcer, the presence of gallbladder disease, and so forth. If pancreatitis has not recurred for a year after the removal of the inciting agent, one can feel somewhat more comfortable about the risk of offering transplantation.

4. Gallbladder Disease

The presence of active infection of the gall bladder, of course, precludes transplantation until the infection has been appropriately treated. Silent gallstones may well be an indication for cholecystectomy prior to transplantation because of the hazard of subsequent obstruction, infection, or both. We recommend cholecystectomy prior to transplantation in such patients.

5. Infection

The presence of any infection is an absolute contraindication to transplantation until that infection has been cleared by appropriate antibiotic and or surgical therapy. The possibility of spreading such an infection under the influence of immunosuppressive drugs is so great that to transplant a patient in the face of infection is unwise.

6. Cancer

Immunosuppressive therapy, through the same mechanisms that allow a kidney to be accepted by the new recipient, may enhance the growth of any cancer. A patient with malignancy must have already undergone therapy that has given him a reasonable chance of cure before transplantation can be contemplated. We arbitrarily evaluate such patients 1 year after definitive therapy for their malignancy. In the absence of evidence of retained tumor or metastatic disease transplantation may then be offered. These patients, however, need to be aware that the chance of tumor recurrence is probably increased by the medications received to prevent rejection of the kidney.

7. Age

Patients over 50 years of age have an increased risk of mortality and morbidity after renal transplantation. Older patients are more likely to have complications after transplant due to immunosuppressive medications and, if a complication occurs, are less able to recover successfully. With currently available immunosuppressive medications patients over the age of 60 years should be actively dissuaded from considering transplantation and should be offered transplantation under only the most unusual circumstances.

8. Diabetes Mellitus

The diabetic patient is at increased risk with all forms of therapy for renal failure. Some centers have demonstrated results after transplantation that are superior to those obtained with dialytic forms of therapy whereas other centers have not attained such improved results. Because dialysis is often such an unsatisfactory form of therapy for the diabetic patient, it may well be most rational to attempt to transplant such a patient before that patient needs dialysis. Such timing of transplant requires considerable cooperation between the transplant group and the nephrologist caring for the patient during the pre-end-stage phase of diabetic nephropathy.

9. Cardiovascular Problems

Although it is often said that patients with coronary artery or other cardiac diseases do better with transplantation than dialysis, the careful pretransplant assessment of these problems is essential to a successful transplant outcome. Symptomatic coronary artery disease must be thoroughly assessed prior to transplantation; such an assessment should include coronary angiography. If correctable lesions are present and demonstrated by angiography, they should be surgically remedied prior to transplantation.

10. Elective Surgery

All patients being considered for transplant should be counseled regarding the need to postpone elective surgical procedures until the maintenance dose of immunosuppression has been reached, usually 8–12 months after transplant. If such a postponement is not desired by the patient, then the elective surgery should be accomplished prior to considering transplantation. After recuperation from the surgery, the patient then can be assessed and plans made for organ replacement therapy.

11. Psychiatric Risks

ESRD patients considering renal transplantation must be emotionally stable enough to tolerate the stresses of the operation and postoperative course. A past history of depression, psychosis, or inappropriate behavior dictates a careful psychiatric evaluation and, if necessary, appropriate treatment before transplantation.

B. Recurrent Disease

It is most important to assess the cause of the potential recipient's renal failure. There are certain disease entities that can recur and cause destruction of the transplanted kidney. It must be kept in mind, however, when counseling the patient that recurrence of the disease does not necessarily herald immediate return to dialysis. The process of destruction of the transplanted kidney may be a gradual one and life-sustaining renal function may remain for many years before dialysis is once again necessary.

1. Amyloidosis

Amyloidosis is a cause of nephropathy which can and does recur posttransplantation (15). Such a recurrence may be very gradual and its progression to renal failure prolonged. Thus, transplantation in such patients is still a reasonable approach toward their therapy.

2. Oxalosis

Renal failure occurs in patients with primary oxalosis due to accumulation of oxalate within the kidney itself. Oxalosis also involves the transplanted kidney. The rapidity with which this oxalate deposition occurs ranges from immediate to several years. The possibility of primary nonfunction of the transplanted kidney because of oxalate deposition is also greatly increased. Because of these factors, the transplantation of a patient with oxalosis must be approached very cautiously and with a clear understanding that the expectations for dramatic and prolonged success are small.

3. Focal Sclerosing Glomerulonephritis

This kind of glomerulonephritis has been reported to recur posttransplant in 20–50% of cases (16). Again, the rapidity with which the disease destroys the transplanted kidney is highly variable and several years of life-sustaining renal function may result despite recurrence of the disease.

4. Anti-GBM Glomerulonephritis

In the past it had been thought that rapidly progressive glomerulonephritis with the presence of specific antiglomerular basement membrane (anti-GBM) antibody was a relative contraindication for transplantation because of the risk of recurrent disease. The present generally adopted procedure involves waiting until this antibody is no longer detectable in the patient's serum before proceeding with transplantation. Most centers suggest bilateral nephrectomy prior to transplantation to remove the antigen source that might have been responsible for the continued levels of antiglomerular basement membrane antibody. Subsequent experience has demonstrated that these patients do quite well after transplantation, although many of them have abnormal urine sediments with significant proteinuria. Nevertheless they seem to maintain good renal function for long periods of time.

C. Evaluation of the Potential Transplant Recipient

1. Psychosocial Factors

The management of the patient posttransplant is a complicated undertaking and depends for its success on patient compliance with the directions of the health care team regarding administration of medications, control of diet, and the observance of clinical factors in order to pick up potential complications should they occur. Assessment of psychosocial factors, including psychiatric consultation when indicated, is an important part of evaluating how well the patient will be able to follow the posttransplant routine. Although a patient who is not compliant on dialysis may prove to be very compliant after transplantation, such is the exception. More likely, a patient who is poorly compliant with the dialysis regimen tends to be careless in posttransplant follow-up as well. The assessment that a patient may not follow the posttransplant regimen is not necessarily an absolute contraindication to transplantation, but it certainly decreases the potential for a successful outcome. This knowledge also puts the transplant team on notice to watch very closely for such behavior. In the extreme case, the assessment of these factors may dictate that transplantation not be offered to a specific patient. Fortunately, such situations are rare.

2. Evaluation of the Lower Urinary Tract

Evaluation of the bladder and urethra is an important step before transplantation to ensure that the patient's lower urinary tract is functional.

In the absence of previous pathology, a voiding cystourethrogram (VCUG) is obtained to document that the bladder has adequate capacity and empties completely upon voiding. Cystoscopy and cystometrogram are reserved for those with an abnormal VCUG or a history of prior bladder probiems. If the bladder proves to be unsuitable for transplantation, the creation of an ileal loop has proved quite satisfactory for the purposes of transplantation. This surgery must be performed 3–4 months in advance to allow complete healing before transplantation.

3. Bilateral Nephrectomy

The indications for bilateral nephrectomy prior to transplantation vary from one transplant center to another. In general, the indications for such surgery include uncontrolled hypertension (renal in origin), persistent urinary tract infection, which is thought to involve one or both of the patient's kidneys, anti-GBM nephritis, and polycystic kidney disease if the size of the diseased kidney is so great that no suitable space is available for the new kidney (a most unusual situation). If indicated, bilateral nephrectomy may be accomplished either prior to or at the time of transplantation. Removing the kidneys at the time of transplant is desirable because the recipient is thus saved an operation and a general anesthetic. We have found that bilateral nephrectomy can safely be performed at the time of transplant if the patient is in good physical condition and if active infection is not present. If the nephrectomy must be accomplished prior to transplant, at least 6 weeks are allowed for recuperation before the transplant operation.

4. Blood Transfusions

Three factors have been demonstrated to improve the results of transplantation (13). These factors include (1) the use of an antilymphocyte preparation for immunosuppression, (2) matching the recipient to the donor with respect to HLA specificities at the A and B locus, and (3) the administration of pretransplant blood transfusions. Factors 1 and 2 of the above will be discussed subsequently as we turn our attention to immunosuppressive measures and to the results after transplantation and the relationship of those results to histocompatibility.

Analysis of transplant data has recently revealed that those patients who have never received a blood transfusion attain a 20–30% poorer graft survival following either living-related or cadaveric transplantation when compared to similar patients who have been transfused. The mechanism of this transfusion effect is unknown as is the type of blood product (frozen blood, packed cells, whole blood, etc.) that is most effective. Also unknown is the most desirable time interval between transfusion and transplantation. It is clear, however, that the preparation for transplant must include assurance that the recipient has received blood transfusions. The recommendations as to the amount of blood to be given and the type of blood to be used varies from transplant center to transplant center. Our policy is to make sure that each patient has received at least four units of some kind of blood (frozen, whole, packed cells, etc.) prior to transplantation. Any kind of blood that the patient has received because of therapeutic indications counts toward this total four units. As the chance of sensitization to HLA antigens is increased in proportion to the content of white cells in the transfusion given, frozen blood is the blood product of choice since it contains the fewest white cells. We have demonstrated the same improvement in graft survival with the use of frozen blood as that reported from centers using whole blood or packed cells (17). If frozen blood is not available, the next best blood product is washed packed red cells.

5. Counseling and Education of the Patient

First, the individual patient's risk factors are evaluated and those procedures that would be required to make the patient a transplant candidate are identified, then the patient, his family, and his nephrologist are informed of the proposed plan. All patients should be given the opportunity to discuss the proposed course of therapy with a member of the transplant team. At times, however, such a counseling session is not possible. In that event, the patient's own nephrologist may be the counselor. Therefore, it is important for the nephrologist to make himself knowledgeable about the approach to transplantation undertaken by the specific transplant program to which he refers patients. Regular communication with refering nephrologists of transplant results, changes in immunosuppression, and views on specialized procedures related to transplant are thus quite important so the nephrologist can feel competent and comfortable in counseling his patients. Pamphlets that describe in lay language what the patient may expect after transplantation and point out potential benefits and hazards are extremely useful and often stimulate questions that the patient ought to have answered prior to transplantation. We currently use a monograph for this purpose which is made available to all patients considering transplantation and to all dialysis facilities which refer patients to our program for transplantation. Since the utilization of this monograph was initiated, we have noted a significant improvement in the degree of patient understanding and knowledge at the time they are admitted for transplant. It is also very important for the patient's family to be aware of many of the aspects of transplantation so that they may assist during the pretransplant period and in medical follow-up after the patient returns home following transplantation.

III. THE EVALUATION OF PROSPECTIVE KIDNEY DONORS

Of equal importance to the assessment of the potential transplant recipient is the evaluation of the donor who provides the kidney to be transplanted. The kidney may come from one of two sources. The best source, because it provides the recipient with a more structured timetable toward transplantation and improved results after transplantation, is the living-related donor. As the name implies such a donor is a family member of the patient with ESRD who desires to give the potential recipient a kidney. If no suitable family member is available to donate, the patient then must rely on the second source, that of a cadaveric kidney. The cadaver donor is a person who donates both kidneys after death for the purpose of transplantation. The majority of patients on dialysis who wish transplantation must rely on this latter source if their desire is to be fulfilled.

A. Immunological Testing

Regardless of the source of the kidney certain immunological assessments of the relationship of donor and recipient must be accomplished before the transplant can take place. It is important to measure the HLA antigen specificities at the A, B, D and DR loci in patients who desire transplantation. The initial selection criteria is to match the tissue antigens of the donor with those of the recipient as closely as possible. It has now been demonstrated in both living-related and cadaveric transplantation that improved results after transplantation can be achieved by improving the HLA match between the recipient and the donor (*10–14*). In living-related transplantation, generally a one-haplotype match (i.e., a one antigen match at the A, B, D, and DR loci) is the minimum degree of match accepted. The situation for the cadaver transplant is more complicated. Although it is known that with this type of transplantation improved matching for HLA antigens will result in improved graft survival, attempting to achieve a superior match can result in a patient waiting a longer period of time to be transplanted. Thus, a balance must be achieved with the help of the patient and the patient's nephrologist that weighs, on the one hand, the amount of waiting time for a specific match with the results to be expected after transplantation, on the other. The clinical assessment of how well a patient is doing on dialysis plays a very important part in the decision of whether the patient can wait for a good match or needs to be transplanted sooner with a poor match. Further complicating the situation is the fact that not all HLA antigens are of equal frequency in the population. Some antigens, such as A2, are present more commonly in the population while other antigens, such as Aw36, are far less frequent.

Since enough data have currently been collected to assess the antigen frequencies in the general population, it is now possible, knowing a patients HLA antigen types, to arrive at a rough estimate of how long that patient is likely to have to wait for a cadaver kidney with varying degrees of antigen match. This information can then be used by the transplant team, the patient, and the patient's nephrologist to arrive at the kind of match that will permit transplantation within a suitable length of time and with the chance of success that is reasonable in the individual patient's clinical situation.

B. Cytotoxic Antibody Testing

In addition to tissue typing, the presence or absence of circulating cytotoxic antibodies directed against HLA antigen specificities is another important consideration in the immunological assessment of the recipient for transplant. Patients who are exposed to HLA antigen specificities different from their own are quite able to form antibody against these specificities. Such antibody formation causes no harm to the individual who forms the antibody. However, should such an individual receive a kidney that contains an HLA specificity to which he has previously been exposed and formed cytotoxic antibodies, there is an 80–90% chance of rejecting the kidney in a hyperacute or accelerated fashion (*18*). It thus becomes very important to detect such antibodies prior to transplantation so that a kidney to which the patient has been sensitized will not be transplanted into that patient. The crossmatch is a method by which detection for such a specific antibody is accomplished. Lymphocytes from the potential donor are exposed to serum from the potential recipient in the presence of complement and evidence of cytotoxic effect is sought. If the cells of the donor are killed by the serum of the recipient, the crossmatch is said to be positive and indicates that the potential recipient has preexisting cytotoxic antibodies directed against some antigens present on the donor's cells and most probably also present within the donor kidney. If no cell death occurs, the crossmatch is said to be negative and it is safe to proceed with the transplant.

Periodic assessment of the potential transplant recipient's antibody level prior to the offering of the kidney is also important to assess likelihood that a crossmatch against a given kidney will be positive. Such an assessment is accomplished through a procedure called antibody screening. This procedure involves the exposure of serum from the potential recipient to lymphocytes from a variety of volunteer cell donors whose tissues represent the known HLA A and B specificities. Usually, such a panel of donors includes lymphocytes from about 25 different individuals. The panel is then tested for reactants as in the crossmatch mentioned above. Results are reported as the percent of individuals whose cells are killed by the potential recipient's serum.

If 10 of 20 cell samples are killed the recipient is said to have a panel reactive antibody level (PRA) of 50%. Extrapolating from this test it is said that the potential recipient has antibody directed against about 50% of the population from which a cadaver kidney might be sought. If the serum kills all of the cells, it is said that the potential recipient has developed cytotoxic antibodies against 99% of the population. Since a positive crossmatch means a kidney cannot be used for that patient, a high antibody level makes it exceedingly difficult to find a compatible kidney. Thus, assessment of the antibody level also is a factor in determining how long a patient is likely to wait for a suitable cadaveric kidney to be found.

Because cytotoxic antibody levels can fluctuate with time, it is important to obtain periodic (usually monthly) serum samples so that an accurate sensitization profile can be maintained. It must be remembered that once sensitization occurs the patient's immune system retains the memory of the event for life, even though the antibody level may fall to undetectable levels after a period of time. Reexposure to such an antigen can result in a rapid rise of antibody titer and destruction of the antigen carrying cells. Thus, crossmatching before transplantation should be performed with all available sera in an attempt to avoid the situation in which antibody has become undetectable but sensitized cells remain that could lead to the destruction of the allograft.

C.   Blood Transfusions and Cytotoxic Antibody

The importance of cytotoxic antibody raises additional questions about the medical management of the patient prior to transplant. Formation of cytotoxic antibodies may result from any exposure to HLA antigens. Such exposure occurs during pregnancy, because of the rejection of a prior transplant, secondary to infections with certain bacteria and, most commonly, because of blood transfusions. The likelihood that antibody will be formed is related to the immunological capacity of the individual to make antibody and to the amount of antigen to which the individual is exposed. In blood transfusions the sources of antigen are the white cells and platelets inadvertently transfused with the blood. The smaller the amount of antigen within the transfusion, the lower the chance that the patient will make cytotoxic antibodies. Frozen blood contains the lowest amount of such antigen and thus has the least potential for stimulating the production of cytotoxic antibodies. The other forms of blood increase in their potential to stimulate antibody formation in proportion to the increase in the amount of antigen present. Paradoxically, as already mentioned, a certain number of blood transfusions have been found by many transplant centers to have a salutary effect on graft survival whether living-related or cadaveric. The reason for this effect is at present unknown. The type of blood thought to be best to attain these improved transplant results is much debated. Because in our program we can achieve improvement in graft survival with the use of frozen blood and appreciate that frozen blood has the least potential for cytotoxic antibody production, it is this form of blood that we favor when transfusion is required.

D. The Living-Related Donor

Current results in most transplant programs with living-related transplantation are superior to all forms of dialysis and to cadaveric transplantation. For the patient who is medically suitable, living-related transplant must be considered the therapy of choice for ESRD. Thus, all patients who are interested in transplantation should undergo family evaluation for potential living donors.

Living-related kidney donation must be a spontaneous and voluntary act on the part of the donor. The observation of absolute confidentiality with regard to the evaluation of the donor is essential to achieve such a coercion-free decision. There are many approaches to achieve this result. Our approach is as follows. When a patient desiring transplantation is identified, we ask if the patient would accept a kidney from a member of the family were it freely offered. If the patient answers affirmatively, we request the telephone numbers and addresses of all family members who would seem to be suitable kidney donors. Following the receipt of this information, each family member is mailed an explanatory letter along with a form to be completed and returned to us in a preaddressed, stamped envelope. The letter explains that the purpose of the communication is to ask whether the family member would like to be considered as a kidney donor and explains the ramifications of such a decision. On the form the family member may check one of three options: The first option is "I am not interested in being considered as a kidney donor"; the second option is "I wish to have more information about kidney donation"; and the third option is "I am interested in being considered as a kidney donor." If the first option is elected by the potential donor, the communication with that individual is terminated at that point. If option two is elected, further information is provided to the potential donor to allow that person to make an informed decision regarding whether to consider kidney donation or not. If option three is elected, we proceed to the next step of evaluation.

Step two of the donor evaluation involves obtaining a blood specimen for histocompatibility testing. When we have received information from all members of the family, we look at the tissue types and the ABO blood type to assess who might be considered the best potential donor from an immunological point of view. In addition to the tissue types which we have already discussed, the donor must be compatible with the recipient in ABO blood type as well. Rules for kidney donation are much the same as for the administration of blood as far as ABO blood types are concerned: a person with O blood can give a kidney to an individual with any other blood type; an A donor can give to an A recipient or an AB recipient; a B donor can give to a B recipient or an AB recipient; and an AB donor can give a kidney to only an AB recipient. If a suitable donor is found within the family, this individual is contacted by telephone and the results of the tissue typing are shared with him. If the individual still wishes to proceed, admission to the hospital for a "donor workup" is arranged.

1. Living Donor Evaluation

The risk to a healthy person of donating a kidney to another individual is very small. Data collected on individuals who have undergone unilateral nephrectomy due to benign renal disorders demonstrate that they have the same survival as the normal population (19). Thus, the hazard of donating a kidney is not in the long-term effects of living with only one kidney, but in the short-term hazard of the nephrectomy operation itself. This procedure usually takes $4-4\frac{1}{2}$ hr, is accomplished under general anesthesia, and requires a postoperative recuperation period of about 1 week before the donor can return home. A further recovery period during which the donor must be unemployed ranges from 3 to 8 weeks depending on the type employment. In order to minimize the hazard the potential donor is admitted to the hospital for a 2 or 3 day stay to undergo an overall assessment of his medical status. During this period of time in the hospital, renal function is measured and an IVP and renal arteriogram are performed in order to ensure that the patient has two normally functioning kidneys with vascular systems that are suitable for transplantation. Any medical problem that could increase the risk of kidney donation for the donor, or any problem with the kidney that would decrease the likelihood of transplant success, rules that individual out as a kidney donor. Generally, kidney donors must be between 18 and 60 years of age. Under extenuating circumstances a donor over the age of 60 might be considered if all other factors are determined to be acceptable. It would only be under extremely unusual circumstances that a donor under the age of 18 could be utilized. These circumstances would involve legal actions to ensure that the minor's rights were not being violated by the donation of the kidney. Once the donor evaluation is satisfactorily accomplished, the date of the transplant is set. If at any time the potential donor decides not to give the kidney, the transplant team has an obligation to provide the donor with a reason that will protect that individual from any possible family pressures. In addition, prospective donors should have the opportunity to discuss any concerns they may have with a psychiatrist who is knowledgeable about renal transplantation. Such a psychiatrist is a valued member of the transplant team.

E. The Cadaver Kidney Donor

Most patients awaiting transplantation must depend on a cadaveric source for a kidney. As with live-related transplantation, in our program improved matching results in better success following the allograft. Obtaining a specific kidney for a particular patient, however, is a complicated undertaking and often involves sharing between various transplant centers.

1. Criteria of Acceptability for the Cadaver Donor

Certain medical criteria must be met for an individual who has died to be considered a kidney donor. Such an individual must be between the ages of 2 and 65 years, must have normal kidney function immediately prior to death, must be free of cancer excepting primary malignancy of the central nervous system, and must have no evidence of systemic infection. Because cancer and infection can be transmitted along with the kidney to the recipient, the presence of these conditions is an absolute contraindication to the use of the kidney for the purpose of transplantation. If the malignancy is of the central nervous system origin, however, such an individual may be considered a kidney donor because in this instance the tumor generally does not spread beyond the brain. If the above criteria are met, such a patient upon death may donate kidneys for use in transplantation.

2. Permission for Donation

A great deal of effort is currently expended by a variety of organizations to educate the public about the possibility of donating organs after death. The Uniform Anatomical Gift Act, which has been enacted in all 50 states, allows a person during life to make a bequest of any or all bodily parts for the purpose of transplantation to take effect after death. When signed by the individual and two witnesses the organ donor card becomes a legal document and authorizes physicians to utilize the specified organs to help others in need. Despite these education efforts most people have not utilized the donor card to express their desires one way or the other regarding organ donation after death. In the event that a signed and witnessed donor card is not present at the time of the potential donor's terminal illness, next of kin may be asked to give permission for organ donation. Because time is of the utmost importance in removing the kidneys, permission must be obtained prior to the donor's death. The family may be approached by the patient's attending physician or anyone else who knows the family and understands what kidney donation is about. Making such a request of a bereaved family is a very difficult task and is perhaps a major reason why the concept of organ donation has not been more widely embraced by the medical profession. Many donations are stimulated by a family member who may have heard of organ donation and appreciates the significance of such a gift. With continued public and professional education, hopefully such donations will increase since the number of patients waiting for cadaveric renal transplantation is large and increases every year. Their only chance for a transplant and a more normal life relies on organ donation.

3. The Kidney Retrieval Procedure

When circulation to the kidney ceases, deterioration rapidly ensues. After 60 min of ischemia the kidney becomes irreversibly damaged and nonviable. Thus, in order to be considered for transplantation the kidney must be removed within 60 min after cessation of circulation. For all practical purposes this means that the potential kidney donor must be alive upon arrival at the hospital. This time limit also explains why permission for kidney donation must be obtained before death occurs. Furthermore, the pronouncement of death must be performed by a physician who is unrelated to the transplant team to avoid any possible concerns about conflict of interest. The criteria for diagnosis of death vary from location to location. Many states in this country have adopted laws that allow death to be pronounced if complete and irreversible cessation of brain function can be demonstrated according to usual and customary medical practice. Such a statute allows a physician to pronounce a patient dead because brain death has occurred even though circulation continues to the kidneys. Patients are supported with respirators until the pronouncement of death. If the individual or his family wishes to donate the kidneys, they can be removed under ideal physiological circumstances at the time of death. Retrieval from "heartbeating" cadaveric donors allows for the least amount of damage and provides a kidney of best quality for transplantation. In those situations where brain death is not diagnosed, cessation of circulation may be utilized as the criterion to pronounce the patient's death. When cessation of cardiac activity is the basis for pronouncement of death, immediately mechanical aeration and closed chest massage are instituted in an attempt to provide some perfusion of the kidneys, which are removed as quickly as possible. However, the retrieval of kidneys from nonheartbeating cadaver donors presents a monumental logistical problem. In an attempt to salvage kidneys from such donors innovative techniques to shorten the retrieval process have been used with varying results. One of the most successful has been the introduction of a triple lumen, double balloon catheter into the aorta immediately upon cessation of circulation. When the upper and lower balloon on this catheter are inflated in the aorta, the renal arteries are isolated. The third lumen of this catheter then may be utilized to perfuse the kidney with a cold, specially prepared solution which initiates the preservation process (20).

The actual surgical retrieval of the kidneys is a procedure that must be accomplished by individuals familiar with this operation. The donor is prepared and draped as if he were having abdominal surgery. Swiftness is imperative as is extreme care not to damage the ureter or the vessels of the kidney. Adequate length of vessels and ureter are essential to insure the transplantability of the kidneys. In addition to the removal of kidneys several lymph nodes and the spleen are also taken from the donor to provide additional material for tissue typing and crossmatching procedures.

4. Preservation of the Kidney

As soon as the kidneys are removed measures designed to preserve them are instituted. The blood is quickly flushed from the kidney with a cold 8°C solution to prevent clotting within the renal vasculature. The flush solution approximates intracellular electrolyte and osmolar composition in formulation. The kidney is flushed with this solution until the effluent from the renal vein is clear of blood. The kidney is then placed in a sterile container, which is sealed and, in turn, placed in an ice filled foam insulated box. Simply packaged in this manner, the kidney will remain viable for 36 hr. If transplantation is anticipated within this period of time, no further methods of preservation need be contemplated. If the time before transplant can occur is to exceed 36 hr, the kidney is placed on a pulsatile preservation machine. Such machines consist of a pump that serves to circulate the perfusate, a membrane oxygenator so that oxygen can be added to the perfusate and thus to the kidney, and a method whereby the perfusate can be cooled to about 8°C. A sterile container for the kidney is provided as part of this apparatus. This method of preservation has been effective in maintaining the viability of the kidney for up to 72 hr. Nevertheless, it is axiomatic that the best preservation device is the human body. Regardless of the form of preservation, the longer a kidney remains *ex vivo* the more damage it will sustain prior to transplantation. It makes sense then to strive toward maximum efficiency in order to perform the transplant as quickly as possible after the kidney is made available.

5. The Logistics of Organ Procurement

The retrieval of kidneys from the cadaver donor and the location of suitable recipients for the retrieved kidneys are quite complicated procedures requiring considerable coordination. Each transplant program accepts responsibility for the retrieval of kidneys in its own geographic area. Many programs establish organ procurement agencies as an administrative base through which the retrieval and sharing activities can be coordinated. Such an "organ procurement agency" may have individuals who specialize in public education, other professionals who are experts in the preservation and sharing of kidneys, and still others who interact with physicians in the community to identify potential kidney donors and cooperate with the donor's physician to attain the goal of kidney retrieval. Key to the goal of finding a suitable recipient for each kidney retrieved is the concept of sharing kidneys between different transplant centers or organ procurement agencies. Several organizations have been established within the United States to facilitate such sharing and to eliminate as far as possible the wastage of viable organs. The South Eastern Organ Procurement Foundation (SEOPF) is a group of 45 transplant centers in the southeastern part of the United States established for and dedicated to the sharing of kidneys in order to maximize utilization. Patterned by the methods established by SEOPF, a nationwide network, the United Network for Organ Sharing (UNOS), is currently also facilitating the sharing of cadaver organs. Utilizing a central computerized listing of patients waiting for transplant, now numbering about 8000, any center that is a member of UNOS or SEOPF can, in minutes, locate a suitable recipient for each kidney that is retrieved. This computerized listing of patients has proved to be of significant benefit in facilitating the sharing of kidneys. Thus, if a kidney cannot be used locally, a suitable recipient may be quickly located and the kidney sent to that center. Data accumulated within the SEOPF have demonstrated that kidneys shared between centers achieved the same degree of success as kidneys transplanted at the same center where they were retrieved. Not only does the kidney donation benefit the person who receives the kidney, but we have found that in many instances the donation of a kidney provides for the family of the deceased the only positive aspect of an otherwise unfortunate situation. Families have often commented that the positive aspects of organ donation help them through their grieving process. The various organ procurement agencies in the country are continuing the work of trying to find enough kidneys to meet the needs of those patients waiting for cadaveric transplantation. Much still needs to be done, however, as the scarcity of kidneys continues to be all too evident.

IV. THE SURGICAL PROCEDURE

A. Introduction

In the conventional medical management and treatment of illness, the patient has one physician who is primarily responsible for this care. Consultants are utilized to supplement this care as needed. In contrast, the optimal management of a patient who has ESRD requires input from several disciplines. The "team" of individuals caring for the patient includes not only physicians, but nurses and other nonphysician professional personnel as well. This "team approach" is utilized when the patient elects to have a kidney transplant as a means of treating his renal disease. Thus, the nephrologist and the dialysis nurse are responsible for seeing that dialysis is appropriate and timely both in the preoperative and postoperative period. The urologist evaluates the genitourinary tract to decide whether a nephrectomy is needed, the bladder functions adequately, or an ileal loop is required. At the time of the operation, the urologist may be involved in reestablishment of the urinary tract. The transplant surgeon is responsible for the preoperative evaluation of the patient and for counseling him about the potential risk and complications involved in the procedure. He also is responsible for evaluating the donor kidney, completing the vascular anastomosis, and following the patient in the postoperative period. The transplant coordinator is responsible for preservation of the cadaver kidney once it has been removed, for transporting it from one center to another, and for helping to match a kidney for a recipient. The transplant immunologist is responsible for the HLA tissue matching necessary to select a donor/recipient combination. A nephrologist whose main interest is in transplantation may follow the patient and help with management of his immunosuppressive regimen. In order to achieve a successful functioning transplant, extremely close follow-up is mandatory in the postoperative period. This requires that the patient know and understand how to take the necessary medication vital to success. A nurse coordinator works closely with the patients and their families to help accomplish this. Thus, each of these individuals has a role in the pre- and postoperative management of a transplant recipient.

B. Surgical Preparation

The source of the donor kidney determines the timing of the operation. If it is a living related donor, the procedure is scheduled on an elective basis. Operations on the donor and recipient are carried out in adjacent operating rooms. This allows the donor kidney to be implanted into the recipient as soon as possible, thereby minimizing ischemic time, which is the time from removal of the donor kidney until revascularization in the recipient. On the other hand, if the kidney is from a cadaver donor, the operative procedure will need to be done expeditiously, again keeping in mind the ischemic time of the kidney. Ideally, this should be as short as possible although, realistically, it often exceeds 24 hours and at times is 36 hr (Fig. 2). Prolonged ischemic time may be necessitated by the distance the kidney must be transported, by becoming available without prior knowledge, or if the patient has not dialyzed in the preceding 24 hr. For the last instance, dialysis may therefore be necessary prior to surgery. In preparation for receiving a renal allograft, the patient needs a thorough evaluation including chest X-ray, electrocardiogram, and an analysis of serum electrolyte concentrations. The presence of hyperkalemia is another indication for preoperative dialysis. This

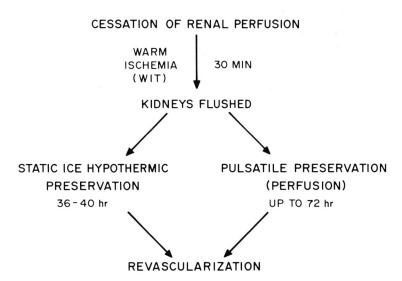

Fig. 2.   Diagram showing limits of ischemic times in cadaver kidney preservation.

should be accomplished prior to the operation rather than afterward because of the possibility of bleeding into the wound as a result of the heparin which is given during dialysis. A general anesthetic agent is preferred when the patient has been dialyzed immediately prior to the operative procedure because spinal anesthesia carries the risk of hemorrhage. However, if the patient did not require dialysis prior to the transplant, a spinal anesthetic can be utilized.

C. Surgical Site

The site selected for the transplant may be either iliac fossa. The right side is preferable because it is easy to mobilize the cecum in order to make an extraperitoneal neohabitat for the transplanted kidney. If this side has been used previously and there is considerable scarring, the left side may be used. Some surgeons prefer to use the left side if the donor kidney is from the right side because this will permit the pelvis of the kidney to be anterior instead of posterior (21). If one has a choice of donor organs, the left kidney is chosen because of the longer left renal vein, which facilitates placing the allograft into the iliac fossa (22). Occasionally, at the time of the transplant concomitant splenectomy and/or bilateral nephrectomy will be considered. If the patient has an enlarged spleen and hypersplenism with leukopenia or thrombocytopenia, a splenectomy may be indicated so that larger doses of azathioprine can be given. In selected patients where hypertension is considered to be of renal origin, we have elected to remove the kidneys at the time of transplant rather than doing the nephrectomy prior to transplant (23). There is no added risk and the patient is spared an additional operation. When there is documented pyelonephritis a nephrectomy should be done prior to transplant (21, 24). If a splenectomy or bilateral nephrectomy is planned, a standard midline xyphoid to pubic symphysis incision is made. After completion of the above procedure or procedures, the right colon is reflected medially to expose the right iliac fossa. However, the standard approach is an oblique incision in the right or left lower quadrant (25) (see Fig. 3). Special care is taken to assure good hemostasis because of the increased incidence of hematoma formation should the patient need dialysis in the postoperative period. The retroperitoneal space is entered by incising the external oblique fascia, elevating the medial side to expose the lateral border of the rectus muscle and incising the anterior and posterior rectus fascia. The incision is carried superiorly to the level just below the umbilicus. After incising the transversalis fascia, the peritoneum is dissected superiorly and medially. Care is taken not to enter the peritoneum. In the female, the round ligament is divided to facilitate exposure. In the male, the cord is dissected free from the peritoneum and placed lateral to the iliac artery and vein. The external iliac artery and vein are identified, and encircled with silastic vessel loops. The perivascular lymphatics are dissected from the vessels and, if they are transected, they are ligated with nonabsorbable suture in order to prevent lymphocele formation at a later time (26). The kidney is then brought into the operating field. If the donor is living-related, little if any attention need to be paid to the vessels or hilar structures. If the kidney is from a cadaver, a thorough inspection should be carried out to make sure

a.

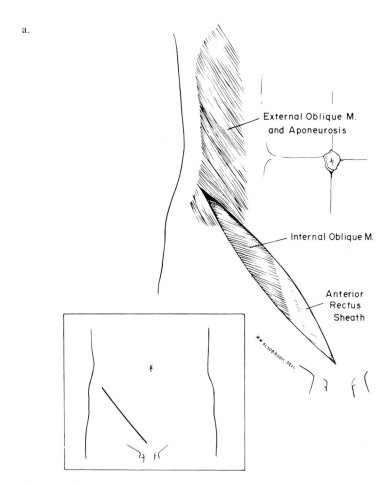

Fig. 3. (a) Incision in right lower quadrant showing incision of the aponeurosis of external oblique muscle. (b) Incision of anterior rectus sheath. (c) Incision of posterior rectus sheath with retraction of rectus muscle medially exposing peritoneum. (d) Peritoneum retracted superiorly and medially to expose external iliac artery and vein extraperitoneally.

b.

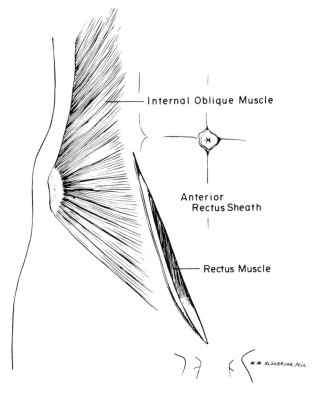

Internal Oblique Muscle

Anterior
Rectus Sheath

Rectus Muscle

External Oblique

Aponeurosis of ext. oblique

c.

Anterior Rectus Sheath

Rectus Muscle

Posterior Rectus Sheath

Peritoneum

Vas Deferens

Fig. 3. (*Continued*)

d.

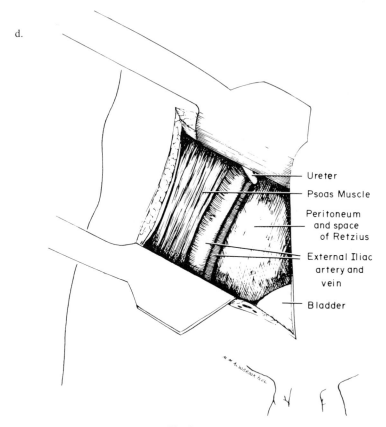

Ureter

Psoas Muscle

Peritoneum
and space
of Retzius

External Iliac
artery and
vein

Bladder

Fig. 3.   (*Continued*)

of the integrity of the artery and vein because, not infrequently, numerous
small vessels will require ligation, and occasionally a small polar vessel
heretofore unrecognized will need attention. The kidney is placed in the iliac
fossa and, depending on the anatomic length of the donor artery, the anastomosis can be carried out in an end-to-side fashion usually with the external
iliac artery or in some instances with the common iliac artery (Fig. 4). Some
surgeons prefer to do an end-to-end anastomosis with the hypogastric artery.
We prefer not to use this vessel in males because diversion of arterial blood
flow has been implicated as a cause of impotence. However, if it is necessary
to use the hypogastric artery, we feel it is important to divide the vessel
proximal to the trifurcation and oversew the distal end so as to permit
adequate collateral circulation between the gluteal and vesical arteries. The

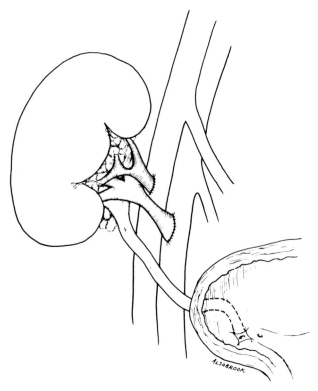

Fig. 4. Diagram showing kidney in right iliac fossa with end-to-side anastomoses of the renal artery to external iliac artery and renal vein to external iliac vein, and ureteroneocystostomy.

venous anastomosis is done in an end-to-side manner preferably to the external iliac vein, although on occasion the common iliac vein is used. Small 6-O nonabsorbable suture material is used for both anastomoses. If there are deviations in the normal anatomy of the vessels to the donor kidney, then anastomotic variations may be necessary. A kidney with two or more arteries can frequently be anastomosed with a cuff of aorta if such is available. If not, the smaller vessel can be attached to the larger one in an end-to-side manner and then the larger one can be sutured to the host vessel (27). If there is more than one vein, the larger one can be used and the smaller one ligated because all the veins drain into a common pelvis in the kidney.

After completion of the two vascular anastomoses, small vascular clamps are placed on the donor vessels and the clamps are removed from the recipient's vessels. This will permit evaluation of the suture line for hemostasis without allowing perfusion of the kidney. After hemostasis is felt to be adequate, the clamps are removed and the kidney is perfused with the recipient's blood. At this point, careful attention is paid to the color and turgor of the kidney. Urinary continuity is established by means of a ureteroneocystotomy. The bladder is distended with a solution of antibiotics to render the urine sterile and thereby prevent contamination of the wound when the bladder is opened. The donor ureter is brought through the bladder using a tunneling procedure and the orifice is sutured to the mucosa near the patient's own ureteral opening. After completing this step, a small polyethylene catheter is passed up the ureter to assure patency. The bladder is closed in layers with absorbable suture. All patients will have received preoperative parenteral antibiotics. We prefer cefazolin sodium, 1 g IV preoperative and 1 g IV daily for 3 days postoperatively. Three hundred mg of azathioprine are given intravenously prior to the completion of the vascular anastomoses. At the completion of the venous anastomosis, 25 g of mannitol are given intravenously, and at the completion of the arterial anastomosis, 80 mg of furosemide are given intravenously, in order to induce a diuresis. The wound is irrigated with a solution containing kanamycin. Suture lines are reexamined for hemostasis. When hemostasis is felt to be secure, the wound is closed with nonabsorbable suture.

D. Postoperative Management

The patient must be monitored very closely in an intensive care unit in order to detect the usual postoperative complications such as bleeding, wound problems, pulmonary dysfunction, and thrombophlebitis. It is essential to evaluate closely the function of the allograft so that one can treat a rejection episode as early as possible. When a prompt diuresis follows the transplant, hourly monitoring of the urinary output is mandatory. There must be adequate fluid replacement in order to ensure that dehydration does not occur. If the kidney was from a cadaver donor, it may be necessary to give a solution of mannitol and furosemide in order to try to initiate a diuresis. Should this not be successful then fluid intake must be restricted so that there will not be an excessive increase in the vascular volume. Concentrations of serum electrolytes are determined. In the presence of significant hyperkalemia and no diuresis, the patient may require dialysis as an emergency procedure.

On the day immediately following the operation, radioisotope studies are done to determine both blood flow and function of the kidney. Fifteen millicuries of technetium pertechnetate are injected intravenously for the perfusion study (Fig. 5). Fifty microcuries of [^{131}I]hippuran are injected intravenously with multiple sequential images being obtained from 0 to 20 min in order to determine renal function (Fig. 6). These studies establish base line renal perfusion and function and may indicate whether acute tubular necrosis or a rejection episode has occurred (Fig. 7). Thereafter, a hippuran renogram is repeated three times a week in order to monitor renal function. Blood chemistries and a complete blood count are obtained daily. Routine daily immunosuppression consists of 60 mg of prednisone and 100–150 mg of azathioprine. The dose will depend on the size of the individual. These medications may be given either intravenously or by mouth. At our center antilymphocyte serum is manufactured and administered to renal transplant recipients by vein as an additional immunosuppressive agent.

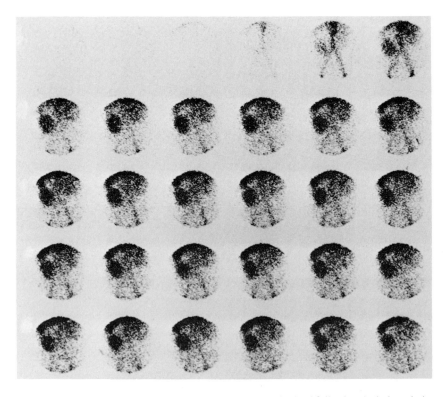

Fig. 5.   Normal renal bolus. Sequential 1.5 sec images obtained following the bolus administration of 15 mCi of TcO$_4$ demonstrate prompt perfusion of a renal allograft.

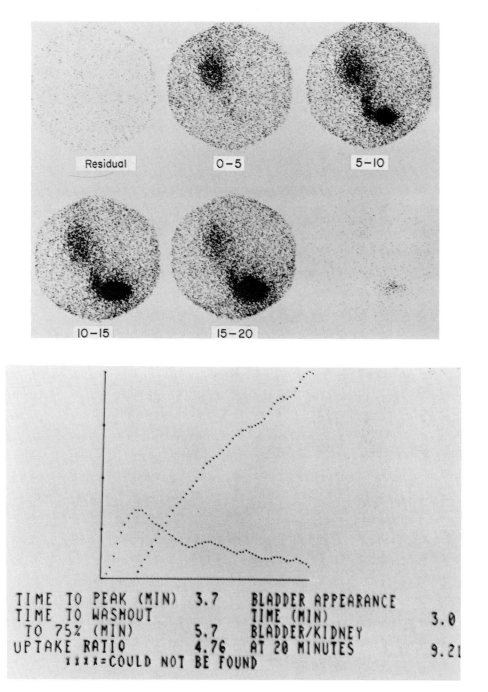

Fig. 6. (a) Normal hippuran renogram. Following the IV administration of 50 μCi of [¹³¹I]hippuran, serial 5 min collections were obtained from 0 to 20 min. There is prompt clearance of hippuran from the plasma with normal transit of the radiopharmaceutical through the renal allograft. (b) Normal hippuran renogram curve.

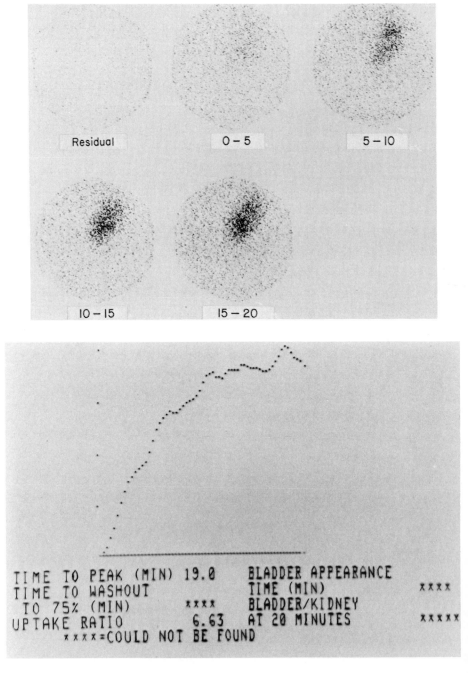

Fig. 7. (a) Acute tubular necrosis. Slow progressive accumulation of the radiopharmaceutical by the kidney with no evidence of "peaking" or bladder activity. (b) Curve consistent with acute tubular necrosis showing uptake but no excretion into the bladder.

E. Rejection of an Allograft

Allograft rejection occurs despite our attempts to prevent or suppress this with tissue matching, pharmacological agents, and antilymphocyte serum. The extent and degree of rejection is highly variable and difficult to predict despite our most sophisticated present day immunological studies. There are three classic types of rejection: (1) hyperacute or a variation often referred to as accelerated rejection, neither of which is reversible; (2) acute rejection, which is reversible with treatment; and (3) chronic rejection, which is nonreversible.

1. Hyperacute Rejection

This type of rejection is usually seen within an hour following revascularization of the kidney. The kidney may look mottled, blue in color, and flaccid. There is obvious lack of cortical blood flow. If this occurs, the kidney must be removed immediately. Hyperacute rejection is caused by the presence of preexisting antibodies against the donor antigens. This phenomenon is rarely seen today because a crossmatch is done between donor cells and

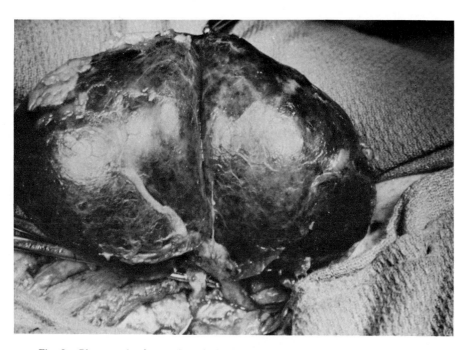

Fig. 8. Photograph of transplanted kidney with accelerated rejection, showing marked enlargement and cortical necrosis despite a patent artery and vein. This kidney had been transplanted 8 days previously. A transplant nephrectomy was done.

recipient serum. If this is positive, the transplant is not done. Accelerated rejection occurs between the sixth and fourteenth postoperative days. The patient develops fever, marked pain, and swelling over the graft, and a sudden cessation of urine output. The renogram indicates lack of blood flow to the kidney. The patient may become toxic and begins to sequester platelets in the kidney with a fall in the peripheral blood platelet count. A transplant nephrectomy is usually necessary (Fig. 8). The pathological lesion seen with these two types of rejection is the result of endothelial cell damage and formation of platelet and fibrin thrombi, resulting in cortical necrosis.

2. Acute Rejection

Acute rejection is exceedingly common and reversible with treatment. It usually occurs from 24 hr to 2 weeks posttransplant and is more common at 6 to 7 days. However, in some patients this type of rejection may be latent

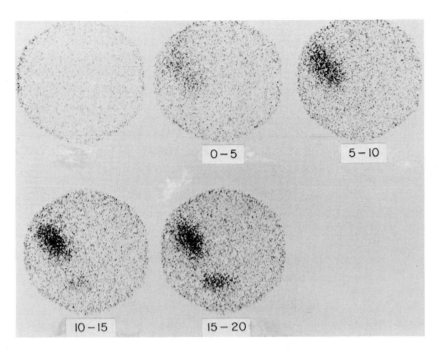

Fig. 9. Chronic rejection. Following the IV administration of 50 μCi of [^{131}I]hippuran, serial 5 min collections were obtained from 0 to 20 min. There is delayed plasma clearance of the radiopharmaceutical with prolongation of the rate of transit through the kidney as evidenced by significant parenchymal retention at 20 min. There is, however, bladder activity.

and is only evident on renal biopsy several months after the transplant. The clinical manifestations are fever, increase in size of the kidney, graft tenderness, oliguria, and decrease in renal function as manifest by deterioration of the renogram and blood chemistries. The microscopic lesion consists of an infiltrate of small lymphocytes with edema in the interstitium. This type of rejection is usually reversible and will respond to treatment with large doses of glucocorticoids and graft irradiation. In addition to this, antilymphocyte serum may be used if available.

3. Chronic Rejection

Chronic rejection is seen from 6 months to many years following a transplant and is independent of the acute reversible rejection episodes (Fig. 9). Usually the patient is asymptomatic and the diagnosis is suspected because the serum creatinine and BUN are elevated. A hippuran renogram will show deterioration of renal function. On biopsy there is a decrease in the size of the arterial lumens due to hyperplasia of the intima and thickening of the media of the vessels. There is also fibrosis of the interstitial tissue. These changes are progressive and will lead ultimately to the loss of function of the kidney. The cause is unknown and there is no specific therapy.

F. Treatment of Rejection

In the case of hyperacute or accelerated rejection, a transplant nephrectomy is the preferred treatment. Any delay will result in the appearance of a generalized toxic state in the recipient which may be life endangering. Prompt removal of the allograft will permit the recipient to return to the pretransplant state. If the rejection is thought to be acute and reversible, treatment with a bolus dose of glucocorticoids and graft irradiation will afford stabilization of the graft and return to a more normal level of function. At our institution, methylprednisolone bolus infusions of 0.5 g are given slowly intravenously, simultaneously with graft irradiation of 150 rads. One course of treatment consists of 2 g of methylprednisolone and 600 rads irradiation in four separate administrations. If there is no clinical response, this is repeated. The total dose of steroids given as a bolus should not exceed 6 g and irradiation should not exceed 1200 rads. If there is no response, then the treatment is discontinued, and the kidney is permitted to progress to complete rejection followed by a transplant nephrectomy. When the diagnosis of chronic rejection is confirmed by biopsy, no definitive treatment is indicated. The patient is followed closely and returned to dialysis when kidney function has deteriorated. The kidney may need to be removed upon return of the patient to dialysis if the patient becomes toxic.

G. Complications

1. Acute Postoperative Complications

As with any surgical procedure, fever may be one of the earliest complications seen following a renal transplant. The most common cause of fever in postoperative patients is retained pulmonary secretions. While this must be kept in mind in the transplant recipient, rejection of the kidney must also be considered. Chest X-ray, hippuran renogram, BUN, and serum creatinine values will help determine the exact etiology of the fever. A difficult differential diagnostic problem occurs in transplant recipients with oliguria and increasing BUN and serum creatinine levels. Here, it is necessary to determine whether rejection or acute tubular necrosis is present. Clinical signs of rejection include fever, tenderness over the allograft, and increased size of the graft. A hippuran renogram will show diminished excretion into the bladder. On the other hand, if acute tubular necrosis is the cause of oliguria the graft will not be enlarged and tender, and hippuran will be taken up by the kidney but not excreted (see Fig. 7a and b). If the latter is the cause, the patient needs to be managed with fluid restriction, renal diet, and dialysis when appropriate and followed closely for signs of improving renal function. If rejection is thought to be occurring, then appropriate treatment consists of bolus steroids and graft irradiation. Complications involving the alimentary tract can be seen at any time following a transplant. Bleeding or perforation from a peptic ulcer may be life threatening (28, 29). The added risk from either of these complications is so great that if a patient has a documented history of peptic ulcer disease, he should be considered as a candidate for a prophylactic ulcer operation prior to receiving the transplant (30). In the presence of an active ulcer, a vagotomy and gastric resection may be necessary. However, if the ulcer has healed, we prefer to employ a proximal gastric vagotomy without resection of the stomach. The development of pancreatitis is not rare and is also associated with an increased mortality (31). Should this diagnosis be made, the dose of steroids is tapered rapidly and the patient treated conservatively with total parenteral alimentation and nasogastric suction. If a patient has a previous history of pancreatitis we assess the pancreas with ultrasound and computerized tomography in order to detect any abnormality. Frequently, we will give the patient a trial of azathioprine prior to placing him on the transplant list. Colonic perforations that occur in the posttransplant period are also associated with an extremely high mortality (28, 32, 33). At our institution, if there is documented evidence of diverticular disease of the colon, we feel an elective resection of the colon should be done prior to receiving a transplant. In addition to the preceding, we have observed complications involving the wound itself, the blood vessels, or the urinary tract.

2. Wound Complications

a. HEMATOMA. In the immediate postoperative period, bleeding with subsequent hematoma formation is frequently seen (see Figs. 10 and 11). This is more common when a cadaver kidney has been used because the patient is frequently taken to the operating room immediately following dialysis. In those instances when the individual has required dialysis immediately following the operation, similar hemorrhage may occur. The clinical features are swelling and tenderness over the allograft with a concomitant fall in hematocrit. Ultrasonography often is helpful in differentiating this from rejection. Occasionally, the patient needs to be taken back to the operating room to have the hematoma evacuated.

b. INFECTION. Infections of the wound are uncommon. If the infection is superficial to the fascia, simply opening the wound and letting it heal by secondary intention will suffice. In some instances, infection is deep to the

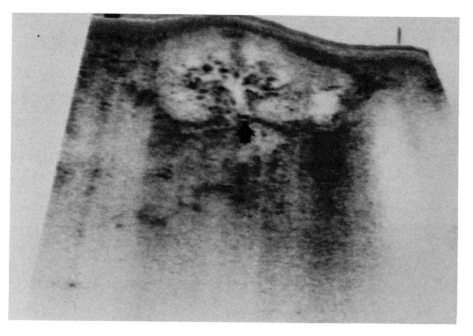

Fig. 10. Normal renal transplant. This static sonogram was obtained down the long axis of the renal transplant. The renal pelvis, infundibula, and calyces can be clearly outlined (arrow). The renal pyramids appear as hypoechoic areas relative to the more echogenic renal cortex. A sonolucent area in the lower pole of the transplant corresponded to an area of focal infarction secondary to sacrifice of a small accessory renal artery.

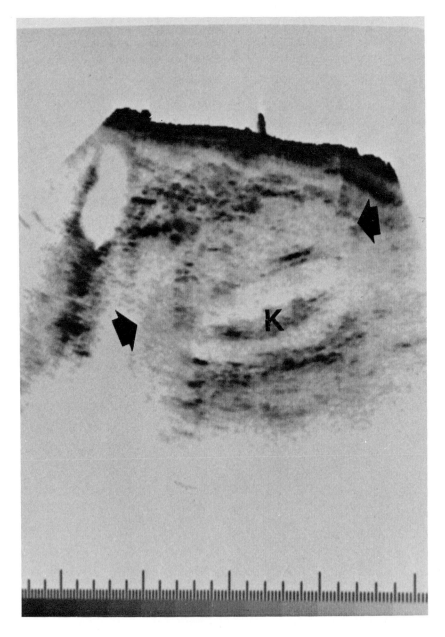

Fig. 11.   Longitudinal sonogram of hematoma (arrow) surrounding renal transplant (K). This mass is echogenic and corresponded to a large hematoma surrounding the transplant.

fascia and around the kidney and in these cases the entire wound must be left open to heal by secondary intention. Once the wound has started to granulate sufficiently, a split-thickness skin graft can be used and placed directly on the kidney. After there is complete healing, the patient can have the skin graft removed and the fascia can be closed over the kidney as an elective procedure.

c. LYMPHOCELE. Some patients will develop a perinephric collection of lymph which is called a lymphocele. The incidence is reported to be from 2 to 18% (*34, 35*). The major clinical manifestation is swelling around the graft. There may be a reduction in renal function due to obstruction. Rarely, the patient will present with unilateral edema of the leg. Ultrasonography can be quite helpful and it is our practice to order this procedure on any patient who develops sudden reduction in renal function (*36*) (Figs. 12 and 13). Methods of treatment include drainage through a small stab wound, open drainage, or intraperitoneal marsupialization. Initially, simple drainage may be successful. However, in a few instances the lymphocele will

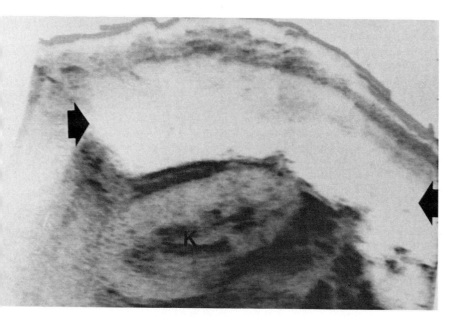

Fig. 12. Longitudinal static sonograms of lymphocele anterior to the transplanted kidney (K). A large echo free mass is seen anterior to the transplanted kidney (arrows). Within the lymphocele are some linear interfaces probably representing synchae.

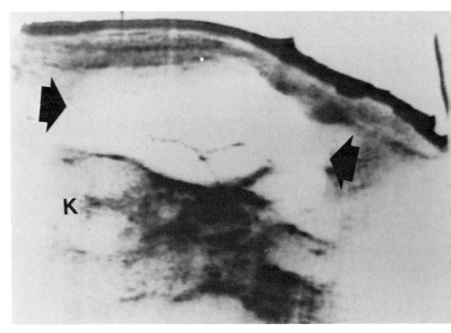

Fig. 13.   Longitudinal static sonogram of urinoma (arrows). The mass has a similar sonographic appearance to the lymphocele depicted in Fig. 12. The mass is anterior to the transplanted kidney (K).

reaccumulate. In these cases we have utilized open drainage permitting the wound to heal by secondary intention.

3.   Vascular Complications

If careful inspection is made at the initial procedure, bleeding from the anastomoses can usually be prevented. We have seen thrombosis of the transplant artery in a few instances. This usually occurs in the first 24 hr, although on one occasion it developed as late as 1 week following the operation. By the time the diagnosis is established, it is usually too late to salvage the kidney. When this diagnosis is suspected, either an arteriogram or a technetium pertechnetate isotopic flow study should be carried out immediately. If either of these studies demonstrates no arterial flow to the kidney, then immediate exploration should be undertaken. Although chances of the kidney being viable are slim, there have been several reported cases of successful revascularization following ischemic times of up to 5 hr. Therefore, exploration is mandatory to determine the precise status of the kidney (*37*). A thrombotic event also indicates the necessity for a very thorough evaluation of the patient's hematological status. Next, the position of the

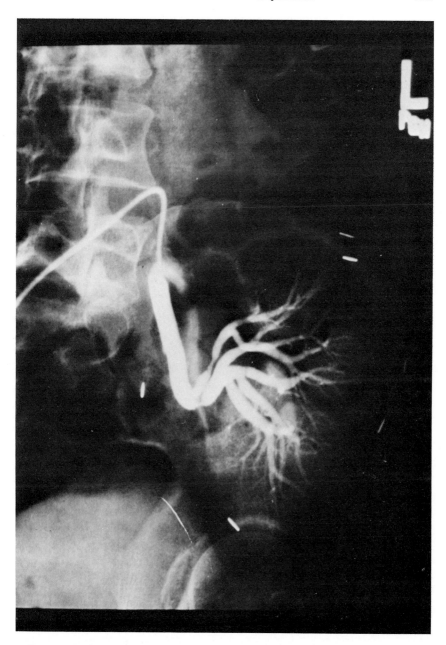

Fig. 14.   Radiograph with contrast material injected into patient's left hypogastric artery. Note stenosis of two of the secondary renal arteries distal to the end-to-end anastomosis of the renal artery with the hypogastric artery.

kidney is important because kinking of the artery may compromise the circulation. This functional stenosis will reduce blood flow and create a "jet effect" leading to subintimal fibrosis with eventual anatomic narrowing of the artery (*38*). The renal artery stenosis may then cause hypertension (*39–41*) (Fig. 14). Finally, thrombosis of the renal vein rarely occurs but can lead to venous hypertension with subsequent infarction of the kidney (*42*). This will necessitate a transplant nephrectomy.

4.   Urinary Tract Complications

Because continuity of the urinary tract must be reestablished, we encounter complications resulting from this procedure (*43*). Extravasation of urine can occur at any time during the first 2 weeks. There can be simple leakage from the ureteroneocystostomy, where the ureter is implanted into the bladder. There can also be leakage from the other cystotomy wound, which is made in order to do the ureteral implant. Leakage from the site of implantation of the ureter can often be treated by catheter drainage of the bladder (Fig. 15).

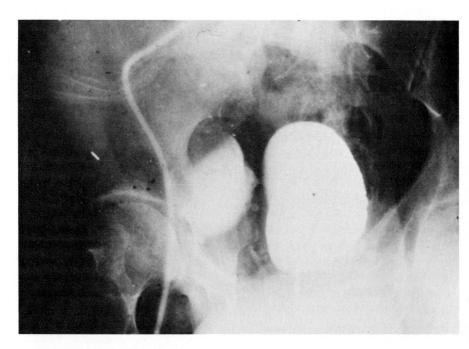

Fig. 15.   Radiograph showing a cystogram in a patient who had been transplanted 10 days previously. Note extravasation of dye outside bladder. A diagnosis of leakage from the ureteroneocystostomy was made and the patient was successfully treated with catheter drainage of the bladder for 10 days.

On the other hand, if the leak is from the breakdown of the cystotomy wound, surgical exploration with closure of the bladder is necessary. In rare instances we have seen necrosis of the ureter and this necessitates an alternate method of reconstruction. Should the patient's own ureter still be available, a ureteroureterostomy or a ureteropyelostomy can be carried out. If the patient has had a bilateral nephrectomy with removal of the ureters, and the donor ureter has become necrotic, a transplant nephrectomy will unfortunately be necessitated.

V. IMMUNOSUPPRESSION

Despite attempts to match the tissues of the donor with the recipient and to thereby decrease the chance of rejection, almost all patients who receive kidney transplants undergo some sort of rejection process. Generally, it is the success with which rejection can be managed with immunosuppressive drugs that dictates the chance of success for the transplant. Although necessary to achieve long-term transplant function, the side effects of these medications provide the major hazard for the transplant patient. Research continues to develop improved methods of immunosuppression with a greater therapeutic index. Currently, certain key drugs are utilized in an attempt to prevent and/or treat rejection.

A. Azathioprine (Imuran)

The immunosuppressive effects of azathioprine were first demonstrated in 1958 by Schwartz and Dameshek (5). It was first used in human kidney transplantation in 1961 and, since that time, has become a mainstay of most immunosuppressive regimens (6). The drug is given orally, is quickly and almost completely absorbed, and depends for its immunosuppressive effects on its metabolism by the liver to various active metabolites. Exactly how these metabolites affect the immune system is not entirely known. It is known, however, that azathioprine is an antimetabolite and inhibits DNA and RNA synthesis, although the immunological effects of the drug are probably not due to this effect alone. In humans, azathioprine's major effect seems to be on the lymphocyte, primarily the T lymphocyte. Through this mechanism, Imuran has been shown to inhibit the antigen recognition phase of the immunological response. Azathioprine side effects include bone marrow suppression, which is generally dose related, and a form of cholestatic hepatitis. This latter hepatic problem sometimes responds merely to a decrease in the dose of azathioprine or may require discontinuation of the drug. Azathioprine is rarely, if ever, given alone as an immunosuppressive drug after renal transplant, but more usually is given in combination with one or more additional immunosuppressive medications.

B. Corticosteroids

The most common steroid used as an immunosuppressant following transplantation is prednisone. When intravenous medication is required, methyl prednisolone (Solu-Medrol) is usually substituted for the prednisone when continued steroid therapy is desired. Prednisone exerts both an immunosuppressant and a very significant anti-inflammatory effect when given to humans. It is unclear which of these actions is primarily responsible for its effectiveness as a part of the immunosuppressive regimen following renal transplantation. Prednisone affects the way lymphocytes, primarily thymus-derived lymphocytes, respond to antigen *in vivo* and *in vitro*. In addition, this medication has the capacity to lyse cytotoxic lymphocytes, that is, those lymphocytes that have been sensitized by antigen and are about to, or have already, invaded the graft as part of the rejection process. Corticosteroids are used in two fashions in renal transplantation. In relatively low maintenance doses, they are effective in maintaining graft function by helping prevent rejection. In addition, once an acute rejection episode has started, higher steroid dosage over a short period of time has proved to be most effective in reversing acute rejection. Unfortunately, prednisone is responsible for the majority of complications seen in the posttransplant patient. It is probable that the multiple metabolic effects of this medication are responsible for the variety of problems that may be seen with its usage. These complications include increased susceptibility to infection, the development of diabetes mellitus, aseptic necrosis of bone, osteoporosis, cataracts, and peptic ulcer disease. Because of these hazards, one should strive to use the minimum amount of steroid necessary to maintain stable graft function. In addition, a maximum level of steroid should be decided on that will not be exceeded in the given patient. The amount of steroid that is reasonable for one patient may be very different from that which is appropriate for another. Steroids, like Imuran, are not effective in preventing graft rejection when given alone. They are always given as part of an overall immunosuppressive regimen, which generally includes azathioprine and may include other therapeutic modalities as well. The dose of corticosteroids used as part of these immunosuppressive regimens is variable. Prednisone in maintenance doses of 1–3 mg/kg/day is utilized initially after the transplant. The dose is tapered according to a varying schedule until a low, stable dose is achieved of 0.1–0.25 mg/kg/day. The dosage used to reverse an acute rejection episode is in the range of 5–10 mg/kg of prednisone or its equivalent given orally or as a single intravenous infusion. This dose may then be repeated every day or on alternate days as seems appropriate to reverse the rejection episode. Recently, because of side effects, there has been a general trend in transplantation to decrease the amount of prednisone given, particularly when a patient is considered to be in the high risk group.

C. Antilymphocyte Serum (ALS)

Antilymphocyte serum (ALS) is a potent immunosuppressive agent that is made by injecting human lymphocytes into animals of certain species and bleeding the animals to obtain serum. This serum contains antibody directed against those lymphocytes and, when appropriately purified, can be injected into humans causing destruction of lymphocytes and significant immunosuppressive effect. The methods of production and purification of antilymphocyte serum vary widely. It is now generally agreed that antilymphocyte preparations that can be demonstrated to have immunosuppressive properties by prolongation of skin graft survival in primates are highly effective in both preventing and treating transplant rejection (17). One commercial preparation, Atgam, is a highly purified globulin fraction of horse serum that is available from the Upjohn Company. We prefer to make our own antilymphocyte serum utilizing the rabbit. This material we believe to be less toxic and more effective than antilymphocyte preparations made in the horse. In addition, we have found that the rabbit protein has the advantage of being less allergenic in man, therefore requiring less purification prior to use. As all of these preparations contain foreign animal protein, the possibility for allergic reaction exists. Should a patient become sensitized to one animal protein, it *is* possible to utilize an antilymphocyte preparation that has been made in another animal. Often, however, the patient who becomes sensitized to one animal protein will also, with time, become sensitized to another. The sensitization of the patient to the protein contained within the antilymphocyte preparation not only increases the chance of (and is probably responsible for) allergic reactions in that patient but, because the foreign protein is rapidly deactivated by such a patient, it probably makes the antilymphocyte preparation ineffective.

Antilymphocyte preparations are generally used as part of an immunosuppressive regimen in combination with azathioprine and corticosteroids. The medication is given as daily injections starting the day of transplant and continuing for several weeks. ALS may also be reinstituted at any time to treat an acute rejection episode. Our ALS regimen entails the administration of nineteen treatments spread out over a 10 week period immediately posttransplant. Any subsequent rejection episode is treated by 14 additional treatments administered over 8 weeks. The antirejection therapy is generally also combined with corticosteroid and azathioprine administration.

D. Irradiation

Total body irradiation was one of the earliest immunosuppressive regimens used in renal transplantation. Although demonstrably quite effective, it is no longer used because leukopenia and fatal sepsis frequently resulted. Local graft irradiation, however, is utilized by numerous transplant programs, generally in conjunction with other antirejection modalities such as steroids and/or antilymphocyte serum. Since excess irradiation itself may injure the kidney, the dosage must be limited to that which can safely be given, about 1200 rads to any individual kidney. This total dose is usually administered in increments of 150 rads on a daily or alternate day schedule according to the dictates of the clinical situation.

E. Lymphocyte Depletion by Thoracic Duct Drainage

Lymphocyte depletion by means of thoracic duct drainage pretransplant has been demonstrated by several centers to enhance allograft survival. Because of the logistical problems related to the cannulation of the thoracic duct and the maintenance of lymph flow during the prolonged period of time required to achieve the desired results, drainage is utilized in only a few transplant programs. Another form of lymphocyte depletion, lymphopheresis, is currently under investigation. Preliminary evidence would suggest that similar salutary immunological effects can be achieved by this method. The advantage of lymphopheresis is that it is less complicated and can be performed during dialysis on an outpatient basis. The methodology is similar to plasmapheresis.

F. Other Immunosuppressive Medications

A variety of additional approaches toward the immunosuppression of the patient either prior to or following transplantation are currently under investigation. *Cyclosporin A* is a drug that was initially used as an antifungal agent but subsequently has been found to have significant immunosuppressive properties. This drug is currently under investigation in several transplant centers around the world. Initial evaluation has demonstrated Cyclosporin A to be a potent immunosuppressive agent, although side effects have included the occurrence of severe nephrotoxicity and a disturbingly high incidence of lymphoma. Hopefully, these side effects are dose related and can be eliminated as more is learned about the administration of the drug. Although not ready for general use this drug shows significant promise for the future. *Total lymphoid irradiation* is a means of immunosuppression attained by irradiating the majority of lymphoid tissue of the body. This is accomplished prior to transplantation and results in significant immuno-suppressive effect. Several centers are investigating this method but their results are too preliminary to determine its potential usefulness in kidney transplantation.

Effective immunosuppression posttransplant, generally involves the judicious use of several immunosuppressive modalities. Since the perfect regimen has yet to be achieved, these immunosuppressive regimens are under constant modification in order to improve results and decrease risk.

VI. LONG-TERM MANAGEMENT

If there are no complications, the usual length of hospitalization after a successful renal transplant is about 21 days. This 3 week stay is necessary because acute rejection is most likely to occur during this period. The earlier acute rejection is identified and treatment instituted, the more likely that the rejection can be successfully reversed. In addition to the close clinical scrutiny which this period of hospitalization affords, a process of patient education is begun to introduce the posttransplant therapeutic regimen. This regimen is in many ways entirely different from that which the patient has utilized during his dialytic treatment.

A. Medication

The posttransplant patient at the time of discharge is faced with a be-wildering array of medications which must be taken at appropriate times during the day every day during his initial posttransplant course. In addition to the immunosuppressive drugs already mentioned (Imuran and prednisone) the patient must also take a variety of other medications. Generally, an antacid is given repetitively during the day and at bedtime in an attempt to decrease the chance of developing peptic ulcer disease. Cimetidine (Tagamet) is prescribed for those patients who are at particularly high risk for the development of peptic ulcer or for those patients who develop symptoms of hyperacidity during their posttransplant course. Vitamins, iron, and usually a prophylactic antibiotic preparation (most commonly a sulfa drug) may be part of the posttransplant medication regimen. Because of the high dose of steroids given initially after transplant, many patients have a tendency to retain salt and water and therefore must take diuretics. There is also a tendency toward high blood pressure after transplantation which may re-quire therapeutic intervention. The critical nature of these medications is such that the patient should be able to demonstrate the ability to take his own medications prior to discharge from the hospital. Toward this end, an intensive education program is utilized so that by 14 days posttransplant the patient should be taking his own medications under the supervision of the nursing staff in the hospital. To facilitate the education process and to assure the correct administration of the medications, each patient is given a notebook listing each medication that he is expected to take and the time that the medication is to be taken each day. He checks off the medications as they are taken and, in that way, is less likely to forget or confuse medication. This process is continued after discharge from the hospital. The accuracy of the medication administration is checked by review of the notebook when the patient returns for regular clinic visits. The process of education and self-medication while still in the hospital has proved to be a highly successful method to train the patient as to the importance of regular medication administration and to ensure accuracy of administration before the patient is discharged from the hospital.

B. Diet

The specifics of the posttransplant diet which is utilized by our program are outlined in detail elsewhere in this volume (Chapter 12). This diet is quite different from that which is consumed during the patient's period of dialytic therapy and therefore must also be learned by him and his family. In general, this diet is high in protein and low in carbohydrates, with the needed calories being made up by adding the appropriate amount of fat. The degree of adherence to this diet, in our experience, determines how effectively the cosmetic side effects of exogenous hypercortisolism can be avoided. Caloric limitation is also important as the steroids utilized after transplant greatly stimulate the appetite. If uncurbed, this appetite will invariably lead to excessive weight gain, usually to the distress of the patient involved.

C. Exercise

Following discharge from the hospital, each patient is encouraged to embark on a regular exercise routine. Because of the hazard of aseptic necrosis, which seems most likely to affect the weight-bearing joints (the hips and knees), we encourage patients to engage in exercises which are non-weight-bearing. A variety of floor calisthenics are utilized, but jogging, running, and even walking for long distances are discouraged for the first year after transplant. Athletic activities, such as tennis, basketball, etc., which may stress the skeletal system, are also discouraged for this period of time. The ideal exercise for the posttransplant patient is probably swimming. This activity exercises most of the muscle groups of the body and yet is virtually free of weight bearing. The use of an "exercycle" in the home is also encouraged to strengthen the legs which may be particularly prone to weakness secondary to the prednisone administration.

D. Clinical Monitoring

During hospitalization, the patient is closely observed for signs and symptoms of rejection as well as infection. Blood pressures are monitored regularly as are the patient's temperature, urine output, and daily weight. While in the hospital, the patient is taught how to measure urine output, to take blood pressure and temperature, and to weigh accurately. These data are tabulated in the transplant notebook. To check for the possibility of gastrointestinal bleeding the patient also learns to test the stool for occult blood. Upon discharge from the hospital these elements of clinical monitoring are continued in the home setting. Ranges of acceptance for each measured clinical parameter are provided for the patient so that results outside these normal ranges stimulate a call to notify the health care team that such an abnormality has been documented. Such an occurrence generally dictates a clinic or hospital emergency room visit for further evaluation. We encourage our patients to check blood pressure twice a day, temperature twice a day, weight every morning, 24 hr urine output daily, and the stool for occult blood twice a week during the initial 6 months posttransplant. Although the degree of compliance with this regimen varies widely, most patients do a remarkably good job in keeping up with their data and in notifying us when a problem is identified by their own clinical monitoring at home. As mentioned previously, patients who are unwilling or unable to comply with the posttransplant regimen place themselves at increased risk of complications after transplant and decreased likelihood of having a successful kidney for very long.

In addition to the above home clinical monitoring, the patients are seen at regular intervals in the clinic. During the first week after discharge, patients are seen twice. Thereafter, they are seen at weekly intervals for a month, and then start coming back to the transplant clinic every 2 weeks for about the next 3 months. Following this, the frequency of visits is dictated by the degree of follow-up care the patient can obtain in his own community and by the clinical status. Whenever possible, the patient's nephrologist is involved in the posttransplant care. Ideally, a situation is arranged where posttransplant follow-up visits are alternated between the patient's nephrologist and the transplant clinic. Good communication between the transplant team and the patient's nephrologist with sharing of laboratory and clinical data ensures that both physicians are aware of all developments of importance during the posttransplant period. After the first year posttransplant, should the patient desire it, the entire responsibility for posttransplant care may be shifted to the patient's nephrologist with only rare visits back to the transplant clinic.

At each clinic visit we obtain certain laboratory tests to evaluate the patient's status. These include a white blood cell count, hematocrit, and platelet count to monitor the azathioprine (Imuran) dose; BUN and serum creatinine to follow renal function; serum potassium if the patient is on a diuretic; serum calcium and phosphorus to observe for evidences of continuing hyperparathyroidism or possible hypophosphatemia, which often occurs after transplantation; serum bilirubin, SGOT, and alkaline phosphatase to observe for possible hepatotoxicity of the azathioprine; and serum uric acid because of the not infrequent occurrence of hyperuricemia in the posttransplant period. Routine urinalyses are obtained at each clinic visit to observe for proteinuria and pyuria. Urine cultures are also obtained at each clinic visit to evaluate for the presence of urinary tract infection. Should such an infection occur, even if asymptomatic, it is treated with appropriate antibiotics.

E. Rehabilitation

Renal transplantation is not a cure for ESRD. It is merely a form of treatment for that medical problem. Patients must continue to take immunosuppressive medications after transplantation for as long as their transplants function. The discontinuation of that medication will, in all likelihood, result in the loss of the grafted organ. It is not unrealistic to anticipate that the successful renal transplant patient will be capable of returning to full time employment 6–8 months posttransplantation. We tend to suggest that such employment not involve strenuous physical activity, at least initially. The watchword is to start slowly and gradually increase the number of hours worked as well as the amount of activity while observing the patient's health. The degree of activity which can be tolerated is frequently determined by the presence or absence of complications during the preemployment, posttransplant period. Generally, a higher proportion of patients become reemployed after successful transplantation than are employed during their time on dialysis.

F. Sexual Function

Impotence in the male and decreased libido in the male and female are commonly reported problems in the dialysis population. Following transplantation a significant number of patients report improvement in these sexual problems. This improvement, however, is far from uniform as many patients report impotence and decreased libido persisting even after successful transplantation. Sexual counseling is as important to the patient and the patient's spouse after transplant as it is during dialytic therapy. The relatively high incidence of hypertension and the necessity of administering antihypertensive agents, which are known to adversely affect sexual function, may complicate the situation in those patients who require these medications.

Most women being treated with dialysis for their ESRD are infertile. Most men on dialysis, because of low sperm counts, are unlikely to father children. Following successful transplantation, both sexes usually return to their pre-renal failure state with regard to their ability to have children. A conscious decision on the part of these patients as to the timing of families or the desire to have children must therefore be made. In the past it has been recommended to patients who have received transplants and who are taking immunosuppressive medications that it would be unwise to have children because of the risk of birth defects. With the experience that has been obtained from patients who elected to have children anyway, such a blanket recommendation against procreation seems inappropriate (44). There is, however, an increased incidence of spontaneous abortion and of teratogenic effects. Patients should be counseled about the effects of these medications on potential offspring and then allowed to decide for themselves whether they feel it is appropriate to proceed with raising a family. Such unknowns as the life expectancy for the posttransplant patient, the quality of life likely to be enjoyed by that particular patient, and the hazard of rejecting the kidney with the resultant return of the patient to dialysis must also play a part in this decision. We strongly recommend to our patients that they should not consider initiating a family until at least 18 months posttransplantation. After this period of time we will have a much better idea of what the future holds for that kidney and patient.

VII. LONG-TERM COMPLICATIONS FOLLOWING TRANSPLANTATION

Although the greatest chance for complications is during the immediate posttransplant period, problems may also occur well after discharge from the hospital. As with early problems, these late complications of transplantation are primarily related to the immunosuppression that is being given to prevent rejection of the kidney.

A. Rejection

The most common complication late after transplantation continues to be rejection. Both acute and chronic rejection can be seen and are pathologically and clinically the same regardless of when in the posttransplant course the process occurs. The need for continued immunosuppressive therapy for as long as the transplanted kidney functions must be stressed repeatedly to patients. Although there are isolated cases of patients stopping their immunosuppression without rejection occurring, such cases are distinctly the exception rather than the rule. It is estimated that the discontinuation of immunosuppressive therapy will result in acute rejection in 80–85% of patients who do so, regardless of how much time has elapsed since the transplant (45). An acute rejection episode long after transplantation must always raise the possibility that immunosuppressive therapy has been stopped. Specific questioning is often rewarding in this regard.

B. Cardiovascular Disease

1. Hypertension

Elevated blood pressure is relatively common following transplantation. Hypertension may be related to excess salt intake, steroid administration with its attendant salt retaining effects, or simply due to the decreased ability of a transplanted kidney to handle volume because of damage sustained during the early posttransplant course. Fluid retention is usually handled satisfactorily with diuretic therapy. Hypertension caused by excessive secretion of renin by the kidney is more difficult to treat. This hyperreninemic hypertension can be due to rejection, usually of the chronic type, or may be secondary to narrowing of the main renal artery (46). This latter condition can usually be corrected surgically or, alternatively, the stenotic lesion may be treated by transluminal dilatation with a balloon catheter (47). Either process is quite successful in relieving the hypertension. Drug therapy is also useful in this situation. Hypertension may also be related to recurrent glomerulonephritis in the transplanted kidney or may be caused by the patient's own kidneys if they have not been removed in preparation for transplant. Severe hypertension caused by the patient's own kidneys may dictate their removal. Control of hypertension is essential since continued elevation of blood pressure will damage the allograft.

2. Coronary Artery Disease Associated
with Hypercholesterolemia

The reader is referred to the chapter on endocrine and metabolic changes in ESRD.

C. Infection with Bacteria and Viruses

As the dose of immunosuppression, specifically corticosteroid, is reduced the patient's susceptibility to infection likewise is lessened. Despite this, late infection with bacterial, viral, or fungal agents occurs with greater frequency than in patients not taking immunosuppressive drugs (48, 49). The treatment of a late rejection episode with increased immunosuppression may further increase the patient's susceptibility to infection. Of the viral infections, cytomegalovirus, herpes zoster, and herpes simplex are the most frequent. The herpes infections are most often localized and usually do not disseminate. Cytomegalovirus infection, however, often involves multiple organs, particularly the lungs and liver (50). Because cytomegalovirus infection can be associated with fever and decreased renal function, it is at times difficult to distinguish from an acute rejection episode. Percutaneous allograft biopsy may clarify this situation and dictate appropriate therapy. If doubt exists, the results of a biopsy should be available to confirm rejection before treatment is instituted because of the severe consequences of giving additional steroids to a patient who has active cytomegalovirus infection.

A wide variety of bacterial infections also may affect the posttransplant patient. Bacteremia is not uncommon. The urinary tract is a likely site of origin; thus, urine cultures at each clinic visit are important for early detection. A sulfa drug, such as sulfisoxazole (Gantrisin) may be given to suppress urinary tract infection. We utilize this form of prophylactic antibiotic coverage in our program.

D.   Fungal and Other Infections

Cryptococcus, Candida, Aspergillus, and Histoplasma infections are seen more commonly in the immunocompromised patient. In addition, nocardiosis and toxoplasmosis are observed with a fair frequency in renal transplant recipients. These unusual infections must be considered in any transplant patient with clinical evidence of infection.

It is axiomatic in transplantation that the occurrence of a significant infection dictates withdrawal of immunosuppressive therapy. Steroid doses must be significantly reduced (usually to the level of 10–15 mg/day) in the face of such infection to facilitate the patient's response to the infection. Often such withdrawal of immunosuppression results in loss of the kidney and the return of the patient to dialysis. Despite this, such a maneuver gives the patient the best chance for survival and therefore must be utilized. Care must also be taken, however, to assure adequate steroid coverage during an infection, since many transplant patients have suppressed adrenal function.

E.   Bone Complications after Transplantation

Virtually all patients with renal failure have some element of bone disease due to secondary hyperparathyroidism. With the reestablishment of normal renal function after transplantation, parathyroid overactivity generally decreases with time. In some instances, however, hyperparathyroidism continues quite long into the posttransplant period and, when this occurs, is termed *tertiary* hyperparathyroidism. Subtotal parathyroidectomy may be indicated when significant hypercalcemia, evidence of progressive bone involvement or extraosseous calcification is demonstrated. The necessity for parathyroidectomy after transplantation is, however, unusual.

The most common bone disease affecting the posttransplant patient is aseptic necrosis (*51*). This lesion occurs in about 5% of posttransplant patients and seems to be correlated with the age of the patient (older patients being more likely to experience this problem) and the amount of corticosteroid administered to the patient during the first 6–8 months after transplant. Higher dose corticosteroid administration in the early posttransplant period increases the likelihood that aseptic necrosis will occur. Generally, this lesion involves weight-bearing joints, most commonly the hips and knees. This condition is associated with pain in the hip and knee which may precede the radiological demonstration of bone pathology. Bone scan will often pick up the evidence of aseptic necrosis early, at times in advance of radiological change. Treatment of the problem includes limiting weight bearing as much as possible and then, when pain and/or bone destruction becomes severe, prosthetic replacement of the affected bone. Such replacement surgery has in our experience proved quite successful in relieving the pain while preserving good mobility in the affected joints.

F. Gastrointestinal Complications

The gastrointestinal complications after transplantation are generally thought to be due to steroid therapy and therefore are also directly related to the dose of steroids being utilized. The most common complication is peptic ulcer disease with bleeding and/or perforation (*52*). Because these complications result in a high mortality, all efforts must be utilized to identify patients with a prior history of peptic ulcer disease and to institute therapy prior to transplantation. All patients are treated aggressively with antacid therapy to lessen the possibility of development of an ulcer. Cimetidine (Tagamet) is utilized at the first development of ulcer symptomatology.

Large bowel perforation is fortunately a rare complication but is devastating when it does occur. Generally, this occurs in previously existing large bowel diverticula. Thus, the presence of diverticula in the transplant candidate is a risk factor that must be considered prior to transplantation. The peritonitis resulting from large bowel perforation is among the most difficult posttransplant problems to manage successfully.

Pancreatitis occurring after transplantation is generally thought to be due to either steroids, Imuran, or the combination of these two drugs (53). All too often pancreatitis is recurrent in nature. It is quite important to identify such patients with a history of pancreatitis prior to transplant so that they may be counseled about their increased risk. When pancreatitis occurs, it is treated in the standard way but is more refractory to treatment than in the patient who is not receiving immunosuppression. Withdrawal of the immunosuppression is critical in the successful management of this transplant complication as it is with all the gastrointestinal complications mentioned above.

G. Liver Complications

Evidence of viral hepatitis is quite common in hemodialysis patients. Thus, the assessment of liver problems after transplantation must be interpreted in the setting of what transpired in that patient prior to transplantation (54). Nevertheless, there is little doubt that azathioprine (Imuran) can cause hepatic injury as can many of the other drugs being administered after transplantation. Regular follow-up of liver function studies is mandatory during the posttransplant period. Progressive deterioration of these liver function tests dictates a withdrawal of potentially hepatotoxic medications including a tapering of azathioprine (Imuran) to that dose at which the liver function abnormalities improve. It is controversial whether the withdrawal of Imuran should be accompanied by replacement with another immunosuppressive drug such as cyclophosphamide (Cytoxan). Because cyclophosphamide has been demonstrated to decrease the numbers of suppressor T cells, we currently do not replace Imuran with this or any other immunosuppressant when decrease of Imuran dosage is necessary. In some instances, this has resulted in the total withdrawal of Imuran and the maintenance of the posttransplant patient on steroids alone. The discontinuation of Imuran alone has been reported to carry about a 25% risk of initiating a rejection episode.

H. Malignant Tumors

Malignancies are about 100 times more frequent in the posttransplant patient than in the population at large (55). This increased incidence of malignancy seems to be due to the immunosuppressive drugs being used since it has also been reported in nontransplant patients receiving these medications for other purposes. Lymphoma is the most common such malignancy and accounts for about a third of all patients who develop malignant tumors posttransplant. Large cell lymphoid neoplasm (reticulum cell sarcoma, histiocytic lymphoma) is the most common cell type of lymphoma being seen. These lymphomas are now thought to be related to post transplant infection, possibly with EB virus. They are quite difficult to treat and carry a poor prognosis. Skin cancers are the second most common tumor type to be described in the posttransplant patient and usually are squamous cell carcinomas. These tumors are amenable to treatment and generally can be resected with cure.

I. Miscellaneous Complications

Various other problems can arise due to the steroid therapy. Cataracts occur in about 5% of patients receiving steroids posttransplant. Diabetes mellitus, not present in the recipient prior to transplant, can also develop in response to corticosteroid therapy and contribute to cataract formation. Often, as the steroids are tapered, the diabetic condition resolves, but not always. The cataracts generally progress until surgical removal is necessary.

It can be seen once again, by the list of potential problems that may afflict the posttransplant patient, that the decision for transplantation should not be arrived at casually. Patients and their families need to be aware of these potential problems and weigh them against those that may occur during other forms of therapy for their ESRD.

VIII. DATA ANALYSIS

Analysis of transplant results is a deceptively simple procedure. The initial inclination is simply to determine the number of patients who are alive and have a life-sustaining renal function at some time point after transplantation. However, this approach is incomplete since it does not reveal information about the number of grafts lost to rejection, those lost for technical reasons (i.e., primary nonfunction of the graft, arterial stenosis, etc.), and those lost because of patient death. If information regarding the *mechanism* of failure is sought, which might be of use in improving results, then it is necessary to critically evaluate each individual component. In the Nashville Transplant Program* almost as many grafts are lost for technical reasons as to rejection (Table I). Thus, improvement in results can be anticipated not only with more effective immunosuppression but also by more thorough evaluation of the grafted kidney and the transplant recipient.

Another difficulty with only considering the overall results is that graft

---

* Includes resources of Vanderbilt University and Veterans Administration Medical Centers and Dialysis Clinics, Incorporated.

TABLE I

Patient and Graft Survival Since Initiation of ALS Utilization (1978–1981), Nashville Transplant Program[a]

Group[b]	Time (years)	Number[c]	Graft survival (%) Rejection[d]	Graft survival (%) Technical[e]	Patient survival all causes[f] (%)	Functioning graft survival[g] (%)
Cadaver donor						
Primary low risk	1	50	88.4	91.8	87.1	71.6
	2	31	88.4	91.8	87.1	67.2
Primary high risk[h]	1	38	78.9	88.9	73.1	52.2
	2	13	78.9	88.9	66.5	47.5
Repeat transplant	1	41	74.5	91.5	89.9	65.9
	2	36	69.4	91.5	78.2	53.1
Total	1	129	80.9	90.8	84.1	64.1
	2	70	77.0	90.8	78.3	56.8
Related Donor						
Low risk only						
2 haploidentical	1	33	92.9	96.8	100.0	90.1
	2	29	92.9	96.8	100.0	90.1
1 haploidentical	1	47	86.6	100.0	95.2	82.1
	2	30	86.6	100.0	95.2	82.1
All (low and high risk)						
2 haploidentical	1	39	93.6	94.7	91.8	81.1
	2	31	93.6	94.7	91.8	81.1
1 haploidentical	1	53	87.8	100.0	86.2	75.1
	2	32	87.8	100.0	86.2	75.1
Total	1	92	90.4	96.2	90.1	77.9
	2	63	90.4	96.2	90.1	77.9

[a] Includes resources of Vanderbilt University and Veterans Administration Medical Centers and Dialysis Clinics, Inc.
[b] Includes only patients transfused sometime prior to transplant (excepting two-haplotype related). Most received ALS following transplantation.
[c] Number of patients at beginning of time interval.
[d] Grafts lost to rejection.
[e] Grafts lost for reasons other than rejection.
[f] Patients dying for any reason.
[g] Patients alive with life-sustaining graft function.
[h] Patients with history of diabetes, pancreatitis, oxylosis, older than 50 years, and foreign nationals.

loss tends to be considered as due to rejection. This is a problem since it could subtly influence the way a patient with a nonfunctioning graft is treated. For example, it has recently been demonstrated that cytomegalovirus infections can mimic rejection symptoms. If one is accustomed to thinking only in terms of rejection, inappropriate therapy could be initiated.

In addition to determining how to categorize the various causes of failure, several decisions regarding patient classification must be made. Should a patient who has initially rejected a transplant and returned to dialysis, but who subsequently dies on dialysis, be considered a transplant death? In this case, choosing a period of time to consider the patient to have been "at risk" of the operative procedure after rejecting the transplant would probably be the most appropriate decision. Another possible circumstance is a patient whose graft is rejected because the immunosuppressive medication has been terminated in an attempt to save his life. How should this patient's graft loss be considered? Although there is probably no absolutely right (or wrong) way to account for such circumstances, the decision should be based on what one hopes to determine from the data analysis and requires a patient-by-patient evaluation.

A question often overlooked in analysis of transplant results is to what should the values be compared. The obvious choice would be results of patients on dialysis. This immediately becomes more involved since several dialytic procedures are now available. Patients may also be deemed too sick or too old for transplantation yet are carried on dialysis registers. Another complicating factor is that transplantation is performed at one central location whereas dialysis occurs at a number of referring locations. Unless data are available from all (or at least representative) locations a direct comparison between these treatment modalities cannot be made.

Transplant data are usually analyzed using actuarial or life-table methods. The formula for calculating survival is as follows:

$$P_{(t)} = P_{(t-1)}(1 - F/N - 1/2WD) \tag{1}$$

with P = proportion surviving; t = time interval post transplant; F = number failing during that time interval; N = number at risk at beginning of time interval; WD = number withdrawn during the time interval (56).

The formula allows for the inclusion of new patients who enter the data pool and also takes into account those patients who have not been "at risk" for the entire time interval. This formula allows for projected survival values. However, in transplantation where the patient population and treatment modalities change with time, this aspect is not useful since these changes cannot readily be identified in this analytic procedure.

As seen in the preceding sections, there are a number of factors that can potentially affect transplant survival results. The general approach to data analysis is to select one variable and ask whether or not altering this variable has an effect on transplant results. This, however, does not take into account the effect of combinations of variables. For example, a variable with a weak positive effect can be overridden by one with a strong positive effect, leading to the erroneous conclusion that the former had no effect at all. Unfortunately, multivariant data analysis is not always possible, either because the data base is too small (as in a single center analysis) or information on all of the appropriate variables is not always available (as in most multicenter analyses). Recently, a prospective study undertaken by the Southeastern Organ Procurement Foundation (SEOPF) has provided clarity regarding this for cadaveric transplants (*14*). Data were collected in a strictly controlled fashion and analyzed to allow for multiple (confounding) variables. The overall 1-year functional graft survival for 942 recipients of primary transplants was 48%, and the corresponding patient survival was 86%. The predominant factor affecting transplant success was whether or not the patient had been transfused prior to transplantation. Those patients who had been transfused had a 1-year functional graft survival of 52% as compared to 28% for individuals who had not been transfused. This dominant transfusion effect was obtained with recipients who had received a well-matched graft, i.e., sharing three or four HLA antigens of the A and B loci with their donor (55%) or a poorly matched graft, i.e., sharing two or less HLA antigens of the A and B loci with their donor (49%). Such data not only demonstrate the importance of transfusions but also suggest the importance of HLA matching. Further analysis revealed that recipients who had no HLA antigens mismatched with their donor had the best functional survival rate of 61% at 1 year. This study, using pooled data, demonstrated for the first time in the United States the beneficial effect of HLA matching on graft survival. Similar results had previously been shown only in single center analysis, presumably because some of the other confounding variables would tend to be more constant within a single center.

Another interesting finding of the SEOPF data was that the ancillary use of ALS also improved transplant survival by approximately 10%. This effect became most apparent when the data were stratified for transfusions and HLA match.

Two overall conclusions regarding this information can be made. First, the best transplant results are obtained in recipients who receive a well-matched graft, have at some point prior to transplantation received several transfusions, and who receive ALS treatment following transplantation. Conversely, the worst results would be expected in individuals receiving poorly matched grafts, who had not been transfused, and who were not treated with ALS. Second, the beneficial effects are roughly additive. Thus, intermediate survival values can be expected in recipients who have two of these three positive variables since the absence of one can be partially overcome by the presence of the other two. A corollary of this is that the effect a variable can have can be manifested at various times after transplantation. Thus, the effect that ALS utilization would have on survival rates would be expected to be seen immediately while the effect of HLA matching would be more long-term.

A number of other variables, such as donor and recipient age and race; pretransplant nephrectomy; incidence of acute tubular necrosis; utilization of diuretics, vasodilators and vasopressors in the donor; cause of donor death; origin of the kidney (i.e., local versus other centers), as well as method and time of preservation of the graft prior to transplantation, were also evaluated in the SEOPF study. Of these, the only factor that appeared to be of importance was pretransplant nephrectomy. Individuals who were ne-phrectomized because of some underlying medical condition (i.e., high blood pressure, etc.) had slightly improved graft survival in comparison to individuals who were nephrectomized only for preparation for transplant or individuals who had not been nephrectomized prior to transplant. Although all aspects of graft failure were not thoroughly analyzed in this study, the importance of multivariant analysis was clearly demonstrated.

One aspect of data analysis which is often overlooked is the type of patient involved. This is especially difficult to analyze since in part it involves a subjective evaluation of the patient. For example, although diabetes mellitus is recognized as a great risk for transplantation, it is readily appreciated that there are degrees of debilitation due to the disease and that these could influence the success of the transplant. In addition, the length of time the patient has had the disease prior to transplantation, as well as the length of time the patient has been on dialysis prior to transplantation, is also known to affect the transplant results. A similar complexity is seen when one critically evaluates patient age. Although most transplant centers would consider patients over the age of 50 to be at increased risk, it is readily recognized that some patients over this age are more physiologically fit than other patients who might be 30 years younger. At this transplant center, patients classified as high risk and who receive a cadaveric transplant have a 1-year functional graft survival of 52.2% as compared to low risk patients who have a 1-year functional graft survival of 71.6%. Approximately half of the losses in the high risk group are due to rejection while the other half is due to increased patient mortality (Table I).

A common observation in transplantation is that recipients of grafts from a living-related donor (LRD) generally have a more successful outcome than recipients of cadaveric transplants. Presumably, this reflects better matching *by chance* of antigens at minor histocompatibility loci than in the cadaveric situation. Confounding variables, i.e., transfusions, age, underlying disease, etc., can also be of significance in affecting results of transplants in recipients of living-related grafts. For example, in this transplant program, the 2-year patient survival of recipients of a living-related graft is 90.1%. However, almost half of the deaths occur in patients with insulin-dependent diabetes.

If such individuals are factored out of the calculations, the 2-year patient survival is 96.0%, making this the treatment of choice for patients with ESRD.

The lowest rejection rate for LRD recipients is obtained with patients who are HLA identical with a sibling donor. Such donor–recipient pairs share two haplotypes since they would have inherited the same two chromosomes from their parents. The rejection rate during the first year for such individuals in this program is 6.4% as compared to 12.2% for recipients sharing only one haplotype with the donor.

As with cadaveric transplants, preoperative transfusions and ALS utilization play a significant role in the transplant success of recipients of grafts from less than ideally HLA matched living-related donors. In addition, a confounding variable that appears to be of importance in recipients of living-related donor grafts is the gender of the recipient. The graft survival with living-related transplants obtained in this program is given in Fig. 16. As anticipated, preoperative transfusions did not influence graft survival in recipients of HLA identical grafts. In addition, blood transfusions did not appear to be of significance in females, although the amount of data is rather limited. Overall, transfused males had a better survival rate than nontransfused males. All recipients of one-haplotype (two antigen) matches also received ALS, which probably accounts for the improved results in this group as compared with the three antigen matched group that did not receive ALS. Surprisingly, females (whether or not they had been pregnant)

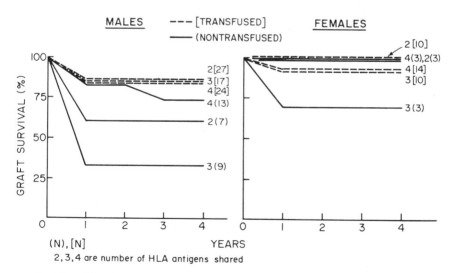

Fig. 16. Effect of gender, transfusions, and HLA antigen match on living related donor grafts in the Nashville Transplant Program, January 1977 through December 1981.

had a better graft survival than males. Whether this is due to differences in the type of original disease leading to the renal failure in those individuals or whether this might point to a basic immunological acceptability of foreign tissue by females needs to be clarified. Regardless of the reason, this emphasizes the need for multivariant analysis of transplant results.

The foregoing emphasizes that in order to make rational decisions regarding transplantation, a number of variables that can affect patient and graft survival must be considered. This type of information is most important in advising patients regarding which type of modality to select for the treatment of ESRD.

If the form of therapy decided on for the patient is transplantation, its successful implementation depends on a continuation of the same team approach that was utilized in deciding on the approach to this patient's therapy. It is also important to reassess therapeutic decisions periodically as a patient's clinical situation changes and as the effectiveness of the alternative therapies is improved by medical research. The problem of adequate organs for transplant will only be solved by the gradual process of public and professional education. This task is immense and will be accomplished only if all involved with ESRD patients and medical staff alike participate.

GENERAL REFERENCES

Alfred, H. J., Graff, L. G., Cohen, A. J. et al. Treatment of renal failure. In "Pathophysiology of Renal Disease" (B. D. Rose, ed.), pp. 475–573. McGraw-Hill, New York, 1981.

Carpenter, C. B., Strom, T. B., and Garovoy, R. M. Renal transplantation: Immunobiology. In "The Kidney" (B. M. Brenner and F. C. Rector, eds.), pp. 2544–2598. Saunders, Philadelphia, Pennsylvania, 1981.

Hollenberg, N. K., and Tilney, N. L. Renal transplantation: Donor selection and surgical aspects. In "The Kidney" (B. M. Brenner and F. C. Rector, Jr., eds.), pp. 2599–2617. Saunders, Philadelphia, Pennsylvania, 1981.

Strom, T. B., Tilney, N. L., and Merrill, J. P. Renal transplantation: Clinical management of the transplant recipient. In "The Kidney" (B. M. Brenner and F. C. Rector, Jr., eds.), pp. 2618–2658. Saunders, Philadelphia, Pennsylvania, 1981.

REFERENCES

1. Carrel, A. Anastomosis and transplantation of blood vessels. Am. Med. 10, 284–285 (1905).
2. Hume, D. M. Early experiences in organ homotransplantation in man and the unexpected sequelae thereof. Am. J. Surg. 137, 152–161 (1979).

3. Merrill, J. P. An historical perspective of transplantation. *Dial. Transplant.* **11**, 32–37 (1982).

4. Hume, D. M., Merrill, J. P., Miller, B. F., *et al.* Experience with renal homotransplantation in the human. Report of nine cases. *J. Clin. Invest.* **34**, 327–378 (1955).

5. Schwartz, R., Stack, J., and Dameshek, W. Effect of 6-mercaptopurine on antibody production. *Proc. Soc. Exp. Biol. Med.* **99**, 164–167 (1958).

6. Murray, J. E., Shoil, A. G. R., Moseley, R., *et al.* Analysis of the mechanism of immunosuppressive drugs in renal homotransplantation. *Ann. Surg.* **160**, 449–473 (1964).

7. Starzl, R. E., Marchioro, T. L., Porter, K. A., *et al.* The use of heterologous antilymphoid agents in canine renal and liver homotransplantation and in human renal homotransplantation. *Surg., Gynecol. Obstet.* **124**, 301–317 (1967).

8. Little, C. C., and Tyzzer, E. E. Further experimental studies on the inheritance of susceptibility to a transplantable tumor carcinoma of the Japanese waltzing mouse. *J. Med. Res.* **33**, 393–425 (1916).

9. Dausset, J. Leuco-agglutinins and blood transfusion. *Vox Sang.* **4**, 190 (1954).

10. Ting, A., and Morris, P. J. Powerful effect of HL-DR matching on survival of cadaveric renal allografts. *Lancet* **2**, 282–285 (1980).

11. Ascher, N. L., Simmons, R. L., Fryd, D., *et al.* Effects of HLA-A and B matching on success of cadaver grafts at a single center. *Transplantation* **28**, 172–178 (1979).

12. Albrechtsen, D., Bratalie, A., Kiss, E. *et al.* Significance of HLA matching in renal transplantation. *Transplantation* **28**, 280–284 (1979).

13. Walker, W. E., Niblack, G. W., Johnson, H. K., and Richie, R. E. Relationship of cadaveric renal transplant results to HLA tissue match. *Transplant. Proc.* **9**, 487–489 (1977).

14. McDonald, J. C., Vaughn, W., Filo, R. S. *et al.* Cadaver donor renal transplantation by centers of the Southeastern Organ Procurement Foundation. *Ann. Surg.* **193**, 1–8 (1981).

15. Helin, H., Pasternack, A., Falck, H., and Kuhlbäck, B. Recurrence of renal amyloid and de novo membranous glomerulonephritis after transplantation. *Transplantation* **32**, 6–9 (1981).

16. Pinto, J., Lacerda, G., Cameron, J. S. *et al.* Recurrence of focal segmental glomerulosclerosis in renal allografts. *Transplantation* **32**, 83–89 (1981).

17. Green, W. F., Niblack, G. D., Johnson, H. K., Richie, R. E. *et al.* Multifactorial analysis of factors influencing graft survival in recipients of living-related renal allografts. *Transplant. Proc.* (in press).

18. Patel, R., and Terasaki, P. I. Significance of the positive crossmatch in kidney transplantation. *N. Engl. J. Med.* **280**, 735–739 (1969).

19. Ringden, O., Friman, L., Göran, L., and Magnusson, G. Living related kidney donors: Complications and long term renal function. *Transplantation* **25**, 221–223 (1978).

20. Garcia-Rinaldi, R., Lefrak, E. A., Defore, W. W. *et al.* In situ preservation of cadaver kidneys for transplantation. *Ann. Surg.* **182**, 576–584 (1975).

21. Hume, D. M. Kidney transplantation. *In* "Human Transplantation" (F. T. Rapport and J. Dausset, eds.), pp. 110–150. Grune & Stratton, New York, 1968.

22. Simmons, R. L., Kjellstrand, C., and Najarian, J. S. Technique, complications, and results. *In* "Transplantation" (J. S. Najarian and R. L. Simmons, eds.), pp. 445–495. Lea & Febiger, Philadelphia, Pennsylvania, 1972.

23. Turner, B. Bilateral nephrectomy concomitant with renal transplantation. Presented at Southeastern Section, American Urological Association, 1981 (personal communication).

24. Freed, S. Z. Bilateral nephrectomy in transplant recipients. *Urology* **10**, Suppl., 16–21 (1977).

306   H. Keith Johnson, Robert E. Richie, and Gary D. Niblack

25. Richie, R. E., Rawl, J. L., and Braren, V. New incision for renal transplantation. *Urology* **9**, 433–435 (1977).
26. Howard, R. J., Simmons, R. L., and Najarian, J. S. Prevention of lymphoceles following renal transplantation. *Ann. Surg.* **184**, 166–168 (1976).
27. Merkel, F. K., Straus, A. K., Anderson, O. *et al.* Microvascular techniques for polar artery reconstruction in kidney transplantation. *Surgery* **79**, 253–261 (1976).
28. Hadjiyannakis, E. J., Evans, D. B., Smellie, W. A. B. *et al.* Gastrointestinal complications after renal transplant. *Lancet* **2**, 781–785 (1971).
29. Moore, T. C., and Hume, D. M. The period and nature of hazard in clinical renal transplantation. *Ann. Surg.* **170**, 1–11 (1969).
30. Spanos, P. K., Simmons, R. L., Rattazzi, L. C. *et al.* Ulcer disease in the transplant recipient. *Arch. Surg.* (*Chicago*) **109**, 193–197 (1974).
31. Tilney, N. L., Collins, J. J., Jr., and Wilson, R. E. Hemorrhagic pancreatitis: A fatal complication of renal transplantation. *N. Engl. J. Med.* **274**, 1051–1057 (1966).
32. Penn, I., Brettschneider, L., Simpson, K. *et al.* Major colonic problems in human homotransplant recipients. *Arch. Surg.* (*Chicago*) **100**, 61–65 (1970).
33. Demling, R. H., Salvatierra, O., and Belzer, F. O. Intestinal necrosis and perforation after renal transplantation. *Arch. Surg.* (*Chicago*) **110**, 251–253 (1975).
34. Schweizer, R. T., Cho, S. I., Kountz, S. L. *et al.* Lymphoceles following renal transplantation. *Arch. Surg.* (*Chicago*) **104**, 42–45 (1972).
35. Braun, W. E., Banowsky, L. H., Straffon, R. A. *et al.* Lymphoceles associated with renal transplantation. Report of 15 cases and review of literature. *Am. J. Med.* **57**, 714–729 (1974).
36. Phillips, J. F., Neiman, H. L., and Brown, T. L. Ultrasound diagnosis of post transplant lymphocele *Am. J. Roentgenol.* **126**, 1194–1196 (1976).
37. Gerard, D. F., Devin, J. B., Halasz, N. A. *et al.* Transplant renal artery thrombosis: Revascularization after $5\frac{1}{2}$ hours of ischemia. *Arch. Surg.* (*Chicago*) **117**, 361–362 (1982).
38. Morris, P. J., Yadav, R. V. S., Kincaid-Smith, P., *et al.* Renal artery stenosis in renal transplant. *Med. J. Aust.* **1**, 1255–1257 (1971).
39. La Combe, M. Arterial stenosis complicating renal allotransplantation in man. A study of 38 cases. *Ann. Surg.* **181**, 283–288 (1975).
40. Vidne, B. A., Leapman, S. B., Butt, K. M. *et al.* Vascular complications in human renal transplantation. *Surgery* **79**, 77–81 (1976).
41. Lindsey, E. S., Garbas, F. B., Golliday, E. S. *et al.* Hypertension due to renal artery stenosis in transplanted kidneys. *Ann. Surg.* **181**, 604–610 (1975).
42. Ehrlich, R. M., and Smith, R. B. Surgical complications of renal transplantation. *Urology* **10**, Suppl., 43–56 (1977).
43. Starzl, T. E., Groth, C. G., Putnam, C. W. *et al.* Urological complications in 216 human recipients of renal transplants. *Ann. Surg.* **172**, 1–22 (1970).
44. Penn, I., and Makowski, E. L. Parenthood in kidney and liver transplant recipients. *Transplant. Proc.* **13**, 36–39 (1981).
45. Zoller, K. M., Cho, S. I., Cohen, J. J., and Harrington, J. T. Cessation of immunosuppressive therapy after successful transplantation: A national survey. *Kidney Int.* **18**, 110–114 (1980).
46. Pollini, J., Guttmann, R. D., Beaudoin, J. G., Morehouse, D. D., Klassen, J., and Knaack, J. Late hypertension following renal allotransplantation. *Clin. Nephrol.* **11**, 202–212 (1979).
47. Sniderman, K. W., Sos, T. A., Sprayregen, S., Saddekni, S. *et al.* Percutaneous transluminal angioplasty in renal transplant arterial stenosis for relief of hypertension. *Diagn. Radiol.* **135**, 23–26 (1980).

48. Rubin, R. H., Wolfson, J. S., Cosini, A. B. *et al.* Infection in the renal transplant recipient. *Am. J. Med.* **70,** 405–411 (1981).

49. Ramsey, P. G., Rubin, R. H., Tolkoff-Rubin, N. E. *et al.* The renal transplant patient with fever and pulmonary infiltrates: Etiology, clinical manifestations, and management. *Medicine (Baltimore)* **59,** 206–222 (1980).

50. Simmons, R. L., Matas, A. J., Rattazi, L. C. *et al.* Clinical characteristics of the lethal cytomegalovirus, infection following renal transplantation. *Surgery* **82,** 537–546 (1977).

51. Nielson, H. E., Melsen, F., and Christensen, M. S. Aseptic necrosis of bone following renal transplantation. *Acta Med. Scand.* **202,** 27–32 (1977).

52. Doherty, C. C., and McGeown, M. G. Peptic ulceration, gastric acid secretion and kidney transplantation. *Dial. Transplant.* **8,** 970–977 (1979).

53. Penn, I., Durst, A. L., Machado, M. *et al.* Acute pancreatitis and hyperamylasemia in renal homograft recipients. *Arch. Surg. (Chicago)* **105,** 167–172 (1972).

54. Sopko, J., and Anuras, S. Liver disease in renal transplant recipients. *Am. J. Med.* **64,** 139–146 (1978).

55. Penn, I. Tumor incidence in human allograft recipients. *Transplant. Proc.* **11,** 1047–1051 (1979).

56. Rimm, A. A., Hartz, A. J., Kalbfleisch, J. H. *et al.* Survival curves. *In* "Basic Biostatistics in Medicine and Epidemiology," pp. 306–314. Prentice-Hall, Englewood Cliffs, New Jersey, 1980.

11

Nursing Care of the Patient with End-Stage Renal Disease

LOWANNA S. BINKLEY

I. INTRODUCTION

The patient who has kidney disease requires treatment planned by a group of highly trained and sophisticated nephrology team members. One member of this team is the nephrology nurse, a skilled professional whose functions and responsibilities have evolved into a subspecialty within nursing.

A nephrology nurse is an integral member of the team, and has chosen this area of specialization because of an interest in and a desire to work with patients and families with kidney disease. This means a commitment to the patient on the part of the nephrology nurse that can last for years because of the chronicity of kidney disease.

309

END-STAGE RENAL DISEASE

Even though nephrology nursing is an area of specialization, it draws on the knowledge and background experiences of medical–surgical nursing. These background experiences are essential for the nephrology nurse, since renal patients, like other patients, can experience a wide range of medical or surgical complications. The professional association known as the American Association of Nephrology Nurses and Technicians (AANNT) provides continuing education for its 3000 members through annual national, regional, and local meetings. In addition, there are publications to update nephrology nurses on changing developments in the field, such as *Dialysis & Transplantation, Contemporary Dialysis, Nephrology Nurse*, and *AANNT Journal*.

By far the greatest concentration of nephrology nurses is in adult dialysis units. However, nephrology nursing covers the spectrum from the outpatient renal clinic to dialysis (hemo- and peritoneal) and transplantation. Nephrology nurses are engaged in clinical research, in patient, personnel, and family teaching, in acute dialysis, in organ procurement, and in public education. There are nurses who work specifically with pediatric patients. A new area of expertise that is being developed by nephrology nurses is the field of plasma exchange therapy or plasmapheresis. When necessary, the patient can be dialyzed and pheresed at the same time by the same personnel.

Because nephrology nurses need a strong background in medical–surgical nursing, most facilities require their nurses to have 1–2 years of general nursing experience prior to applying for a position within a nephrology program. Depending upon the characteristics of the patient population (in-center, acute, outpatient), 1 or more years of experience in an intensive nursing setting, such as an intensive care unit or emergency room, may also be required.

All nurses receive on-the-job training; some orientation programs are quite sophisticated and formalized. It usually takes 3 months of intensive orientation, study, and practice before a beginning nephrology nurse can become a contributing member of the team. Coping with chronic illness is a very taxing undertaking, and can take its toll on nurses, as well as patients and family members. Therefore, the nurse who chooses to work with renal patients must find rewards in dealing with the challenges of a chronic illness.

The nephrology nurse's function in the renal clinic, dialysis, and transplantation will be described.

II. THE RENAL CLINIC

Nursing responsibilities within the setting of a renal clinic are based on the philosophical approach that the patient who is knowledgeable about his illness will be better able to care for himself. Therefore, nursing efforts are directed toward educating the patient to accept, as far as possible, the responsibility for following the recommended therapeutic regimen (*1, 2*).

Patients attending renal clinic generally fall into three categories: the patient with varying degrees of kidney function, pre-end stage; the patient undergoing dialytic therapy; and the patient with a renal transplant. The first significant encounter the patient has in clinic is with the nurse.

The nurse begins by assessing the patient, eliciting a history of physical or emotional problems, changes noted by the patient or family, and ascertaining the need for further laboratory or radiological studies to rule out or confirm physical findings. This assessment period gives the nurse an opportunity to determine patient understanding of the disease process and the rationale behind his therapeutic regimen, the diet, and medications. Important patient and family teaching takes place within the confines of the clinic setting. Areas such as the impact of illness and the physical manifestations of kidney disease, as well as expectations of the patient and family, are reviewed. Because of the chronicity of kidney disease, much of the patient and family teaching is repetitive but necessary (*1*).

General physical assessment involves eliciting any complaints or problems that the patient identifies, as well as any changes that the nurse recognizes from previous visits. Because the nurse is always present, he or she is able to assess changes in the patient. Thus, the nurse becomes a very familiar face to the patient and generally a source of considerable support. Usual vital signs of weight, temperature and apical pulse are determined on all patients. Any cardiac or pulmonary abnormalities, or changes detected when listening to the chest, are followed up with EKG and chest X-rays, if indicated. Patients are informed of any changes, which provides an excellent opportunity to teach patients the relationships between sodium, fluid, weight, edema, and blood pressure. By doing three positional blood pressures, further patient teaching can be conducted with respect to the relationship among position, blood pressure, and antihypertensive medications (*3, 4*).

Patients are taught that detectable edema represents 5–10% of their body weight as excess fluid, and that 500 ml of fluid equals a pound of weight. In reviewing possible causes for excessive fluid weight gain, it may be important to do a brief dietary history. If such questioning reveals that the patient is indeed having some problems either in understanding dietary restrictions or in adherence, a referral to the dietitian may be appropriate (*2*).

The nurse in the renal clinic can serve as a coordinator making referrals to the appropriate disciplines. Utilization of the dietitian for help in understanding dietary restrictions is very important, since the diet is often considered the patient's most important medication. If the nurse perceives depression or emotional strife brought on because of medical or social problems, the appropriate referral is made to either the psychiatrist or to the social worker, or to both, depending on the nurse's assessment of the situation. Evidence of dental problems, problems in eating, or difficulty surrounding oral hygiene warrant referral to the dentist for follow-up and recommendations for appropriate intervention. It is particularly important to get any needed dental work completed before the patient reaches end-stage renal disease (ESRD) so that a potential source of bacteremia can be eliminated. By noting inadequate oral hygiene or poorly fitting dentures that might interfere with good nutritional intake, it may be possible to take corrective action that would prevent long-term problems. The nursing role is one of a facilitator and organizer, so that the patient need not make unnecessary trips to the hospital.

An important concept that is implemented in the renal clinic setting is the recognition of the need to involve the family and significant others in the teaching and planning of the patient's medical care. While the emphasis is on the patient accepting the responsibility for his own care, it is extremely important to involve family members, as they can provide considerable support to the patient (2, 4). They also can become a valuable resource in noting physical and psychological changes occurring within the patient. Family members and others who are involved in the patient's care provide integral components of the patient's support system. If, at any time, they withdraw from the support system, for whatever reason, it may become necessary to restructure the support system, with the clinic personnel assuming a more active participant role.

Thus, patient and family teaching includes aspects of coping with chronicity of illness and the importance of the therapeutic regimen. Not only are they taught about the medications, what they are for, and how to take them, but also the side effects of the drugs. With so many drugs on the market, patients no longer need to suffer silently with intolerable side effects. There are several choices currently available to treat various medical problems, such that many alternative combinations can be found that can be quite satisfactory.

Dialysis patients are followed in the renal clinic at 4–8 week intervals. Some patients may be seen more frequently, while others may be seen only quarterly depending on individual patient needs and the distance the patient must travel. In addition to a general physical assessment of the dialysis patient, the nurse also reviews with the patient his dialysis records and associated problems. In order to assure comprehensive follow-up of the patient, it is useful to maintain a log or flow sheet on the front of the chart (Fig. 1). Complications arising during dialysis are discussed until satisfactory solutions are mutually determined. If the patient has been ill and not eating properly, he may lose muscle mass, thus dropping his ideal weight (also called dry weight). When this happens, the patient usually replaces his good weight with fluid and aims at his ideal weight for a postdialysis weight. Not realizing that he has lost muscle mass or good weight, the patient can easily go into pulmonary edema because of the excess fluid retained.

Immunizations   Date:

Diphtheria-Tetanus

Influenza

Pneumovax

Blood Work

Hepatitis Associated Antigen (HAA)

Parathyroid Hormone (PTH)

Blood Urea Nitrogen (BUN)

Creatinine

Packed Cell Volume (PCV)

Genitourinary Tract (GU)

Rectal Exam (Prostate)

Voiding Cystourethrogram

Eyes and Ears (EENT)

Visual acuity

Hearing

Other

Electrocardiogram (EKG)

Chest X-Ray (CXR)

Hand Films

Baseline Electroencephalogram (EEG)

Speech Evaluation

Echocardiogram

Fig. 1.   Renal health maintenance flow sheet.

Most home dialysis patients do exceptionally well. They are in control of their therapeutic regimen, as well as their personal lives. Most of them are engaged in activities that are quite meaningful to them and their families. Many find that dialysis can be arranged to fit into their lives without too much disruption. With a little planning, vacations and vacation dialysis can be satisfactorily arranged (5, 6). The home dialysis patient is an extremely knowledgeable individual, and it behooves the nurse to listen closely to the patient in clinic.

The patient who has received a renal transplant will be monitored very closely in renal clinic. Many areas need to be evaluated in the renal transplant patient, and all of them are important. The patient will be questioned regarding symptoms of graft rejection: sudden weight gain, decrease in urinary output, fever, graft swelling and tenderness, and hypertension (7, 8). Symptoms of infection (urinary tract and other systems) can be particularly troublesome during the first 6 months following transplantation. In addition, the patient may experience side effects from the medication that he takes. Steroid medication may cause GI bleeding, mood swings, moon facies, acne, hirsutism, multiple purpuric lesions, and herpes infection. Long-term side effects include phlebitis, cataract formation, diabetes, or asceptic hip necrosis (9).

Throughout the critical first year, the patient may require considerable support from the nurse, particularly in view of a changing self-image. Should the patient require hospitalization during this time because of complications, he will want information about prognosis and the chances of rejecting the kidney. Care must be taken to advise the patient realistically and to point out that, should the patient reject and lose the kidney, dialysis is an effective treatment until another renal transplant becomes possible (8-10).

Thus, in the clinic setting, the nurse assesses the patient, makes necessary referrals, schedules appropriate diagnostic studies, and engages in patient and family teaching, in preparation for the patient to be seen by the physician. In some facilities, only those patients who are having problems are seen by the physician after initial screening by the nurse. Other institutions adhere to the philosophy that all patients should be seen by the physician as well as by the nurse, since each functions differently in relation to the patient and family.

III. HEMODIALYSIS

Patients undergoing dialysis may be either "acute" or "chronic," depending on the cause for the renal failure. A patient on chronic maintenance dialysis may become acutely ill because of superimposed medical problems or complications. Acute and chronic patients require very different nursing care (*11*).

A. The "Acute" Dialysis Patient

A patient who is undergoing acute hemodialysis therapy must be closely monitored throughout the procedure. Hemodialysis may be accomplished by a femoral or Shaldon catheter, via a surgically placed external shunt, or by means of a subclavian vein catheter. All accesses need to be monitored to assure patency and to make sure that they do not continue to ooze or bleed around the exit site.

If a patient is so acutely ill as to warrant "after hours" dialysis, or dialysis outside the regular dialysis schedule, that patient should have a physician in attendance throughout the dialysis procedure. Examples are the patient who has taken an overdose of a dialyzable drug or who has hyperkalemia or pulmonary edema resistant to simpler therapy.

The "acute" dialysis patient is not placed on a regular dialysis schedule, but is evaluated daily during rounds to determine the need for dialysis (*11*). In many cases it is preferable to bring the dialysis equipment to the patient's bedside, especially if the patient is housed in an intensive care unit. This eliminates potential problems associated with transporting a seriously ill patient, and assures the patient and staff of sufficient aid during time of crisis. It may also be preferable to dialyze the patient in his own room if he is considered "contaminated" or requires isolation. The dialysis unit also is considered a "dirty area." Further contamination is undesirable, since introduction of new organisms by a grossly infected patient will put all patients in the unit at risk. The decision to dialyze the patient "at place" versus in the dialysis unit is a team effort after consultation with the physician and the head nurse of the dialysis unit, who can best ascertain the capabilities of the dialysis unit and the best utilization of the talents of the nursing staff.

If the patient has a BUN greater than 150 mg/dl, care must be taken to avoid the dialysis disequilibrium syndrome which may occur with the use of too efficient a dialyzer. A "slow" dialysis (blood flow 100–150 ml/min for 2–3 hr on a less efficient dialyzer) will result in a gradual fall in serum urea levels, thereby avoiding the dialysis disequilibrium syndrome of headache, nausea, and vomiting (Fig. 2).

Nursing responsibilities will include initiating and terminating hemodialysis; administering intravenous medications as ordered; and frequent blood pressure monitoring and determining whether to administer normal saline, plasmanate, or hypertonic sodium chloride for hypotension. Patients

Patient starting dialysis for the first time or for the first time after an interval of several weeks (transplant patients in rejection) need to be dialyzed slowly to prevent dialysis disequilibrium syndrome.

This can be accomplished by any of several methods:

Slow blood flow rate (BFR): less than 150 ml/min

Short dialysis: 2–3 hr

Little or no ultrafiltration

Use of less efficient dialyzer, such as Gambro 17

Unless otherwise ordered, these new patients will be dialyzed according to the following schedule:

First Dialysis:	17 μm Gambro dialyzer
	BFR of 100 ml/min
	For 3 hr
Second Dialysis:	13.5 μm optima Gambro dialyzer
	BFR of 125 ml/min
	For 3 hr
Third Dialysis:	Gambro Major dialyzer
	BFR of 166 ml/min
	For 3–4 hr
Thereafter:	Begin the regular schedule
	BFR of 200 ml/min
	For 4 hr

Fig. 2.   Example of a new patient protocol.

taking antihypertensive medications, especially methyldopa, are prone to develop hypotension during dialysis. Acutely ill patients, particularly if they are hypercatabolic, will be losing muscle mass; thus, their optimum or "dry" weight may be lower than initially estimated. This is important in determining whether fluid overload is present. For these patients, it may be desirable to use "dry ultrafiltration" for the first 2 hr of hemodialysis in order to remove excess fluid without causing rapid shifts in fluid compartment.

"Dry ultrafiltration" is achieved by occluding one port of the dialysate compartment while connecting the other port to a vacuum. Several hundred mm Hg of negative pressure can be applied to the dialysate compartment. As the blood passes through the dialyzer, fluid can be literally sucked out of the blood at the rate of up to 50 ml/min. In the patient with massive fluid overload, it is possible to ultrafilter as much as 3 liters of excess fluid per hour without hypotension. Because the ultrafiltrate is readily visible in the vacuum bottle, it is quite simple to determine at a glance how much fluid has been removed. The term "drying the patient out" takes on new meaning when one sees this procedure. Of course, the amount of fluid removed must be modified to approximate the amount present in excess. Often more than one treatment may be required.

Routine monitoring of the patient throughout dialysis always involves checking the blood pressure, regulation and recording of venous pressure (blood compartment of the dialyzer), recording and regulation of negative pressure (dialysate compartment pressure), determination of heparin usage, clotting times as indicated, and any other elements that are pertinent to that particular patient for that particular dialysis. Hourly monitoring/ recording is the accepted practice for routine dialysis. However, an acute dialysis patient may need almost continuous monitoring with frequent adjustment of the dialysis parameters to prevent rapid fluid shifts.

An acutely ill patient will require cardiac monitoring, and will also probably have several different sources of intravenous medications. If the patient is ill enough to warrant a respirator, then it would be preferable to dialyze the patient in the intensive care unit. The only requirement is that the patient be located near a water source and a drain in order to accommodate the dialysis equipment.

A very sick patient may be hypotensive and thus present a formidable challenge to the nurse, as efforts to maintain the blood pressure through use of medications, fluid, or colloidal expanders are balanced with the need to correct fluid overload (*12*). Because the nurse understands what is happening and possesses the skills to successfully dialyze the patient, the physician rarely needs to specify all the parameters of the planned dialysis. However, the physician may want to identify specific fluid replacement, and whether or not the patient needs to be kept "tight" in the area of anticoagulation, that is, the patient's clotting time kept close to normal with minimal heparinization. This is especially important if the patient has a bleeding problem. "Regional" heparinization is performed by the nephrology nurse when the patient has a bleeding site, e.g., a peptic ulcer. This involves constant infusion of equimolar amounts of protamine into the venous line of the dialyzer to neutralize heparin administered on the arterial side. The nurse checks clotting times for both patient and dialyzer.

B. The "Chronic" Dialysis Patient

Ideally, a patient who will be undergoing chronic dialytic therapy has been followed in renal clinic for a period of time prior to the institution of dialysis. Thus, this patient and family should have received considerable teaching about the disease process, the therapeutic regimen appropriate for the specific disease, treatment modality options, and information about dialysis and renal transplantation (*2, 4*). This cannot all be accomplished within the confines of clinic itself. As much teaching as possible is conducted during the period of nursing assessment, as well as during the time the patient/ family are with the physician.

At the VA Medical Center in Nashville, Tennessee, one approach that we have utilized for patient and family teaching is to put aside one hour of renal clinic time and designate this as "Kidney Talk." "Kidney Talk" is held during the noon hour, before renal clinic meets at 1PM.

"Kidney Talk" is structured not only to provide information to patients and family, but also to encourage discussion among the participants. Topics are varied but cover many aspects of kidney disease and its treatment (Fig. 3). These topics are repeated at 3 month intervals.

When the patient has been followed in clinic for a period of time prior to the initiation of chronic dialytic therapy, the way is paved to direct the patient on a smooth treatment course. It is extremely important to get to know the patient, to establish a working relationship with the patient and family, and to identify the patient's support system. Identification of a patient's support system is crucial to enable a return to maximum health. For example, a patient with no family and very little community support will require considerable intervention from the nephrology team if that patient is to survive for long (5, 10).

Should a patient enter the chronic dialysis program after acute renal failure or as a transfer from another institution, a different approach to the patient's care is required. More teaching on dialysis will be necessary, and the patient's apprehension and anxiety can prove to be a real barrier to learning. Every patient requires basic information in order to survive on chronic dialysis. Our philosophy is to teach the patient as much as he is capable of learning. Thus, while one patient may be quite capable of absorbing the intricacies of mass transfer during dialysis, another patient may be able only to respond to the alarms of the machine.

A data base needs to be established on every patient entering a dialysis treatment program. Whenever possible, base line electrocardiogram, chest X-ray, and hand films are obtained on the patient (bone changes of renal osteodystrophy can be detected with hand films) (see Fig. 1). If the patient

What Is Depression?
Common Medical Problems in Kidney Disease
Dialysis Past, Present, and Future
Skin Problems Associated with Renal Failure
Dental Care in Renal Disease
Diet and the Restaurant Menu
How a Kidney Transplant Is Done
Medications
How the Kidney Works
Summer Fruits and Vegetables
Why a Transplant?

Fig. 3.   Topics of discussion at kidney talk.

is a home dialysis candidate, speech and hearing data are necessary to determine the patient's capacity to read the dials of the dialysis machine and to hear the alarm system. Because of the adverse effects of poor oral hygiene and dental problems, we believe it is important to have any necessary dental work completed as soon as possible.

C. The Home Dialysis Patient

Our experience has shown us that patients do better (live longer) on home dialysis. Therefore, we make every effort to encourage the patient to dialyze at home. While most patients will manage well on home hemodialysis, there will be some patients for whom home peritoneal dialysis will be indicated. If the patient starts hemodialysis, he will first be dialyzed in a center unit until (a) a slot opens up in the home training unit (i.e., a new class starts) and/or (b) the patient and his assistant are emotionally ready to start learning about dialysis. It is during this time prior to starting home training that the nurse and patient spend considerable time together. Nursing assessment involves evaluation of the vascular access, with determination of the type of needles to use and potential puncture sites. Care must be taken to assure long life of the access. Therefore, in order to give a fistula every opportunity to mature before it is used, an external shunt will sometimes be placed as a temporary vascular access. The astute dialysis nurse can make a rough estimate of shunt longevity based on blood flow, venous pressure, and changes occurring during dialysis itself. Any decrease in blood flow through the access, or sudden venous pressure changes that indicate potential vascular access failure, should immediately be brought to the attention of the physician. A shuntogram will provide the physician with information about the internal characteristics of the vascular access, and identify areas where surgical intervention would be of benefit.

Although the internal fistula is preferable to the external shunt, we generally do not remove the external shunt even when the fistula has matured and is ready to be punctured with large bore needles. Therefore, the external shunt is usually placed in a lower leg rather than sacrifice the vessels of the upper extremities. Planning around an individual's needs can assure a longer shunt life. For example, most people drive a vehicle using their right foot for accelerator and brake. An external shunt in the right ankle would be subjected to a considerable amount of stress, thereby compromising the shunt. Thus, a shunt in the left ankle might be preferable.

Once a fistula has been constructed, a period of 10–14 days may be required for healing to take place. It is preferable to place the fistula in the non-dominant arm, thereby encouraging self-venipuncture. After that, the patient will be instructed in fistula exercises: The placing of a tourniquet in the upper arm to restrict venous blood flow while squeezing a rubber ball to promote distention of the venous system of the fistula. These exercises should be done 5 min out of every hour or a minimum of several times each day. This will toughen the vessels as well as distend them, thus hastening the maturation of the fistula and allowing the use of large bore needles. A fistula that is fragile will "blow out" when punctured and hematoma formation will cause deterioration of the fistula. Thus, the longer one can wait for a a fistula to mature, the better the chance for a long-surviving access. However, if after faithfully performing the fistula exercises the patient still has a poorly functioning fistula at the end of 2 months, another access should be attempted. Should a hematoma develop, warm soaks the following day will ease the soreness and encourage resolution of the hematoma. A whirlpool is useful for resolving the hematoma and for fistula exercises. Once the acute bleeding has stopped, a whirlpool treatment 20 min twice a day can turn a very nasty swollen and ecchymotic arm into a useful limb again.

If the patient is destined for home hemodialysis, he will be taught to perform all of the procedures necessary in order to successfully dialyze at home. However, the patient will dialyze in-center until he is stabilized and ready to enter the home training class. If home hemodialysis is planned, the patient must be able to insert fistula needles on a consistent basis before training begins (Fig. 4). During this stabilization period, which may take several weeks to months, considerable nursing time is spent teaching the patient and family, as well as developing a strong interpersonal relationship with them. Having this basis of trust, patients on home dialysis feel comfortable in calling the home unit nurse whenever a question or a problem arises (2, 5, 13). A phone call can sometimes save a trip to the hospital and can allay the anxiety of dialyzing at home.

Once the patient enters home training, a regular routine is established. The home training course itself is usually 6 weeks long, but will depend on the patient and physical problems that may develop. Patients usually dialyze Monday, Wednesday, and Friday, with formal classes on Tuesday and Thursday. A class of four patients is a good size in which patients can learn from each other and yet not be such a large group that two nurses cannot readily work with them. Because emphasis is on patient accountability and responsibility, we prefer that the patient undergo the first half of the training period without his assistant. Then, we bring the assistant in for the last 3 weeks of training, with the patient teaching the assistant.

Not only is the patient taught about the function of the kidney, kidney disease, and the various dialysis procedures, but also how to cope with problems that may develop while on dialysis. Hypotension is the most important and may induce nausea and vomiting. This will respond to intravenous saline administration. Patients who are prone to develop intradialytic hypotension are encouraged to ingest sodium-containing foods in the forms of pretzels, saltines, or pickles while they are being dialyzed. Another problem is fluid overload. This can lead to pulmonary edema, which may manifest initially with nocturnal dyspnea. Many patients have had to dialyze in the middle of the night to remove excessive accumulations of fluid. Headaches, especially frontal, can occur in some patients who try aggressive ultrafiltration techniques during dialysis. In these patients, headache is usually due to fluid shifts. Persistent headache, not associated with dialysis, warrants investigation to rule out subdural hematoma. Occasionally, a patient will experience a dialyzer blood leak. In most instances, the patient need not lose the blood in that dialyzer, because it can be returned to the patient prior to changing the dialyzer. If the blood leak occurs early in dialysis, then a new dialyzer can be exchanged for the one with the leak. If it should occur late in dialysis, then the patient can return the blood, terminate dialysis, and make up the time at the next dialysis. Patients are encouraged to call the dialysis center personnel should any problems arise while they are dialyzing at home. Diabetic patients who have taken their insulin but have not eaten may become hypoglycemic while on dialysis

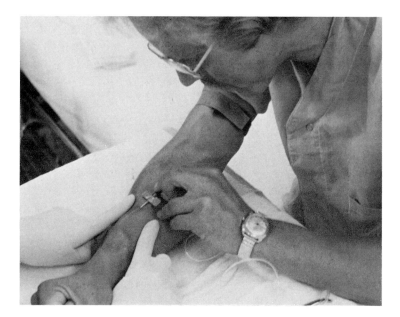

Fig. 4. Patient performing self-venipuncture.

	Date covered in class	Date reviewed	Quizzed	Demon-strated by patient	Patient signa-ture	Nurse signa-ture	Comments
A. Can verbally define hemodialysis							
B. Has some understanding of anatomy and physiology of normal kidneys							
C. Can relate function of normal kidneys							
D. Has understanding of his diagnosis, and can relate this to his physical symptoms							
E. Knows the symptoms of uremia							
F. Can demonstrate taking vital signs, and verbalize relationship of Na, water, and blood pressure							
G. Can verbalize principles of hemodialysis							
H. Understands that there are different types of shunts or access to circulation							
I. Can relate and demon-strate shunt care:							
1. Internal							
a. Check for bruit							
b. Note infection							
c. 5 min scrub with betadine prior to dialysis							
2. External							
a. Check for infection							
b. Check for clotting							
c. Clean and redress everyday							
J. Satisfactorily demonstrates dialysis procedures:							
1. Preparation of equip-ment							
2. Initiating dialysis							
3. Monitoring dialysis							

Fig. 5. Hemodialysis patient education record.

	Date covered in class	Date reviewed	Quizzed	Demon-strated by patient	Patient signa-ture	Nurse signa-ture	Comments
4. Terminating dialysis							
5. Clean up of equipment							
6. Sterilization of equipment							
K. Demonstrates adequate record keeping							
L. Has understanding of medical problems and can relate symptoms, cause, prevention and treatment for these:							
1. Cardiovascular problems							
a. Hypotension–hypertension							
b. Fluid balance, pulmonary edema, fluid overload							
c. Edema							
d. Pericarditis							
e. Hyperkalemia							
2. Bone disease—calcium, phosphorus metabolism							
3. Skin problems							
4. Neuropathy							
5. Anemia							
6. Sexual problems							
M. Can relate cause, treatment and prevention of complications during dialysis							
1. Nausea, vomiting							
2. Hypotension							
3. Headache							
4. Muscle cramps							
5. Infection, fever, and chills during dialysis							
6. Air embolus							
7. Convulsions							
8. Bleeding postdialysis							
9. Arrhythmias							
10. GI bleeding							

Fig. 5. (*Continued*)

	Date covered in class	Date reviewed	Quizzed	Demon- strated by patient	Patient signa- ture	Nurse signa- ture	Comments
11. Blood leak							
12. Needle problems— heparin lock							
a. Hematoma—how to recirculate							
b. Collapsing							
c. Accidental removal— how to return blood through artery							
13. Power failure							
14. Water failure							
N. Can relate normal values for blood chemistries, causes, and symptoms of abnormalities							
O. Can verbalize and recognize medications and proper doses, schedule, purpose, and side effects							
P. Has understanding of, and can relate, prescribed diet							
Q. Has been educated about the transplant program							
R. Understands medical followup in renal clinic							

Fig. 5. (*Continued*)

versus a glucose-free dialysate. Hypoglycemia can cause profuse sweating and a decreased level of consciousness. These patients are advised to have a meal before commencing dialysis.

Repetition is the basis of learning, and patients have reading assignments and quizzes. They will cover all material several times before the nurse and technician determine that the patient can safely dialyze at home, and before the physician releases the patient to dialyze at home. The patient signs his course outline as his statement that he indeed did learn the material presented to him. This becomes a permanent part of the patient's chart (Fig. 5). After going on home hemodialysis, the patient returns regularly to renal clinic for his routine follow-up care. Occasionally, a patient may need to return to the home training unit for a refresher course or in order to perfect certain procedures.

A major goal of chronic dialytic therapy is to improve the sense of well-being sufficiently to permit an individual a reasonable return to activity. The dialysis schedule should be worked into the day-to-day activities, rather than trying to fit life around a dialysis schedule. Therefore, a distinct advantage to home dialysis is that it permits dialysis scheduling that will promote independence. Long weekends can be arranged through alteration of the dialysis schedule, as long as the patient gets his usual weekly hours of dialysis.

Patients and families are taught how to assess medical complications, what steps they can take to prevent or abate problems, and how to respond to emergencies. Probably most importantly, they are taught how to describe the problems they are experiencing so that assistance is only a telephone call away.

IV. PERITONEAL DIALYSIS

Some patients may start peritoneal dialysis without ever experiencing hemodialysis. If this is the case, the patient may not dialyze in-center, but proceed into the home training unit to learn about peritoneal dialysis. There are a few in-center peritoneal dialysis units, but most patients perform peritoneal dialysis at home. Home chronic intermittent peritoneal dialysis (CIPD) training takes approximately 3 weeks. Patients need to learn about the machine and the ramifications of the illness. Continuous ambulatory peritoneal dialysis (CAPD) can be safely taught within a week or 10 days. However, it will take longer to learn about all the medical implications, especially if the patient has not had prior formal teaching about kidney disease.

There are three general types or categories of peritoneal dialysis: CIPD, CAPD, and CCPD (Continuous Cycling Peritoneal Dialysis).

CIPD can be performed manually with bags or bottles, or via automated machine. CIPD refers to peritoneal dialysis on an intermittent basis, such as the 48 hr sessions conducted for acute dialysis. It can also refer to the regular three, four, or five times a week dialysis schedule via machine. The automated peritoneal dialysis machine pumps concentrated peritoneal dialysate that is mixed with reverse osmosis water and delivers essentially pyrogen free dialysate to the peritoneal cavity. Two such devices are currently available: the Drake–Willock peritoneal machine and the Physio Control machine. Both utilize a proportioning system with a conductivity meter as a backup for assurances of correct proportioning. Most patients require at least 40 hr of peritoneal dialysis for "adequate dialysis." This can be divided into four or five sessions per week. Because of the inherent safety of these machines, most patients prefer to dialyze at night during sleep, arising in the morning after the completion of dialysis to pursue work or other daytime activities.

Some patients use an automated device that propels commercially prepared dialysate from 2 liter bags/bottles into the peritoneal cavity. Called a cycler, this simple machine requires no water source or drain, only an electrical outlet in order to run.

CAPD is gaining popularity because it allows dialysis without the need for cumbersome equipment. This method of peritoneal dialysis involves four or five exchanges per day, with each exchange remaining in the abdomen anywhere from 4 to 8 hr. This allows continual dialysis without tying the patient down to a machine. Thus, the term "continuous ambulatory peritoneal dialysis." While CAPD permits freedom, it also entails another kind of dependency, i.e., the need to be dialyzing and exchanging 24 hours per day, 7 days per week, every week. There is no respite. Some patients soon weary of the chronicity of this type of peritoneal dialysis. Other patients actually have an overall physical improvement, as well as an increase in their sense of well-being, probably due to the slower and thus more physiological action of peritoneal dialysis.

With CAPD and its accompanying breaks in the dialysate system, perito-

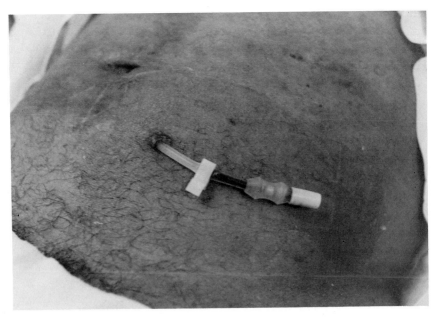

Fig. 6. Permanently implanted peritoneal catheter with Betadine barrier in distal portion.

nitis can be an ever present problem. Strict aseptic technique cannot be stressed enough, including the use of mask and sterile gloves.

CCPD is an attempt to utilize the best features of the cycler and CAPD. It entails three exchanges at night utilizing the cycler, with the fourth exchange in the morning left in the peritoneal cavity throughout the day until time to dialyze overnight. This eliminates the frequent breaks in an otherwise closed system, and still provides for continual 24 hr per day dialysis.

The most important and probably the most difficult concept to teach patients on peritoneal dialysis is the principle of asepsis and the importance of sterile technique in caring for the permanently implanted catheter (Fig. 6). Practice is crucial to perfecting the technique. It has been said that the less educated patient learns this concept better because he does exactly as he is told, whereas the more educated patient believes he does not need to do everything as instructed and can "do it better."

Patients on peritoneal dialysis must be aware of the signs and symptoms of peritonitis. In some, a cloudy outflow from the peritoneal catheter may be the first indication of infection. Alternatively, there may be abdominal pain including rebound tenderness, fever, and malaise. Peritonitis can often be treated at home with instillation of appropriate antibiotics at the time of peritoneal exchange. However, hospitalization is frequently required.

	Date covered in class	Date reviewed	Quizzed	Demonstrated by patient	Patient signature	Nurse signature	Comments
A. Can verbally define peritoneal dialysis							
B. Can verbalize normal functions of kidneys							
C. Can verbalize his diagnosis and can relate this to his physical symptoms							
D. Can demonstrate taking vital signs and verbalize relationship of Na, water, and blood pressure							
E. Can verbalize principles of peritoneal dialysis							
F. Demonstrates proper care of catheter							

Fig. 7.   Peritoneal dialysis patient education record.

	Date covered in class	Date reviewed	Quizzed	Demon- strated by patient	Patient signa- ture	Nurse signa- ture	Comments

G. Verbalizes and demonstrates
   dialysis procedures:
   1. Bag exchange (as
      appropriate)
   2. Changing transfer set
   3. Catheter care
H. Can verbalize signs and
   symptoms of peritonitis
I. Demonstrates adequate
   record keeping
J. Can verbalize complications
   of peritoneal dialysis;
   causes and treatment
   1. Line separation
   2. Air accumulation
   3. Leakage of fluid
   4. Failure to outflow
   5. Depletion syndrome
   6. Abdominal fluid retention
   7. Unable to inflow
   8. Pain on inflow
K. Has understanding of
   related medical problems
   and can relate causes and
   prevention for them.
   1. Peritonitis
   2. Pulmonary edema
   3. Cardiovascular problems
   4. Hypotension
   5. Pericarditis
   6. Hypo- and hyperkalemia
   7. Bone disease
   8. Anemia
   9. Sexual problems
   10. Neuropathy
   11. Skin problems
   12. Fever
   13. Fluid overload
L. Can verbalize and
   recognize medications and
   proper doses, schedule,
   purpose, and side effects

Fig. 7. (*Continued*)

An important technical problem that may accompany confinement to bed is a decrease in the rate of outflow from the peritoneal catheter. Constipation appears to be one contributing factor. Use of stool softeners, suppositories, or enemas often assures optimal catheter functioning during such periods. Daily care of the peritoneal catheter is essential to obviate infection. Soaking in a tub of bath water that covers the catheter is inadvisable and can lead to infection. We advise cleansing the outside of the catheter by washing it with soap and water while taking a shower. Some advise dressing the catheter, whereas others leave it open. Because of its simplicity, peritoneal dialysis home training is shorter and less detailed than hemodialysis (Fig. 7).

V. IN-CENTER DIALYSIS

Some patients dialyze in a center as outpatients. These patients and their families develop very close relationships with the dialysis center nurses. The nurses know the patients and are attuned to changes, both physiological and psychological, that may develop. Nurses will alert the physician or other appropriate team members to the observed change.

Even after a patient receives a renal transplant, he will return to the dialysis unit for dialysis backup during rejection episodes and when there is the eventual loss of a functioning graft (9). Thus, the dialysis community is likened to a large family, were everyone is concerned about the well-being of all members. In time of family crises, the nursing staff becomes a very real source of support for the patient or his family. Although scheduling of dialysis times necessarily is structured, attempts are made to accommodate special needs of a patient or his family.

Nurses can support patients in their decisions to work or not work, when to dialyze, and other plans of daily living. It is possible to arrange dialysis on vacation in another facility, or to encourage the patient to take the equipment in camper or van. It may be necessary to dialyze the patient in-center in order to give the spouse a well-deserved vacation. It is important to do whatever is necessary to enable that patient and family to live as productive a life as possible. This can only be accomplished when all members of the health team work together toward the common goal.

VI. RENAL TRANSPLANTATION

Following transplantation, when the course is uncomplicated, a patient can expect to be in the hospital for a minimum of 3–4 weeks. Some institutions have a separate transplant ward, but most facilities house the patient on a surgical floor. Nursing care includes activities that are routine for any postoperative patient, and some that are specific for the patient who has undergone renal transplantation. Probably the most critical function that the nurse performs is accurate recording of fluid intake and output and patient weight. Protective mask and individual room isolation are important measures during the postoperative period. Most patients accept this confinement without question once they understand the rationale. Patients may, however, become very irritable while in isolation and may display emotional outbursts over apparently trivial matters. Nurses should be encouraged to spend time with the patients at regular intervals throughout the day. Patients, particularly those who have received cadaveric transplants, may experience renal shutdown due to acute tubular necrosis. This is common in the early postoperative period. Other patients may have an episode of acute rejection. During each of these complications the patients may require dialysis. A factual explanation of what is occurring is an essential facet of the approach to the patient, and the nurse can give support to the patient at these times (6–10).

The nurse should encourage the patient to participate in self-care postoperatively. He can be taught to keep daily records of body weight and fluid intake and output. The patient should be made thoroughly familiar with the medications which are essential for graft survival. The mode of action of the medications, the dosages, the frequency of administration, and their side effects should be explained to the patient. Some side effects, such as acne and moon facies, may unduly alarm the patient unless forewarned. Patients are instructed about the importance of carbohydrate restrictions to prevent or minimize these side effects. Certain other side effects, such as phlebitis and gastrointestinal bleeding, require immediate medical intervention. Patients are instructed to be alert for any indications of infection and/or rejection. Dangerous signs include sudden weight gain, decreased urinary output, tenderness and swelling of the allograft, fever, malaise, and increase in blood pressure.

The average hospital stay is about 4–5 weeks. Patients are discharged when the transplant team is satisfied that the kidney is functioning well and all vital signs are within normal limits. Following discharge from the hospital, the patient must be encouraged to adhere to his medical regimen and maintain regular follow-up visits with his physician. The patient should be given a list of transplant team members and their telephone numbers, and should be encouraged to contact them should the need arise.

VII. CONCLUSION

The responsibility of the nephrology nurse in caring for patients with ESRD have been reviewed. The role of the nurse as an integral part of the nephrology team is described in four specific settings: renal clinic, the hemodialysis center, the home training unit for hemodialysis or peritoneal dialysis, and in the postoperative care of patients following renal transplantation. The nurse plays a pivotal role in patient education, an important facet of clinical duties. The nurse provides continuity of care and has the opportunity to observe patients in various settings and will often be the first to detect physical and/or emotional changes in the patients. Nursing observations are of critical importance to the team involved in the care of patients with ESRD.

GENERAL REFERENCES

Aspinall, M. J., and Tanner, C. A. "Decision Making for Patient Care Applying the Nursing Process." Appleton, New York, 1981.

Garfield, C. A. "Stress and Survival." Mosby, St. Louis, Missouri, 1979.

Hekelman, F., and Ostendarp, C. A. "Nephrology Nursing Perspectives of Care." McGraw-Hill, New York, 1979.

Jackle, M., and Rasmussen, C. "Renal Problems: A Critical Care Nursing Focus." Robert J. Brady Company, Bowie, Maryland, 1980.

Lancaster, L. E. "The Patient with End Stage Renal Disease." Wiley, New York, 1979.

Sachs, B. L. "Renal Transplantation: A Nursing Perspective." Medical Examination Publishing Company, Flushing, New York, 1977.

REFERENCES

1. Coppola, B. B., Watson, G. B., McWilliams, M., and Eccles, P. Renal clinic modality. *Nephrol. Nurse* 3(2), 40–42 (1981).

2. Ulrich, B. Adherence to the prescribed therapy for chronic renal failure. *Nephrol. Nurse* 3(4), 14–21 (1981).

3. Coover, D., and Lewis, S. Pre-treatment patient education for dialysis. *Nephrol. Nurse* 3(3), 12–18 (1981).

4. Stephenson, T., and Hayes, C. J. Toward personalized education for adult ESRD patients. *AANNT J.* 9, 39–46 (1982).

5. Butram, V. O. Dialysis—The nephrology nurse-patient relationship. *Nephrol. Nurse* 3(3), 45–54 (1981).

6. Leinweber, B. The hemodialysis client: Nursing focus on self-care. *Nephrol. Nurse* 3(2), 8–10 (1981).

7. Buszta, C. Patient evaluation pre- and post-transplant. *Nephrol. Nurse* 3(3), 38–42 (1981).

8. Butram, V. The nurse-patient relationship when the kidney rejects. *Nephrol. Nurse* 3(6), 33–34 (1981).

9. Moffatt, A. K. Ernie: A case study of a renal transplant patient. *Nephrol. Nurse* 3(6), 26–32 (1981).

10. Frauman, A. C. Health care for the child with a renal transplant. *AANNT J.* 9, 33–46 (1982).

11. Thompson, P. Acute renal failure—A challenge for all nurses. *Nephrol. Nurse* **3**(5), 4–8 (1981).
12. Wells, J. M. Hypotension during hemodialysis: Physiological mechanisms involved. *Nephrol. Nurse* **3**(3), 20–27 (1981).
13. Morris, J. E. Patient education as a nursing intervention for control-seeking behaviors. *Nephrol. Nurse* **3**(5), 20–23 (1981).

12

The Role of Nutrition
in End-Stage Renal Disease

VICTORIA R. LIDDLE

I. INTRODUCTION AND GENERAL PRINCIPLES

Nutrition is an important aspect of care for patients with renal disease. Many of the associated complications of renal disease and dialysis, such as neuropathy, hyponatremia, hyperkalemia, loss of lean body mass, hypertension, and edema, are influenced by the quality and quantity of food and water intake and may be ameliorated by good nutritional management.

333

END-STAGE RENAL DISEASE

Copyright © 1983 by Academic Press, Inc.
All rights of reproduction in any form reserved.
ISBN 0-12-672280-3

Dietary restriction of protein, potassium, sodium, and fluid while maintaining an adequate caloric intake should be initiated at an early stage in the management of end-stage renal disease (ESRD). Acceptance of these restrictions with good dietary compliance is a necessary and important part of the treatment of ESRD.

Protein intake is very important in the patient with ESRD. The Food and Drug Administration's Recommended Daily Allowance (RDA) of protein for a normal person is 0.8 g/kg/day. When a normal person develops ESRD, his protein requirements vary greatly. If he is managed conservatively, his protein intake may decrease to 0.5 g/kg/day. When dialysis is initiated, his requirement may be as high as 1.5 g/kg/day depending on the type and frequency of dialysis. If he receives a kidney transplant, his protein requirements will increase to 2 g/kg/day (1).

The patient with ESRD can usually be managed by medication and diet, as long as sufficient kidney function is present to maintain a creatinine clearance (C_{cr}) of greater than 7–10 ml/min. It is important in patients with kidney disease to prescribe diets that meet as nearly as possible the recommended nutritional allowances for normal individuals. Because some nutrients, such as protein, sodium, and potassium, must be restricted in patients with renal failure, the diet may become inadequate in vitamins, iron, and calcium content. Accordingly, it is usually necessary to supplement the diet with vitamins, iron, and calcium. Conversely, patients with renal failure retain phosphorus. Since it is extremely difficult to prescribe a diet low in phosphorus, phosphate-binding gels are given at meal times and prevent the absorption of phosphorus from the gastrointestinal tract.

II. PREDIALYSIS AND DIALYSIS: INDIVIDUAL COMPONENTS OF THE DIET

A. Protein Requirements

1. Protein Intake in Predialysis

The patient with chronic renal failure has difficulty in eliminating the products of protein catabolism. This is reflected chemically by elevations in blood urea nitrogen (BUN) and serum creatinine concentrations. Many other products of metabolism also accumulate and exert toxic effects on the patient. Accordingly, it is imperative to control the patient's intake of protein. Low protein diets have been shown to be helpful in the management of patients with chronic renal failure (2).

Proteins vary widely in their amino acid composition and, therefore, they vary in their efficacy in supporting normal tissue growth and turnover. The protein prescribed for the patient with ESRD should provide all the essential amino acids in a proper ratio to ensure adequate synthesis of tissue protein. These dietary proteins, known as high biological value proteins, are contained in milk, eggs, and meat. The proteins contained in fruit, vegetables, and legumes have a lower biological value, since they are deficient in one or more of the essential amino acids. These low biological value proteins are a source of calories that should be avoided in ESRD patients because they add to the total amount of the end products of protein metabolism, the excretion of which is compromised in ESRD. Thus, only high biological value protein will efficiently maintain nitrogen balance, and this is of particular importance when total protein intake must be restricted. A decrease in dietary protein intake should be accompanied by an adequate caloric supply from other sources (carbohydrate and fat).

The amount of high biological value protein allowed in the diet will vary with the degree of renal failure. When the creatinine clearance is 15 ml/min, 40 g of protein per day is usually well tolerated. When the C_{cr} falls to 10 ml/min, the patient usually only tolerates 30–40 g per day. If protein intake is excessive at this level of renal function, the result may be aggravation of uremic symptoms, including anorexia, nausea, vomiting, and diarrhea. When urinary protein loss is heavy, intake of protein should be augmented by an amount 1.5 times that of the urinary loss. With the above regimen, supplemented by sufficient calories from nonprotein sources, nitrogen balance can be maintained in ESRD. In 1970, Rubini and Kopple (3) compared isocaloric diets of 20 g protein, 40 g protein, and 1 g/kg protein intake per day in more than 70 nondialyzed uremic patients. They concluded that the patients receiving 20 or 40 g protein diets did well, but those taking 1 g/kg body weight of protein quickly deteriorated and developed uremic symptoms. The patients receiving 20 g protein diets were, however, in negative nitrogen balance.

Bergström et al. (4) added essential amino acid supplements to a 20 g protein diet for predialysis patients and reported that this was acceptable. Walser (5) administered a 20 g per day protein diet supplemented with the ketoacids of several essential amino acids (leucine, isoleucine, and valine) to a group of patients with ESRD. This diet was acceptable to most patients, and they preferred this rigid dietary regimen to chronic dialysis. However, chronic dialysis was eventually required as renal function worsened.

2. Protein Intake in Hemodialysis

The protein requirement increases when hemodialysis is initiated, due to loss of amino acids and peptides in the dialysate. In a 6-hr dialysis, average loss of amino acids is 16–20 g (6). Shinaberger and Ginn (6) demonstrated that patients who were hemodialyzed twice weekly maintained nitrogen balance with a protein intake of 0.8 g/kg of ideal body weight when all the protein ingested was of high biological value. Rubini and Kopple (3) recommended 0.63 g/kg/day of high biological-value protein for patients who were on twice weekly hemodialysis. In our experience most patients on hemodialysis three times per week do well if the protein intake is 1 g/kg of ideal body weight per day and if 80% of the protein is of high biological value. For example, a 70 kg man would receive 70 g of total protein of which 56 g is of high biological-value protein and 14 g of low biological value.

Table I displays a typical meal pattern for a 70 kg man. The proteins are prescribed in "exchange lists" from the two exchange lists of high biological value proteins (HBV) I and II. These are identified in footnotes a and b to Table I. Footnotes also detail exchange lists for starch, fruit, vegetables, and fat.

Table II presents average values of protein, sodium, potassium, phosphorous, and total calories for exchange lists of protein, starch, vegetables, fruit, and fat.

3. Protein Requirements in Peritoneal Dialysis

Patients on intermittent peritoneal dialysis or continuous ambulatory peritoneal dialysis (CAPD) require larger amounts of protein than patients on hemodialysis. Protein loss into effluent dialysate ranges from 6 to 7 g/day and can reach 9–11 g/day in patients with a history of peritonitis (7). The dietary prescription should be 1.2 g of protein per kilogram of ideal body weight per day for maintenance of nitrogen balance. This should be increased to 1.5 g/kg of ideal body weight per day when protein repletion is required and in those patients with peritonitis. Obese patients should receive 1 g/kg of ideal body weight per day.

Protein supplements may be needed to achieve adequate intake in patients on chronic peritoneal dialysis. Most of the protein (at least 50%) should come from high biological value sources such as meat, eggs, and milk. Table III displays some of the commonly used protein supplements and their protein content. There are commercially available products such as Amin-Aid formula and Aminess tablets. If only a short period of therapy is required to supplement the patient's intake, preparations such as electrodialyzed whey or special home recipes such as milkshakes made with eggs, ice cream, and cream can be used.

TABLE I

Meal Pattern for 70 kg Man

Exchange list	Amount	HBV Protein (g)	LBV Protein (g)	Sodium (mg)	Potassium (mg)	Calories
Breakfast						
HBV protein I[a]	1	7		30	120	70
HBV protein II[b]	2	8		120	320	150
Starch list[c]	1	0	2	120	30	70
Fruit list[d]	1	0	0.5	2	200	40
Unsalted fat[e]	2				5	100
Lunch						
HBV protein I	3	21		90	360	210
Starch list	2 (1 unsalted)		4	120	60	140
Vegetable list I[f]	1		1	10	125	25
Vegetable list II[g] (salted)	1		1	240	175	25
Fruit list	0					
Fat list	3 (2 unsalted)			50	15	150
Dinner						
HBV protein I	3	21		90	360	210
Starch list	2 (1 unsalted)		4	120	60	140
Vegetable list I[d] (salted)	1		1	240	125	25
Vegetable List II (unsalted)	1		1	10	175	25
Fruit list	0					
Fat list	3 (2 unsalted)			50	15	150
Total		57	14	1292	2145	1530
Snacks						
Unsalted fats (3)						150
Sugar or hard candy						200
Starch list from meal pattern as high calorie (2)						400
Salt ($\frac{1}{4}$ tsp.)				500		
				1792		2280

[a] **High biological value protein list 1.** One serving contains average values: HBV protein, 7 g; sodium, 30 mg; potassium, 120 mg; phosphorus, 85 mg; calories 70.

Food	Amount
Beef, veal, pork Chicken, turkey, lamb	1 oz.
Fish, shrimp	1 oz.
Eggs	1 med.
Organ meats, liver, etc.	1 oz.

(*Continued*)

TABLE I (*Continued*)

[b] **High biological value protein list II**. One serving contains average value: HBV protein, 4 g; sodium 60 mg; potassium, 160 mg; phosphorus, 105 mg; calories, 75.

Food	Amount
Milk, whole	$\frac{1}{2}$ cup
Milk, canned	
Evaporated	$\frac{1}{4}$ cup
Condensed, sweet	3 tbsp.
Yogurt	$\frac{1}{2}$ cup
Ice cream	$\frac{3}{4}$ cup
Ice milk	$\frac{2}{3}$ cup

[c] **Starch list**. One serving contains average values: LBV protein, 2 g; sodium 120 mg, potassium, 30 mg; phosphorus, 30 mg; calories 70.

Food	Amount
Bread	1 slice
Cooked cereal	$\frac{1}{2}$ cup
Dry cereal	$\frac{3}{4}$ cup
Crackers (no salt on outside)	5
*Cakes and cookies	Size of 1 slice bread
Rice, noodles, etc.	$\frac{1}{2}$ cup
Starchy vegetables	$\frac{1}{2}$ cup

* Higher in calories. Low sodium starches same as above except sodium = 2 mg.

[d] **Vegetables list I**. One serving contains average value: LBV protein, 1 g; sodium, 10 mg; potassium, 125 mg; phosphorus, 37 mg; calories, 25. Use fresh or frozen and prepare and soak 2 or more hours.

Food	Amount
Beans, green	$\frac{1}{2}$ cup
Beans, wax	$\frac{1}{2}$ cup
Beets	$\frac{1}{2}$ cup
Cabbage	$\frac{1}{2}$ cup
Carrots	$\frac{1}{2}$ cup
Celery	$\frac{1}{2}$ cup
Cucumber	$\frac{1}{2}$ cup
Eggplant	$\frac{1}{2}$ cup
Endive	$\frac{1}{2}$ cup
Lettuce	$\frac{1}{2}$ cup
Mushrooms	$\frac{1}{2}$ cup
Onions	$\frac{1}{2}$ cup
Peppers	$\frac{1}{2}$ cup
Squash	$\frac{1}{2}$ cup
Tomatoes	$\frac{1}{2}$ cup

(*Continued*)

(**TABLE I** (*Continued*))

e **Vegetables list II.** One serving contains average value: LBV protein, 1 g; sodium, 10 mg; potassium, 175 mg; phosphorus, 37 mg; calories, 25. Use fresh or frozen and prepare and soak 2 or more hours.

Food	Amount
Asparagus	$\frac{1}{2}$ cup
Broccoli	$\frac{1}{2}$ cup
Brussels sprouts	$\frac{1}{2}$ cup
Collard greens	$\frac{1}{2}$ cup
Mustard greens	$\frac{1}{2}$ cup
Okra	$\frac{1}{2}$ cup
Green peas	$\frac{1}{2}$ cup
Turnip greens	$\frac{1}{2}$ cup

Seasoned or canned vegetables add 240 mg sodium.

f **Fruit and fruit juice list.** One serving contains average value: LBV protein, 0.5 g; sodium, 2 mg; potassium, 2 mg; phosphorus, 20 mg; calories, 40–80.

Food	Amount
Apples	$\frac{1}{2}$ cup
Applesauce	$\frac{1}{2}$ cup
Apricots	$\frac{1}{2}$ cup
Blackberries	$\frac{1}{2}$ cup
Blueberries	$\frac{1}{2}$ cup
Cherries	$\frac{1}{2}$ cup
Fruit cocktail	$\frac{1}{2}$ cup
Grapefruit	$\frac{1}{2}$ cup
Grapes	$\frac{1}{2}$ cup
Melons	$\frac{1}{2}$ cup
Oranges	$\frac{1}{2}$ cup
Peaches	$\frac{1}{2}$ cup
Pears	$\frac{1}{2}$ cup
Pineapple	$\frac{1}{2}$ cup
Plums	$\frac{1}{2}$ cup
Raspberries	$\frac{1}{2}$ cup
Strawberries	$\frac{1}{2}$ cup
Tangerines	$\frac{1}{2}$ cup
Watermelon	$\frac{1}{2}$ cup
Apple juice	$\frac{1}{2}$ cup
Grapefruit juice	$\frac{1}{2}$ cup
Grape juice	$\frac{1}{2}$ cup
Orange juice	$\frac{1}{2}$ cup
Pineapple juice	$\frac{1}{2}$ cup

(*Continued*)

TABLE I (*Continued*)

g **Fat list.** One serving contains average value protein, 0; sodium, 50 mg; potassium, 5 mg; phosphorus, 5 mg; calories, 50.

Food	Amount
Margarine	1 tsp.
Mayonnaise	1 tsp.
Butter	1 tsp.
Cream cheese	1 tsp.
Sour cream	1 tbl.
Salad dressing	1 tbl.
French dressing	1 tbl.
Oils, unsalted margarine, unsalted butter and lard (same as above but sodium is 0)	1 tsp.

TABLE II

Average Values for Each Exchange List[a]

	HBV protein (g)	LBV protein (g)	Sodium (mg)	Potassium (mg)	Phosphorus (mg)	Calories (kcal)
HBV protein list I	7	0	30	120	85	70
HBV protein list II	4	0	60	160	105	75
Starch list	0	2	120	30	30	70
Vegetable list I	0	1	10	125	37	25
Vegetable list II	0	1	10	175	37	25
Fruit and fruit juice list	0	0.5	2	200	20	40–80
Fat list	0	0	50	5	5	50

[a] The table is a simplified breakdown of the composition of each of the dietary exchange lists employed in constructing a meal pattern. This can be used as a food composition guide, but is not intended for use as a diet instruction sheet. HBV = high biological value; LBV = low biological value.

TABLE III

High Biological Value Protein Renal Supplements

	Amount	Protein	Calories
Whey proteins	100 g	35.0	390
Amin-Aid	148 g	6.6	670
Aminess Tablets	30	20.0	93
Meritene	1 oz.	9.9	100
Citrotene	1.18 oz.	7.7	127

B.   Caloric Requirements: Carbohydrates and Fats

The intake of calories for a patient with ESRD should be 35–40 cal/kg body weight per day. The carbohydrate intake should be liberal in the face of restricted protein intake. This ensures that endogenous protein sources are not employed for the supply of energy. There are a number of high caloric, low protein, low electrolyte supplements available (Table IV). Most commonly used are specially prepared low protein starches, liquid glucose polymers, unsalted fats, nondairy creamers and whipped toppings, plain candies, and jellies. Footnote c to Table I displays exchange lists for starches in the construction of a diet.

It should be recalled that patients on peritoneal dialysis receive additional calories because of glucose absorption from the dialysate. An average of 15–17 g of glucose is absorbed during a peritoneal dialysis. The calories derived from this glucose (1 g = 4 cal) should be subtracted from the prescribed daily diet. Failure to recognize this source of calories can lead to excessive weight gain over a prolonged period of time. Conversely, hemodialysis patients may lose calories into the dialysate, especially if it is glucose-free.

Fat is an excellent source of calories for the patient with ESRD. Butter, vegetable oil, whipping cream, cream cheese and mayonnaise all yield high caloric values and are therefore useful in the diet. The type of fat used in the diet should be polyunsaturated because of the high prevalence of cardiovascular disease in patients with chronic renal failure, as well as in kidney transplant recipients. Footnote e to Table I provides exchange lists for fats in the construction of a diet.

TABLE IV

High Calorie, Low Protein, Low Electrolyte Supplements

	cal/ml	Amount	Manufacturer
Microlipid	4.5		Organon
Controlyte	2		Doyle
Polycose	2		Ross
Sumacal	2		Organon
MCT[a] oil	7.7		Mead Johnson
Wheatstarch products			Henkle
Low protein bread	83 cal/slice	1 slice (32 g)	Henkle
A-proten rusk	42 cal/slice	1 slice (10 g)	Henkle
Wheatstarch noodles	100–200	1 cup	Henkle
Wheatstarch flour	100	1 oz.	Henkle

[a] MCT = medium chain triglyceride.

C. Electrolytes

1. Sodium Requirements for Patients with Chronic Renal Failure

Sodium requirements vary with different types of renal disease and should be individualized for patients with some residual renal function. The 24-hr urinary excretion of sodium while the patient is receiving a diet of known composition is a good guide for determining the sodium requirement in patients who are neither edematous nor dehydrated. Otherwise, the dietary content of sodium should be adjusted in order to achieve optimal hydration.

The patient who is stabilized on dialysis usually requires about 2 g of sodium per day to maintain blood pressure during dialysis treatment. This provides a palatable diet by allowing seasoned foods, but the patient should avoid salt at the table and foods that are processed or cured with sodium. Table V provides a list of foods with high sodium content.

2. Potassium Requirements for the Patient with Chronic Renal Failure

Potassium restriction is usually not necessary until the C_{cr} falls below 15 ml/min. A daily intake of 50–70 mEq is allowed on maintenance dialysis with a dialysate potassium concentration of less than 3 mEq/liter. Table V provides a list of foods with high potassium content. If vegetables are soaked to leach out the potassium, and high potassium fruits and vegetables are avoided, the dietary potassium will be derived primarily from meat and dairy products (see footnotes a and b to Table I). Patients should be cautioned

TABLE V

High Potassium and High Sodium Foods

High potassium foods[a]	
Brewer's yeast	Meat extracts
Wheat germ	Molasses
Chocolate	Salt substitutes
Lite salt	
High sodium foods	
Salt	TV dinners
Baking soda	Gravy mix
Baking powder	Packaged dinners
Meat tenderizers	Worcestershire sauce
Monosodium glutamate (Accent)	Pot Pies
Soy sauce	Processed meats
Steak sauce	Sauerkraut
Pickles	Kitchen Bouquet

[a] Read labels for all low sodium diet foods to see if potassium has been used in place of sodium (e.g., low sodium bouillon cubes).

against using salt substitutes, low-sodium baking powder, and low-sodium cheese, all of which may be high in potassium.

D. Fluid Requirements

Prior to starting dialysis, the uremic patient should limit fluids to about 1000 ml/day or the 24-hr urine volume. Some patients may require more rigorous restrictions. Following the initiation of chronic dialysis, fluids should be restricted to the 24-hr urinary output plus 500 ml/day for a weight gain of 1 lb per day. The fluid contained in the food itself is about equal to insensible losses. If this restriction is not heeded, excessive weight gain will occur during the interdialytic period and may result in pulmonary edema and uncontrolled hypertension.

E. Calcium–Phosphorus

Because menus for patients with renal failure contain reduced quantities of dairy products and meat, the diet is low in calcium and phosphorus. Vitamin D deficiency further contributes by decreasing fractional absorption of calcium from the gut. A supplement of at least 1.0 g of elemental calcium and active metabolites of vitamin D are required by most dialysis patients to

TABLE VI

Phosphorus Binder Equivalents

Preparation	Basic dosage	Elemental aluminum content[a] (mg)	Approximate equivalent dose to 30 ml Amphojel
Alternagel	30 ml	1260	15 ml
Amphojel liquid	30 ml	665	30 ml
Amphojel (5 g tablet)	1 tablet	104	6.4 tablets
Amphojel (10 g tablet)	1 tablet	208	3.2 tablets
Alucap [475 mg Al(OH)$_3$]	1 capsule	166	4.0 tablets
Alutab [600 mg Al(OH)$_3$]	1 tablet	210	3.0 tablets
Basaljel tablet	1 tablet	173	4.0 tablets
Basaljel capsule	1 capsule	173	4.0 capsules
Basaljel liquid	30 ml	852	23.5 ml
Extra-strength Basaljel liquid	30 ml	2080	9.6 ml
Nephrox	30 ml	660	30 ml
Dialume	1 capsule	173	4.0 capsules

[a] Elemental aluminum constitutes 35% by weight of aluminum hydroxide.

maintain calcium homeostasis. Doses of each must be individualized, however, depending on the serum calcium, serum phosphorus, type of bone disease, and extraskeletal calcification. Conversely, even on restricted phosphorus intakes, most ESRD patients will be hyperphosphatemic. Until the C_{cr} decreases to less than 30 ml/min, it is possible to diminish phosphorus intake in proportion to the fractional loss of renal function and maintain balance. Below this level of renal function, a palatable diet cannot be constructed because of the ubiquitous presence of phosphorus in all food groups. Therefore, patients with a C_{cr} below 30 ml/min depend on aluminum hydroxide gels to bind dietary phosphorus in the gut and prevent its absorption with resultant hyperphosphatemia. Based on aluminum content, available phosphate binders are listed in Table VI. There is a wide variation in phosphate binder requirement so that doses must be individualized. Preferably, these binders should be given with meals, but the daily dosage should be the same even if meal is omitted.

F. Vitamins

If a balanced diet is consumed, no unusual requirements occur until the patient begins chronic dialysis. However, a daily multiple vitamin tablet containing US RDA levels of C and B complex, including B_6, could be administered to chronically uremic patients nearing dialysis. When chronic dialysis regimens are instituted, losses of water-soluble vitamins increase. Evidence is greatest that pyridoxine (B_6), ascorbate (C), and folate supplementation should be increased (8–10). Excessive consumption of vitamins,

TABLE VII

Some Vitamin Supplements and Their Content[a]

Product and manufacturer	Thiamine	Riboflavin	Pyridoxine	Niacinamide	Calcium pantothenate	Ascorbic acid
Allbee with C (Robins)	15	10	5	50	10	300
Probec-T (Stuart)	15	10	5	100	20	600
Thex-Forte (Ingram)	25	15	5	100	10	500
Vio-Bec (Rowell)	25	25	25	100	40	500

[a] All doses are in milligrams.

especially those products containing vitamin A and ergocalciferol (D), must be avoided. Vitamin A can accumulate in toxic quantities, and large ergocalciferol stores cause refractory hypercalcemia in patients receiving a renal transplant. It is our policy to give chronic dialysis patients one B complex–C (see Table VII) tablet, 25 mg pyridoxine, and 1 mg of folate daily. Requirements of chronic peritoneal dialysis patients have been less well documented than for those on chronic hemodialysis. A regimen similar to that for chronic hemodialysis is suggested.

III. TRANSPLANTATION

Dietary therapy for the patient who has received a kidney transplant is radically different from that prescribed during dialysis (*11*). The diet is constructed in an endeavor to control some of the metabolic aberrations caused by corticosteroids (prednisone and methylprednisolone), which these patients routinely require, often in high doses.

Steroids are catabolic agents and tend to deplete all body tissues of protein. By using a high protein diet, 2 g/kg/day, nitrogen wasting is minimized. Because appetite is increased by steroids, it is usually possible for the transplant recipients to ingest large quantities of protein with little difficulty. Under the influence of steroids, a high carbohydrate diet encourages excessive insulin secretion, and this may contribute to the centripetal obesity as seen in iatrogenic Cushing's syndrome. In our experience, the use of a low carbohydrate diet (1 g/kg body weight per day) has averted the development of Cushingoid features in patients following transplantation.

As discussed above, fats are an important source of calories. However, because of the prevalence of cardiovascular disease in patients who have received a transplant, polyunsaturated fats are recommended. The amount of fat is unrestricted and is determined by the total number of calories required to maintain ideal body weight.

Sodium, potassium, calcium, and phosphorus requirements must be individualized. Calcium and phosphorus intake are each usually between 800 and 1200 mg/day. This may vary, however, if the subject has severe osteitis fibrosa or frank hypercalcemia. A sodium intake of 2 g (85 mEq) per day is usually satisfactory. Sodium may need to be more rigorously restricted in the early posttransplantation period or if the patient becomes hypertensive. Initially, poor transplant function and/or very high doses of corticosteroids lead to diminished excretion of ingested sodium. When the dosage of steroids is decreased, usually 6 months after transplantation, the distribution

TABLE VIII

Suggested Diet Prescriptions

Nutrients and ions	Initial renal failure	Hemodialysis	Peritoneal dialysis and CAPD	Transplantation
HBV protein	30–40 g	Adult 1 g/kg (child 1.5 g/kg)	1.2–1.5 g/kg	2 g/kg
LBV protein	10 g or less	15 g or less	15 g or less	Limited by CHO
CHO	Unrestricted	Unrestricted	Unrestricted	1 g/kg
Fat	Unrestricted	Unrestricted	Unrestricted	Unrestricted
Calories	35–40 kcal/kg/day (children 80 kcal)	45–50 kcal/kg/day (children 80 kcal)	45–50 kcal/kg/day (children 80 kcal)	To maintain ideal weight
Sodium	Individualized	Individualized (usually 2000 mg)	3000–4000 mg	Usually restricted (2000 mg)
Potassium	Individualized (40–70 mEq)	Individualized (50–70 mEq)	Normal	Usually unrestricted
Calcium	RDA (800–1200 mg)	RDA (800–1200 mg)	RDA (800–1200 mg)	Individualized (no less than RDA)
Phosphorus	Less than 600 mg	Less than 600 mg	Less than 600 mg	Individualized

of dietary constituents becomes less critical. Improved renal function may allow more liberal sodium intake at this time, and the need for protein is reduced. However, it remains important to maintain the patient at ideal body weight. Should rejection occur, the recurrence of chronic renal failure will necessitate drastic dietary changes.

Table VIII provides an overview of dietary prescriptions in ESRD for predialysis, hemodialysis, and after transplantation. Table IX lists nutrient requirements for similar patient groups. Table X lists acceptable ranges of blood chemistries for patients who are on dialysis.

TABLE IX
Nutrient Requirements for Normals vs. Adult Chronically Uremic Patients and Patients Undergoing Maintenance Hemodialysis or Peritoneal Dialysis

	Recommended daily allowance (RDA) normal	Chronically uremic	Hemodialysis (HD) and peritoneal dialysis (PD)
Protein (g/kg/day)	0.8	Most men: no less than 40 g/day (0.55–0.60 g/kg/day) Women and small men: no less than 35 g/day	HD: 1.0–1.2 PD: 1.2–1.5
Calories (kcal/kg/day)	45	35	35
Vitamins			
Thiamine (mg/day)	1–1.5	1.5	1.5
Riboflavin (mg/day)	1.2–1.7	1.8	1.8
Pantothenic acid (mg/day)	10	5.0	5.0
Niacin (mg/day)	13–18	20	20
Pyridoxine HCl (mg/day)	2–2.2	5.0	10
Vitamin B_{12} (μg/day)	3.0	3.0	3.0
Vitamin C (mg/day)	60	70–100	100
Folic acid (mg/day)	0.4	1.0	1.0
Vitamin A (RE/day)[a]	800–1000	?	?
Vitamin D (μg/day)	5	Variable	Variable
Vitamin E (αTE/day)[b]	8–10	15	15
Minerals			
Sodium (mEq/day)	Variable	Usually 40–120	Usually 85
Potassium (mEq/day)	Variable	Generally no more than 70	No more than 70
Phosphorus (mg/day)	800–1200	600–1200	600–1200
Calcium (mg/day)	800–1200	1000–2000	1000–2000
Magnesium (mg/day)	300–350	200–300	200–300
Water (ml/day)		Up to 3000 as tolerated	Usually 750–1500

[a] RE = retinol equivalent.
[b] TE = α-tocopherol equivalent.

TABLE X

Acceptable Ranges of Blood Chemistries for Patients on Dialysis[a]

Substance	Normal values	Dialysis patients	Function	Diet changes
Sodium	136–146 (mEq/liter)	Same	Found in salt and many preserved foods. A diet high in sodium will cause thirst. Too much fluid may dilute the sidium and it will look low. Too much sodium and not enough water make it too high. Too much sodium and water raise blood pressure.	High: Eat less salt and salty foods. Make sure there is a weight gain about 1.5 kg between runs and there is not dehydration. Low: Probably drinking too much fluid. Limid weight gains to 1.5 kg between runs and eat less salt and salty foods.
Potassium	3.8–5.1 (mEq/liter)	Same	Found in most high protein foods, and vegetables. It affects muscle action, especially the heart. High levels can cause the heart to stop. Low levels can also cause symptoms such as weakness.	High: Avoid foods over 250 mg/serving and limit daily intake to 2000 mg. Consult dietician. Low: Add one 250 mg potassium food/ day and recheck blood level.
Chloride	100–108 (mEq/liter)	Same	Usually associated with amount of sodium in blood.	No dietary changes
Total CO_2	23–29 (mEq/liter)	Lower than normal	Total carbon dioxide is a measure of how acidic your blood is. Kidneys normally keep this normal. When they fail, blood becomes more acidic and CO_2 is lower.	No dietary changes

Creatinine	0.5–1.5 0.5–1.5 (mg/dl)	F: 10–15 M: 10–18	A normal waste product of muscle breakdown. This value is controlled by dialysis and is a higher amount because the artificial kidney is not working all the time like the normal kidney does.	Normally, dialysis controls creatinine
Glucose	66–110 (mg/dl)	Same (higher for diabetic)	This sugar in blood is made from starches and sugar in the diet. The body uses glucose for energy. For diabetics: A high blood sugar can cause thirst.	You need a *minimum* of four servings of breads/starches or cereals, and two to three servings of fruit to provide energy. For diabetics: avoid concentrated sweets unless the blood sugar is low.
Calcium	8.6–10.7 (mg/dl)	Same	Found in dairy products, meats, and green vegetables. It is used by the body to make bone and help muscle movement. It is closely related to phosphorus: vitamin D is needed for absorption. Calcium and phosphorus are two minerals needed for strong bones. They have a "seesaw" relationship, so when phosphorus is up, calcium is down.	High: Eat fewer meat products. Check to see if taking calcium supplement or vitamin D (DHT, Rocaltrol). Low: Increase calcium in diet (if phosphorus is normal) by adding milk products or may need calcium supplements.
Phosphorus	2.0–4.5 (mg/dl)	2.5–4.5	Found in milk products, dried beans, peas, nuts, and meat. It is also used to build bones (see above). It is important to keep phosphorus within normal range for strong bones.	High: Limit milk and milk products to one serving per day. Take phosphate binders as ordered. Low: Add one serving milk product or other high phosphorus food per day or decrease phosphate binder.

(Continued)

TABLE X (*Continued*)

Substance	Normal values	Dialysis patients	Function	Diet changes
Urea nitrogen (Blood urea nitrogen or BUN)	6–20 (mg/dl)	80–100	Waste product of protein breakdown. Unlike creatinine, this is affected by the amount of protein in your diet. Dialysis removes urea nitrogen.	High: Limit intake of fish, meat, chicken, and dairy products to about three servings per day and contact dietitian. Low: May decrease if not eating and losing weight. May also increase with loss of muscle. Eat more HBV protein.
Uric acid	2.5–8.0 (mg/dl)	Same	A waste product of purine. Purine is found in a variety of foods. A high level may be related to symptoms of gout.	Few diet changes. Since purines are found in most foods, you would have to stop eating! Omit gravies and vegetables containing purine.
Alk Phos (alkaline phosphatase)	30–115 (U/liter)	Same	Found in normal bone. Released from bone when calcium is being removed.	See calcium/phosphorus section. Keep calcium and phosphorus within normal limits.
Cholesterol	150–250 (mg/dl)	Often lower	Found in high fat foods from animal sources: meat, milk, eggs. Body can also make its own if there is not enough in the diet. Within normal levels, cholesterol is not harmful.	Usually no diet changes are necessary except to omit egg yolks and use polyunsaturated fats.

	Normal values	Dialysis patients	Description	Recommendation
Total protein	5.2–8.0	Same	Proteins make up all body cells. Albumin is a type of protein. Both are needed by the body. Protein is lost by dialysis. Peritoneal dialysis protein loss is much more than hemodialysis. If albumin is low, fluid will "leak" from vessels into tissue causing edema. When fluid is in the tissue, it is difficult to remove on dialysis.	Low: Increase intake of protein-rich foods: meat, fish, eggs. Ask dietitian for high-protein recipes. He may recommend a protein supplement to increase protein intake.
Albumin	3.4–4.6 (g/dl)	Same		
HCT (hematocrit)	35–45%	Usually lower	The percentage of red blood cells in blood. Red blood cells carry oxygen to the cells. Everyone's value is different. Learn what is normal for individual.	If hematocrit is dropping, check with your doctor.
Ferritin	123 (men)	Same	This is the way iron is stored in the liver. If iron stores are low, you cannot make new red blood cells.	Iron in food is not well absorbed. Consider an iron supplement. Do not take with phosphate binders.
	56 (women)	Same		

^a This guide is to help understand lab reports. The normal values are for people with good kidney function. Acceptable values for dialysis patients are given in the next column. Values should fall within the range for dialysis patients. Many factors affect blood values; diet is one of these. Understanding chemistries will help control diet.

IV. SPECIAL CONSIDERATIONS

A.   The Diabetic Patient

Chronic renal disease is a common complication of diabetes mellitus. When kidney function begins to decrease in the diabetic patient, it is important to prescribe a diet that will minimize the uremic symptoms while controlling blood sugar and optimizing the general nutritional status. With progressive renal disease, insulin requirements for the insulin-dependent diabetic may decrease. Similarly, the dosage of oral sulfonylurea drugs must usually be lowered (*12*).

Diabetic patients in the early stages of chronic renal disease are managed in a manner similar to that employed for nondiabetics. Dietary protein is curtailed and caloric intake is complemented from carbohydrate and fat, i.e., the carbohydrate intake is usually greater than that prescribed for diabetics who have good renal function. The use of low protein starches, such as wheat starch products, is valuable in this situation. Since both diabetes mellitus and chronic renal disease predispose to atherosclerosis (*13*), fat intake should be from vegetable sources high in polyunsaturated fats. Protein intake should be virtually exclusively of high biological value. Caloric intake should be adequate to maintain nitrogen balance. Davis *et al.* (*12*) recommend 25–35 cal/kg of ideal body weight.

1. Hemodialysis

When the diabetic patient is started on hemodialysis, the diet must be increased to allow for loss of nutrients into the dialysate. Davis and associates (*12*) recommend that diabetics who undergo hemodialysis three times a week should receive 1 g of protein per kilogram of body weight per day. Proteinuria must also be considered and compensated for when present. Caloric needs remain about the same as they were prior to the beginning of dialysis. Mineral content of the diet does not differ from that of the nondiabetic hemodialysis patient. The sodium intake should be about 2 g and potassium intake should be restricted to about 70 mEq/day. Phosphorus can be controlled by the use of phosphate-binding gels. Strict attention should be paid to control of the diabetes during hemodialysis. The blood glucose should be maintained between 120 and 250 mg/dl. Glucose (usually 200 mg/dl) must be present in the dialysate, or hypoglycemia will be produced.

2. Peritoneal Dialysis

Protein and amino acid losses are greater in peritoneal dialysis than in hemodialysis. An intake of 1.5 g of protein per kilogram of body weight per day to maintain nitrogen balance in the diabetic undergoing peritoneal dialysis is generally recommended. Calories and insulin dosage should be adjusted to maintain proper diabetic control. The extra calories received from the glucose (1 g = 4 cal) absorbed from the dialysate should be taken into consideration when prescribing the diet. Sodium and potassium intake can be liberalized. The diabetic undergoing peritoneal dialysis may be able to tolerate normal amounts of potassium and 3–4 g of sodium per day.

B.   Total Parenteral Nutrition in End-State Renal Disease

Patients with chronic renal failure will occasionally have episodes of illness that require partial or total parenteral nutrition (TPN) in order to meet their nutritional needs.

In the early 1970s, TPN was administered by several investigators to renal failure patients. Dudrick *et al.* (*14*) using a formula containing 6.35 g of essential amino acids per 100 ml and 750–1000 ml of 50–70% glucose obtained good results. Abel (*15*) successfully employed a formula containing 750 ml of water, 375 g of glucose, 13.1 g of essential amino acids (FreAmine-E), and vitamins. Meng and colleagues (*16*) added 250 ml of a 5.25% essential amino acid solution (FreAmine-E) to 600–650 ml of a 70% glucose solution, containing vitamins and appropriate amounts of electrolytes. They found this helpful in both acute and chronic renal failure patients. Finally, Kopple and Blumenkrantz (*17*) have exhaustively reviewed and made suggestions for TPN under a variety of circumstances.

There are presently several commercially available products listed in Table III. If only a short period of supplemental therapy is required, such preparations as electrodialyzed whey or home recipes for milkshakes or eggnogs may be used effectively. Enteral nutrition is always the preferred means, whenever feasible.

V.   COMPLIANCE

It is important to have a dietitian work closely with the physician, the patient and the patient's family in order to achieve dietary compliance. The patient must realize that the diet is an essential aspect of treatment. The relationship of blood chemistries to dietary intake should be stressed.

There are many strategies that can be used to increase dietary compliance, such as behavior modification and teaching the patient how to adjust the diet to his life-style. The dietitian must be aware of the patient's educational level, his socioeconomic background, and his personal eating habits and beliefs.

Compliance will improve once the patient learns to understand the rationale for the diet. Involving the patient in teaching sessions about food content and preparation will often enhance compliance. Having the dietitian regularly review all chemistries with the patient is an excellent teaching tool and helpful in gaining compliance.

VI. CONCLUSION

This chapter reviews the role of the diet in the management of patients with chronic ESRD. The specific requirements of the diet of patients during the predialysis period, during chronic hemo- and peritoneal dialysis, and following transplantation are described. In addition, special consideration is given to the diabetic patient and to total parenteral nutrition.

REFERENCES

1. Liddle, V. R. Nutrition for the patient with end stage renal disease. *In* "The Patient with End Stage Renal Disease" (L. E. Lancaster, ed.), pp. 123–40. Wiley, New York, 1979.
2. Giovannetti, S., and Maggiore, Q. A low-nitrogen diet with proteins of high biological value for severe chronic uremia. *Lancet* 1, 1000–1003 (1964).
3. Rubini, M. E., and Kopple, J. D. Dietary management of end-stage uremia. *Bull. N.Y. Acad. Med.* [2] 46, 850–868 (1970).
4. Bergstrom, J., Furst, P., and Noree, L. G. Treatment of chronic uremic patients with protein-poor diet and oral supply of essential amino acids. I. Nitrogen balance. *Clin. Nephrol.* 3, 187–194 (1975).
5. Walser, M. Does dietary therapy have a role in the predialysis patient? *Am. J. Clin. Nutr.* 33, 1629–1637 (1980).
6. Shinaberger, J. H., and Ginn, H. E. Low protein, high essential amino acid diet for nitrogen equilibrium in chronic dialysis. *Am. J. Clin. Nutr.* 21, 618–625 (1968).
7. Harvey, K. B., Blumenkrantz, M. J., Levine, S. E., and Blackburn, G. L. Nutritional assessment and treatment of chronic renal failure. *Am. J. Clin. Nutr.* 33, 1586–1597 (1980).
8. Kopple, J. D., and Swendseid, M. E. Vitamin nutrition in patients undergoing maintenance hemodialysis. *Kidney Int.* 7(S-2), 79–84 (1975).
9. Stone, W. J., Warnock, L., and Wagner, C. Vitamin B_6 deficiency in uremia. *Am. J. Clin. Nutr.* 28, 950–957 (1975).
10. Werb, R., Clark, W. F., Lindsay, R. M. Jones, E. O. P., and Linton, A. L. Serum vitamin A levels and associated abnormalities in patients on regular dialysis treatment. *Clin. Nephrol.* 12, 63–68 (1979).
11. Liddle, V. R., and Johnson, H. K. Dietary therapy in renal transplantation. *Proc.—Clin. Dial. Transplant Forum* 9, 219–220 (1979).
12. Davis, M., Comty, C., and Shapiro, F. Dietary management of patients with diabetes treated by hemodialysis. *J. Am. Diet. Assoc.* 75, 265–269 (1979).
13. Lowrie, E. G., Lazarus, J. M., Hampers, C. L., *et al.* Cardiovascular disease in dialysis patients. *N. Engl. J. Med.* 290, 737–738 (1974).
14. Dudrick, S. J., Steiger, E., and Long, J. M. Renal failure in surgical patients. Treatment with intravenous essential amino acids and hypertonic glucose. *Surgery (St. Louis)* 68, 180–186 (1970).

15. Abel, R. M., Beck, C. H., Abbott, W. M., Ryan, J. A., Barnett, G. O., and Fischer, J. E. Improved survival from acute renal failure after treatment with intravenous essential L-amino acids and glucose *N. Engl. J. Med.* **288,** 695–699 (1973).

16. Meng, H. C., Sandstead, H. H., Walker, P. J., Ackerman, J. R., and Johnson, H. K. The use of essential amino acids for parenteral nutrition in patients with chronic and acute renal failure. *Acta Chir. Scand., Suppl.* **466,** 94–95 (1976).

17. Kopple, J. D., and Blumenkrantz, M. J. Total parenteral nutrition and parenteral fluid therapy. Section I. Total parenteral nutrition. *In* "Clinical Disorders of Fluid and Electrolyte Metabolism" (M. H. Maxwell and C. R. Kleeman, eds.), 3rd ed., pp. 413–498. McGraw-Hill, New York, 1980.

13

End-Stage Renal Disease: An Integrated Approach

WILLIAM J. STONE and PAULINE L. RABIN

When a patient's renal function has diminished to end-stage [creatinine clearance (C_{cr}) of 10 ml/min or less], he may reach the attention of a nephrologist in one of two ways. First, there may be periodic visits to the nephrologist's office or clinic in the early stages of renal disease where blood pressure, fluid balance, and blood chemistry values were monitored and regulated. Progressive loss of renal function is charted, a vascular access for future hemodialysis is placed when the C_{cr} decreases to 15–20 ml/min, any correctable causes of this deterioration are addressed (e.g., bladder outlet obstruction), and the patient is educated about health maintenance and dialysis. During this time the patient also becomes acquainted with the nephrology team consisting of the nephrologist nurse, social worker, dietitian, and psychiatrist experienced in the multiple problems encountered by end-stage renal disease (ESRD) patients. Dialysis is begun in an orderly fashion before the patient becomes even moderately ill with symptoms of renal failure. The second manner of presentation to the nephrologist is at end-stage renal function. This is often unavoidable because the patient has not sought medical attention earlier. Unfortunately, late referrals to nephrologists still occur in patients who have presented themselves to physicians in a relatively well state with C_{cr} values of 15–30 ml/min.

The team will make an initial assessment of all new patients, their families, and other resources. Plans will be made for immediate and future care. If the patient is deemed a suitable candidate for renal transplantation, the nearest transplant center will be contacted and the patient referred. There the patient

357

END-STAGE RENAL DISEASE

will undergo tissue typing and family members will be confidentially inter-viewed about possible organ donation. Willing donors will be evaluated in the hospital if they are normotensive and have no signs of renal or systemic diseases. The patient himself will have tests of bladder function and other indicated procedures performed. Timing of the transplant will be decided as a joint venture, involving the patient, family, nephrologist, and transplant team. Should clinical and laboratory indications suggest that dialysis must begin immediately, in the absence of a vascular access, acute peritoneal dialysis or hemodialysis via a venous catheter will be instituted. At the earliest possible time, a more permanent access such as Brescia–Cimino fistula or Tenckhoff peritoneal catheter will be inserted.

During the early days of treatment it is critical that all members of the team become actively involved with the patient. Here the nephrology nurse plays an important educational as well as therapeutic role. The psychiatrist should be routinely consulted even in currently asymptomatic patients. If the psychiatrist is pictured by the patient as part of a team of professionals participating in his care, the usual stigmata ("they think I'm crazy") are avoided. The psychiatrist brought in "on the ground floor" will have a much easier time dealing with future psychiatric or psychological difficulties. The nephrology social worker must keep in touch with the patient and his family on a daily basis as they adjust to the demanding new life-style and its effects on every aspect of their routine. The renal dietitian instructs the patient and his family in a much more structured food plan and monitors the compliance by following the serum chemistries. Continuing education about diet is often necessary. Finally, the nephrologist must be the orchestrator not only of the patient's direct medical care but also of the integration of input from other team members. He must decide on the amount and frequency of the dialysis regimen and on the timing of transplantation or home dialysis training. A flexible approach concerning the type of dialysis is necessary especially for those patients who tolerate the prescribed treatment poorly. The nephrologist must adjust to disruptions such as poor dietary compliance, crises in the patient's family, superimposed medical complications, and the onset of psychiatric illness. However complex this appears, the usual result is a patient who has been returned from the brink of death to a reasonable state of health.

Subject Index

DATE DUE